Contents

Preface   v

Section 1 – Planning Care for the Individual Patient   1

Section 2 – Breathing   8

Section 3 – Eating   40

Section 4 – Drinking   116

Section 5 – Sleeping   160

Section 6 – Mobility   189

Section 7 – Religion   247

Section 8 – Social Role   269

Acknowledgements

Our particular thanks go to:

Mary Armstrong who, while District Nursing Officer in City and Hackney Health District, initiated the idea for this book.

Ana Ireland and Maureen Theobold who helped shape its early development.

The nurse educators in Bristol, Edinburgh, Leeds, Newcastle upon Tyne and Oxford who ranked the initial problem lists, so we could focus on those considered most likely to be seen in groups of patients assigned for care to student nurses.

Patricia Humpherson, District Dietitian for Tower Hamlets Health Authority and Martin Palmer of the International Consultancy on Religion, Education and Culture, who so willingly supplied information and read the relevant chapters.

The hospital pharmacists, physiotherapists and occupational therapists who answered our questions.

The many staff nurses, students and pupil nurses who tested sections for us.

The staff of Edward Arnold (Publishers) Ltd.

This book is dedicated to all the staff in the many disciplines in Tower Hamlets Health Authority who have helped in the development of individualised patient care.

Preface

This book is intended for use by student nurses when planning nursing care. It will also be of interest to trained nurses who have not used a problem orientated approach to nursing their patients.

Medical disorders affect people in many different situations and are not confined to designated 'medical wards'. The general problems outlined may be shared by patients at home as well as in hospital wards of all types. This book is intended to provide easy reference in hospital wards or the patient's home.

Each person is an individual. Part of the skill of nursing is the ability to identify how the individual is responding to the disease both physiologically and psychologically. Whenever possible, the patient's view of the situation should also be sought. In using this book the nurse must therefore assess the patient and select from the suggested nursing actions those which seem appropriate. The care planned should be tailored to suit the individuality of the patient.

The current state of the art does not allow many precise references to substantiate the nursing actions suggested. They have been derived from practical experience combined with wide reading. The contents contain much that is still based on custom and practice. Each suggested nursing action is followed by suggested review information which may allow the effect of the action to be identified. Nurses have not traditionally sought to review their care in this way. Experience has been limited but the method appears to offer a useful route to evaluating the effect of nursing care.

Traditional nursing textbooks start either from the medical diagnosis or the nursing procedure. This book is divided into main themes which have been found helpful in planning patient care in busy wards and departments. It covers breathing, eating, drinking, sleeping, mobility, religion and social role. The focus is on the commoner problems which may occur due to a variety of medical disorders. Instead of reading the book section by section, it will be more helpful to refer to the likely problem(s) of the patient. Later, as confidence grows, the health maintenance information can be used as a basis for teaching patients about self-help for healthier living.

Each section follows the same layout for easy reference:

1. A general description of HEALTH MAINTENANCE relevant to the theme, which it is hoped will provide a basis for simple health education in whatever setting the nurse is in contact with patients or their relatives.

2. A list of GENERAL ASSESSMENT AREAS to help the student check for problems.

3. A list of the PROBLEMS and POTENTIAL PROBLEMS described in the section for rapid reference.

Each problem is then dealt with under the following headings:

a. Likely **Assessment findings** which may be present and help identify the problem.

b. **Information for the patient** written in simple English to help the student explain the situation to the patient and relatives.

c. **Nursing action** which could be used to help the patient cope with the problem. Review (RE.) suggestions are given to help the student check the effect of the action.

d. **Further action** includes treatments and drugs prescribed by a doctor which require help from the nurse with the procedure, drug administration, advice or observation for side effects.

e. **Associated medical diagnoses** list some of the possible underlying medical disorders which can give rise to the problems experienced by the patient.

Each problem with its nursing and further action is complete in itself and this produces some repetition. However, it is hoped that the book will provide an easy-to-use source of ideas for helping patients to cope with common problems.

The problem-solving approach requires careful assessment and thought. Each individual will have a mix of problems during illness and the problems may interact to give a complex situation. Selecting or adapting the most effective nursing actions may be difficult. Ingenuity and partnership with the patient and relatives has more to offer than trying to make the patient fit the traditional routine care. The interactions and modifications required for complex combinations of problems are beyond the scope of this book.

The authors believe that patients are able to participate actively in the decisions about their care and to suggest new ways of providing it. Given sufficient information, patients are also able to improve their health through changes in their lifestyle. Educating other adults for health requires tact and a developing skill in selling new or different ideas. Happily such communication skills are described in a growing number of texts so this aspect has not been included. It is also hoped that students will also accept responsibility for self-help and developing independence. Useful addresses and sources for further information about each main theme have therefore been included.

1 Planning care for the individual patient

Patients are people, a fact that sometimes seems to be lost in the busy hospital. Each person is a unique blend of physical and psychological reactions and collects a range of experiences through daily living and mixing with others. Illness, especially if serious enough to require hospital admission, adds to the way each person looks at life and tries to cope with the changes it brings.

Nurses are people, another fact that gets forgotten in the rush to get 'all the work done'. Professional education provides a broad range of experience. Each new patient who is cared for can add to professional learning and development. No two nurses share exactly the same nursing experience. It comes as no surprise then that nurses and their patients may interpret the needs for nursing care in very different ways. No two nurses agree on the exact nature of the patient's difficulties and the most effective nursing action.

In the past nursing has sometimes followed rigid routines, with the doctor's diagnosis forming the starting point, and every patient with the same medical label receiving a 'routine pattern' of nursing care. As few patients ever resemble simple textbook examples, it meant nursing procedures would be carried out even though they were not necessary.

Assessment

The current pattern for nursing starts with the patient. Four of the five senses are used to assess the state of the patient. Fortunately the sense of taste is rarely required. Assessment of the patient's condition involves careful observation. Some medical disorders have symptoms that are so subtle that to detect any change from the patient's normal pattern requires skills worthy of the legendary Sherlock Holmes. Some of the problems which result from illness tend to follow a familiar pattern. It is these patterns which help to make sense of a sometimes overwhelming mass of data. The assessment findings listed beside each problem heading may or may not be observed in an individual patient. There may be other findings from the assessment which we have missed. If so, do let us know. Nursing knowledge can only be developed by nurses who are willing to share their views and to comment constructively on the work of others.

The patient may also be able to add a great deal to the assessment information. If the patient's view is not sought then the nurse can only guess at the level of pain, discomfort or despair felt. Research is already highlighting how inaccurate some of these nursing guesses can be.

It can be easy to leave out a part of the assessment and so miss important clues or signs. Hospital and community nursing services are developing check lists and printed frameworks to provide a systematic approach. Ordering the assessment from the head down to the toes or examination of the body systems, such as the respiratory and cardio-vascular systems, may be used. Others use the work of *Nancy Roper (1980) or Virginia Henderson (1978)* to help organise their thoughts. These schemes are often called models. They try to organise information and provide a theory to describe the real world. A model is a description of a reality which tends to be neat and tidy rather than the true, complex, messy one in which we actually live. It is therefore simpler to understand and can act as a clear path to follow while trying to unravel what is happening to the individual patient.

It is a complex world. Some models make better sense in some situations than in others. Knowledge and experience of their use help the nurse to choose the most useful framework for a particular situation. There is no one right answer and no well tested model that has proved all embracing.

Assessment means getting to know about some aspects of the patient or client in considerable detail. Revealing intimate secrets to a stranger within a few minutes of meeting is normally considered odd behaviour. Trust between nurse and patient must be built up quite quickly, far more quickly than normal. Talking about personal affairs produces a feeling of closeness and also a sense of vulnerability. The relationship between the nurse who carries out the initial assessment and the patient often seems closer and deeper than that with other nurses. It may remain so, even if others later spend much more time caring for the patient.

One of the skills which helps in the development of trust is the ability to really listen to what is said. It requires the nurse to hear what words are said and at the same time to notice the tone of voice used, the emphasis on some words and not others, and the non-verbal gestures which accompany the words. The patient needs to know that the nurse really is listening. This requires further questions or checking that what was heard was correctly understood.

The nurse's own body position and non-verbal gestures will also leak information back to the patient. Most of us can sense whether or not someone is genuinely interested in what we are saying, or if they are feeling embarrassed.

Recording a summary of the assessment makes the information available to other nurses, and prevents the often ill and weary patient having to repeat the whole or part of their story to every nurse who looks after them. It is unethical to ask questions and record information which the nurse does not intend to use in her care for the patient. Judgement must be used to filter out useless information and to limit what is recorded to the important items. In the early stages of learning to assess the patient's needs it is common to write far more than is really needed. As judgement develops so the filtering becomes more precise. It then becomes possible to see 'the wood for the trees'.

Planning nursing action

The care that is planned will depend on the patient's individual problem. A precise description of how the problem affects that particular patient makes the selection of nursing action much easier. It also aids in the setting of the goals to be achieved through the nursing care. A detailed analysis of the patient's condition before the illness occurred may aid in describing the desired outcome for the patient.

Nursing action often has to be divided into a series of steps, each one laying a foundation for the next development. The format of the nursing care plan can help or hinder this process. A flow chart format highlights these sequential nursing actions.

Busy people need to take in information quickly so the care to be given is described briefly and uses action words. In the suggestions for nursing actions for the patient problems given in these sections more information is included than would normally be written in a care plan. This should help the reader to select and adapt the suggested action to fit in with the individual patient assessment. Individualized patient care cannot be taken straight out of a book as it has to be tailored to fit the individual patient. There will also be times when the resources available, in the ward or at home, will be less than ideal. Then the selected nursing action also has to be adjusted even further so it becomes realistic in the circumstances.

Setting goals/ outcomes

The outcome of the nursing care prescribed for the patient should be based on the initial problem described, the likely resources available to implement the selected nursing actions and the patient's normal state. The assessment should include information about what was normal for the patient before the illness. The patient's opinions should be taken into account and when possible the outcome described should be mutually agreed. Research in Michigan has shown that this can lead to more effective attainment of goals and greater patient satisfaction, (Horsley, 1982.) Setting a target date may be important, for example when preparing the patient for transfer home. At present there is little research evidence to guide the nurse in predicting the likely rate of progress. It is therefore important to explain to the patient that the date is a guess based on professional experience.

Each nursing action prescribed should have an intended effect on the patient's condition. It would not normally be necessary to record each one in a care plan although learners may be asked to do so for their tutors so that knowledge and understanding can be demonstrated. To aid understanding for the nursing action suggested in this book most nursing action prescriptions are followed by review information. In the ward this information would be used to decide what details of the patient's response to the nursing action should be recorded in the progress notes.

The subsequent rate of progress of the patient's response to nursing care and medical treatment can be compared with the desired outcome set for the problem. If the outcome is described in terms of the physical changes required or what the patient will do, feel or say it becomes easier for those unfamiliar with the patient to assess the speed of progress. For some problems the changes may occur quite quickly and a written note of the patient's response to nursing action may be recorded four or more times in a day. As the rate of change slows so the frequency of the written notes can be reduced. Other problems may not require daily or more frequent comments. For example the leg ulcer being dressed once a week could be described only after the dressing had been removed, so the review comment would be expected on the day the dressing was to be done.

Evelution of the effect of nursing care

The speed with which problems are solved will vary; some, such as recovery from a 'stroke' require weeks of effort rather than days. Evaluation of the effect of the nursing care is important to confirm that the nursing action is having the intended effect and at a speed acceptable to both nurse and patient. Evaluation involves making a judgement about the value of the nursing action and the change achieved. It is more than a description of the patient's response although such information will be needed in making the judgement. Weekly evaluation of all the current problems may be helpful for the acutely ill patient; in the elderly and those with chronic problems, a monthly evaluation may be sufficient.

3

Planning for review and evaluation.

When describing the desired outcome to be achieved for each problem it is helpful to set a frequency for the review comments on the response to care. These then provide information on which to base the evaluation. The frequency of the evaluation should also be set at this time; it may be at regular intervals or relate to a target date for resolution of the problem.

It is also helpful to evaluate the whole of the patient's care just before the patient leaves the hospital ward. Where the nursing service in the hospital is transferring responsibility for the patient's care to the community nurse, additional information may be required. Some problems associated with medical disorders may be chronic. The patient and/or relatives may be able to undertake the necessary treatment and nursing action.

Planning teaching

Teaching patients and their relatives how to carry out nursing care is not the same as merely telling them. It should be carefully planned. The nurse should assess with the patient and relatives how much is known and understood already. Discussing which methods of teaching have been most helpful in the past can guide the nurse in the methods to be used. Some people are visual thinkers. They usually find one of the following helpful: diagrams, drawings, models they can see and handle, equipment they can try for themselves. Others may be able to absorb and understand information only by repeating things several times. A few people can absorb ideas and explanations without other aids, while many prefer to take notes.

In the stress and worry of coping with illness a lot of information may only be held in short-term memory. If the patient is to be nursed at home, this will not be sufficient. A teaching programme should build in small steps and include frequent checks to assess how much has been understood. Information which will be important for care at home has to be firmly fixed in long-term memory. Asking if the patient or relatives have any questions may elicit a request for clarification. It is hard to express what one does not know. Demonstrating what has been remembered is easier. It is therefore important to ask the patient or relative to demonstrate the whole procedure to confirm that it can be correctly carried out.

When the person being taught has difficulty remembering, the procedure or information should be stripped to the bare essentials, as too much information can overload the ability to absorb it all.

It helps to build confidence if a procedure is first demonstrated with a commentary and then tried under supervision. In time the patient or relative should feel able to manage alone, and it is obviously better to reach this stage before the transfer home. The community nurse may well be continuing the care but delays can occur. Confidence is also boosted if any potential difficulties are also discussed. Written instructions can help by providing back-up in case the memory falters. Sometimes just knowing the back-up is there increases confidence, as does permission to telephone for advice, if it should be necessary.

Written information sheets may prove useful for other aspects. Health education is a responsibility shared by nurses in every field in which they work. Most people are curious about how their bodies work and how they can look attractive. The cult of physical fitness and well-being can be useful in moderation. Patient teaching can be extended to education about general health. Relatives appreciate general information about the disease suffered, they may feel unable to express fears that their behaviour has contributed to its development or that there is an increased risk of getting the same disease. Supplies of leaflets and posters can be obtained through the District Health

Education Officer. Most will welcome the opportunity to help in the production of information sheets and leaflets for patients. Writing in a readable, easy-to-understand manner about health care is not always as straightforward as it looks.

The nurse often needs to translate into everyday words the medical terms used by the doctors. It may also be advisable to write down simple explanations which the patient can keep for later reference. Teaching the patient about their condition may require a step by step planned programme within the care plan.

Planning for potential problems

Some medical disorders carry with them an increased risk of additional problems developing. Medical treatments and investigations may also have potential problems. If the patient is aware of these, active participation in their prevention becomes possible. In some instances however, knowing all that could go wrong would worry the patient unnecessarily. The description of the potential problem should include those factors which are present and increase the risk for the individual patient. For example, the number of cigarettes smoked each day would influence the degree of risk of a chest infection developing.

The goal for the nursing care of potential problems will often be focussed on what the nurse hopes to achieve on the patient's behalf rather than a description of the outcome for the patient. Such goals may include early detection of particular changes such as bleeding or limits above or below which medical aid should be sought. An example of these limits would be the maximum blood pressure beyond which the doctor wishes to be called. The nursing action to achieve such goals often includes observation for particular signs or symptoms. The frequency for reviewing the results will change as the risk decreases or increases.

General information in the progress notes

Progress notes are kept to provide assessment information about the patient's condition. Alongside these needs to go more general information which may help to explain the background. Care which has not been given in the way requested in the nursing care plan should be noted together with the reason. There will be times when there is a sudden change in the patient's care. Immediate action is required. To write a plan of care for the future would not be appropriate. The nursing action should be taken and the entry in the progress notes should then give the assessment information, and describe the problem which occurred with the action taken. The result of the action should be assessed. In some instances the immediate problem requires further care to be planned. This then goes into the care plan in the usual way.

Up-dating the care plan

The nursing action section of the care plan should be changed in line with the patient's response to the nursing action. When the problem is considered solved the plan should record this together with the date of resolution.

Sometimes there may be little or no progress or the problem may even have worsened. The patient's condition should be reassessed to check if signs have been missed. New clues may be present and the problem description may be found to be incorrect. The nursing care prescribed in the care plan may not have been carried out, or it may not have been the most effective action to choose. Another reason for the apparent lack of progress is that the outcome described and against which progress has been measured is not realistic and achievable within the time limit that was set.

Nursing care plans require judgements to be made on the basis of professional knowledge, experience and intuition. One way of learning and developing judgement is by weighing up the success of the planned care.

Evaluation of the whole care plan

Making judgements about how effectively the planned nursing care has influenced the patient's problems and potential problems requires a broad range and depth of knowledge. It is often difficult to decide what aspects of change in the patient's condition can be attributed to nursing action. Health care involves team effort with the patient very much part of the team. In the past, the patient's view of what improvement was required has rarely been sought. However health education and the acceptance of individual responsibility for keeping healthy is changing the patient's expectations of involvement.

To evaluate, the nurse needs to know the initial problem for the patient, the available nursing actions, and the patient's desired outcome together with the nurse's assessment of what was desirable and possible. The outcome agreed between the patient and nurse should have been recorded in the goal. It may differ from the individual goals of nurse and patient. The nurse then needs an assessment of the current state of the problem area.

The judgments to be made include whether the desired goal was achieved or even surpassed. The route used to achieve the result needs to be considered to identify whether there may have been more effective or efficient choices. Was time wasted by starting off on an unrealistic pattern of nursing action or did it need to be revised? Did the patient share the same view of the problem or was it imposed by the nurses? Was the result of the action influenced by this?

In developing nursing knowledge the evaluation of care may help to decide which nursing actions are most effective in dealing with specific or new problems. Again the patient's views need to be taken into account. It becomes important to agree criteria for effectiveness. There is a tendency to concentrate on the procedures rather than the outcome. Procedure manuals tend to reinforce the assumption that the process of giving care is more important than the result of that care for the patient. This has led to ineffective procedures being continued — sometimes long after they have been shown to have no effect or even to be dangerous, the handful of salt dissolved in the bath being an excellent example.

The review information can be scanned to provide information for the evaluation of nursing action. This activity may in itself highlight weakness in the choice of frequency set for recording progress or in the amount of detail recorded. Each problem area which required nursing action can be evaluated and its contribution to the total nursing care be considered. A discussion with the patient of the results of the nursing care can help the nurse assess whether there are gaps in her knowledge or skills which led to care that appeared ineffective to the patient. Thinking about the results of nursing care together with the patient helps the nurse assess personal development and knowledge. It can stimulate further study, change assumptions and help to build up new knowledge. It helps to make nursing an exciting activity. Nursing actions cease to be mundane, routine or menial when thought and skill are involved.

References and further reading

Henderson, V., Nite, G. 6th edn. (1978). *Principles and Practice of Nursing.* Macmillan Publishing Co. New York

Horsley, J.A. (1982). *Mutual Goal Setting in Patient Care Conduct and Utilization of Research in Nursing Project.* Michigan Nurses Association/ Grune and Stratton Inc., New York. Distributed in the UK by Academic Press Inc. (London) Ltd.

Roper, N. (1980). *The Elements of Nursing.* Churchill Livingstone. Edinburgh.

2 Breathing

Optimum environment

Most people take the act of breathing for granted, unless perhaps they suffer from a chest disease. The common cold, or sudden exercise such as swimming can temporarily make one aware of the actual effort required to warm and moisten the air ready for the lungs to extract oxygen.

The composition of the air has recently been the subject of concern because of the local increases in carbon dioxide and sulphur products from industrial chimneys, especially those that burn coal or oil. The air is composed mainly of inert nitrogen (79%) and oxygen (20%) with carbon dioxide and tiny quantities of other gases making up the remaining 1%. The air we breathe also contains small particles of dust and water vapour. Rain can wash out some of this material, the sulphur products falling as dilute sulphuric acid which, with nitric acid, in time erodes stone. Acid rain, as this is called, has recently been implicated in killing trees and fish in many lakes in the northern hemisphere. In general humans seem to adapt although the lungs of town dwellers are black with trapped soot.

Healthy lungs contain tiny sacs or alveoli at the ends of fine tubes. They have thin walls with a net of tiny blood vessels on the outside. Inside the alveoli are lined by a detergent-like material called surfactant which helps them distend easily with each breath, and prevents them from collapsing at the end of each expiration.

The air is brought down to the sacs by a system of tubes which change in size from the two large bronchi which join to the trachea down to tiny bronchioles. Partial rings of cartilage in the walls of the larger tubes keep them open. They are lined with tiny hairs or cilia, and cells which produce sticky mucus. Particles of dust which find their way into these tubes can get caught in the mucus and are slowly passed up towards the top of the trachea by the wafting of the cilia. These bend and straighten, rather like a field of corn in the wind, and sweep the particles along.

The larynx or voice box is found between the upper part of the trachea and the root of the tongue. The vocal cords relax opening up the passage during quiet breathing. By a narrowing of the space between these cords as air passes out during phonation the voice is produced.

To protect the larynx, and the lungs, from fluid or food spilling in during swallowing, a leaf-like flap, the epiglottis, closes over the larynx so that food is passed from the pharynx to the oesophagus (gullet).

The air breathed in through the nose is warmed, moistened and filtered by passing over blood vessels lying close to the surface, and by the hairs which line the first part of the nose. Mucus and tiny cilia trap smaller particles. Blowing the nose after doing a dirty job quickly illustrates how efficient a dust trap they are. Air breathed in through the mouth is dryer, colder and unfiltered.

Movement of the ribs outward and upward helps to draw air in. The lungs and the inside of the chest wall have linings known as pleura which stick together with a thin film of fluid. Each lung has its own pleural lining, the visceral pleura. Between the lungs lie the heart, the gullet and part of the trachea.

The lungs not only help oxygen enter the body, they also help get rid of carbon dioxide, a waste product from cell activity. If the lungs suffer chronic damage from repeated, severe attacks of bronchitis, then the carbon dioxide may not be moved out of the body so easily. Chronic bronchitis means a persistent cough with a lot of phlegm (sputum) for 3 or more months each year over successive years. (Grenville-Mathers, 1983.) It is very common in Britain, especially among smokers. The lining of the lungs thickens, and its cells produce extra mucus which narrows the tubes through which air and oxygen enter, and carbon dioxide leaves.

The raised level of carbon dioxide in the body fails to trigger the normal response of faster breaths to expel it and take in more oxygen. The face and lips take on a bluish colour and the ankles and legs swell. Each time the bronchitis gets worse the lungs and heart get damaged still further. Treatment with oxygen becomes more difficult as the brain gets used to higher and higher levels of carbon dioxide. Every cold then carries a risk of serious illness.

The common cold

This unpleasant condition is caused by a virus, of which there are several species. It multiplies within the mucous membrane lining the nose and throat, destroying the infected cells as the new virus particles break out to infect other cells. The irritated membranes get sore and produce mucus in large quantities giving a runny nose. The lining swells as its blood supply increases to bring in the body's defences to fight off the virus and any bacteria which might get a foothold on the damaged surface.

The virus is spread as droplets. A forceful sneeze can spread infected droplets for some distance. Trapping a sneeze in a thick paper tissue helps to prevent spread. Paper tissues which can be used to blow the nose once and then be disposed of (into a plastic bag for burning) also help. Unless it is possible to wash the hands after each sneeze or blow, viral particles may be passed on by the hands. It is wise for the sufferer to stay at home for two days until the worst has passed.

Breathing through the mouth while the nose is blocked dries the mucous membranes. A warm room and lots of warm drinks will help. Aspirin or paracetamol every four hours may be taken for a high temperature or headache (adults only).

Some people believe that taking extra vitamin C during the winter helps to prevent colds. A dose of 500 mg to 1 gram twice a day with food may be taken. Soluble flavoured tablets can be bought from health food shops.

Coughing

The cough is sudden, explosive movement of air from the lungs to remove foreign particles. It may be triggered by dust, irritating gas or smoke, sputum and infected tissues.

If the lining of the trachea and bronchi become infected, for example after a common cold, then mucus production increases. The cough then brings up mucus, dead bacteria and the white cells which have crossed from the blood vessels to fight the infection. The sputum becomes creamy or even green in colour. If possible it should be coughed out into the mouth so it can be spat into a paper tissue or disposable pot. If it is swallowed in large quantities it may irritate the stomach lining.

A cough medicine for such a cough should contain an expectorant to loosen and liquify the sputum, and should not suppress the cough. Extra fluids up to 4 litres a day should also be taken to help keep the sputum moist. The body loses a lot of water when there is productive coughing, particularly if there is associated fever.

Rest and sleep may be less disturbed by the cough if all the loose secretions are cleared out before settling. The patient can achieve this in the following way:

1. Sit up, tissues at hand.
2. Breathe in deeply three times.
3. 'Huff' out in short sharp breaths.
4. Try to cough if the 'huffing' has not triggered the cough.

Repeat until all the loose material has been coughed up.

A dry cough can be exhausting. No phlegm is produced and there may be an irritating tickling sensation. A cough mixture based on codeine may be used to calm down the cough, and allow undisturbed rest.

A persistent cough lasting more than a couple of weeks should be investigated by a doctor as it could be caused by a number of things.

Cigarette smoking Tobacco smoke destroys the tiny cilia which line the trachea and bronchii, when it is inhaled. The irritation can lead to mucus production. During sleep mucus drains from the bronchii while the body is horizontal, and on waking and sitting upright the amount may be enough to trigger the early morning smoker's cough. The tars from the tobacco smoke help colour the phlegm, and may eventually lead to cancer.

On average someone who smokes 20 cigarettes a day will shorten their life by five years. The effects of smoking on the lungs include narrowing of the bronchioles, reduced exchange of gases between the alveoli and the blood and changes in the lining of the lungs. The heart is also affected, and the pulse rate rises as does the blood pressure. The carbon monoxide in the smoke links with the oxygen carrier, haemoglobin, in the red cells of the blood. It therefore reduces the amount of oxygen which can be picked up for transport to other areas of the body. At the same time it makes the lining of the arteries more permeable to cholesterol. Over time, such fatty deposits narrow the blood vessels.

The nicotine carried in the smoke stimulates the nervous system in small doses. In large doses it depresses it, and produces a sedative effect in the regular smoker. It is addictive so stopping smoking leads first to withdrawal symptoms, which include depression, irritability, anxiety, a feeling of tension or restlessness. Some people find it harder to concentrate for several weeks after giving up smoking.

The lining of the lungs (the cilia) can recover, so with an active system a smoker's cough may actually get worse as the debris which has collected is swept up into the trachea once more.

Smoke tends to dull the sense of taste, which apart from sweet, sour, bitter and salty, actually comes from cells in the nose. Once the smoke stops blocking the sense of taste, food becomes more attractive and this increases the temptation to eat more in place of smoking. Smokers lose their sensitivity to smoke so they are unaware that their clothes smell of smoke, as does their breath, hair and skin.

Giving up smoking is not easy, and it needs determination and perseverance to overcome an addiction. The following points may prove helpful:

1. Observe the pattern of cigarette smoking for two days. It may help to note down what activities go with smoking. For many people it may be linked to meals, or to leisure activities.

2. Plan a change of habit to avoid a gap at the time cigarettes are usually smoked, for example at coffee time.

3. Decide to stop smoking on a definite day. Forewarn relatives and friends and ask for their support.

4. Avoid places or situations where the temptation to smoke may be too great, for instance when a lot of other people are smoking. This is particularly important when first giving up.

5. Buy no more cigarettes. Throw out any that remain on the day you are to stop.

6. Put the planned change of habits into action.

7. Concentrate on getting through each day or hour without smoking.

8. Put the money aside that used to be spent on cigarettes, and buy a reward at the end of each week without cigarettes.

Some people find nicotine chewing gum helps. Others use a gum containing a chemical that produces an unpleasant taste when a cigarette is smoked. Support groups may run locally. The anti-smoking group ASH can provide useful addresses.

The Health Education Council provides free information packs on smoking and how to give it up.

Non-smokers can avoid passive smoking by avoiding rooms where smokers congregate, and by using non-smoking coaches, areas in restaurants, cinemas and other public places. Pressure is still needed for an increase in these facilities. Breathing in other people's smoke can increase the level of carbon monoxide linked to the haemoglobin in the blood, so reducing the oxygen available to the body.

Hayfever

Summer can be a misery for those allergic to pollen in the air. Tree and grass pollen are the commonest causes, and they can also trigger asthma in susceptible people.

In a hayfever attack the eyes become red, sore and watery. The nose becomes blocked and produces copious mucus, and the chest may feel tight. Tiredness and the constant discomfort can lead to irritability and loss of concentration.

Some family doctors are willing to give a course of desensitizing injections during early spring, before the pollen count rises. Once the symptoms occur they can be treated by anti-histamine drugs and by reducing exposure to pollen. The anti-histamine drugs help by drying up the nasal secretion and reducing itching, but they also dry up the throat and increase the feeling of tiredness. Care must be taken with activities requiring a quick reaction as drowsiness may occur. Few people are able or willing to have filtered air to breathe but most can limit the time they spend outdoors when the pollen count is high. The radio and some newspapers give the daily pollen counts, although these may be 24—48 hours old.

People who have a tendency towards hayfever are described as being atopic. Atopy runs in families, and the affected person produces large amounts of antibodies to certain antigens — for example pollen in hayfever. They may be prone to other allergies, such as to animal fur, and they may suffer from eczema and asthma.

Sinusitis

The resonance of the voice comes in part from the sinus cavities within the skull. These air-containing bony boxes have small openings which connect with the air passages within the nose. Their mucous membranes can swell with a common cold and so block the openings. Bacteria may infect the static mucus, and give rise to acute pain, fever, swelling over the site and a feeling of heaviness. Once drainage restarts the mucus is thick and yellow or green, being made up from dead bacteria and white cells. The material drains into the nose or down the back of the throat as catarrh. This can give bad breath (halitosis) and nausea.

If the infection is not dealt with by antibiotics it may become chronic. The mucous membrane is swollen due to inflammation and may obstruct the free flow of air through the nose.

Occupational hazards

The Health and Safety at Work Act has made people more aware of their responsibility to use safety equipment properly. Dust and particles in the air inhaled over a long period of time can lead to disease such as coal-workers' pneumoconiosis from coal dust, silicosis in quarrymen, nasal tumours from sawdust in the furniture trade and asbestosis from contact with asbestos fibres. Farmers risk 'farmers lung' (aspergillosis) from fungal spores on hay.

Face masks, breathing apparatus and machine shields should be used to reduce the risk. Dust may be prevented from escaping into the general work area by good design, placing hoods over the dirty process with a powerful fan to suck the air and dust into ducts. Dust cleaning may then be used to prevent the polluted air being spread outside the factory. Such ventilation equipment should be used when supplied. Not only has the employer a duty to provide the equipment but also the employee has a duty to use it and use it properly.

General assessment areas

Rate, rhythm and depth of respirations
Breathing sounds
Shape of thorax, presence of scars
Dyspnoea in relation to activity
Influence of body position
Presence, type and quantity of sputum
Colour of sputum
Pain related to respirations
Use of accessory muscles

Problems

	Page
Unable to expel air adequately (due to bronchospasm)	15
Exhausted by rapid respirations	17
Unable to breathe deeply due to pain, muscle weakness or pressure on diaphragm	20
Unable to expel thick, tenacious sputum	21
Unable to expel sputum due to muscle weakness	24
Uncomfortable from dry cough	26
Hyperventilation/overbreathing	27
Dependent on oxygen therapy	29
Secreting excessive pleural fluid	31

Potential problems

Risk of airway obstruction	32
Risk of pulmonary oedema due to fluid overload	35
Risk of cross infection from infected sputum	37

Problems

Problem	**Unable to expel air adequately (due to bronchospasm).**

Assessment findings	Marked wheeze when breathing out Laboured breathing with prolonged effort to breathe out Coughing spasms Anxious Rapid pulse Exhaustion Thick sputum
Information for the patient	The smaller tubes in the lungs have gone into spasm making it difficult to clear all the used air from the lungs. Any phlegm present gets thick and sticky which makes matters worse. The treatment will help to relax the tubes and loosen up the phlegm.
Nursing action	1. Support the patient with a backrest and pillows in a comfortable sitting position, or leaning forward over a firm bedtable covered with a pillow (orthopnoeic position). Check the patient is not allergic to feathers. RE. Check that the position is comfortable. Foam or flock pillows should be substituted for feather if allergy is suspected. 2. Provide small, frequent drinks to start rehydration. An intake of 2000 ml in 24 hours may be required, depending on fluid balance and the estimated continuing fluid loss in sweat and exhaled air. Avoid ice-cold drinks which may induce further bronchospasm. RE. Record fluid intake and output to measure progress in rehydrating the patient. 3. Stay with the patient if they are distressed. Try to reduce anxiety due to admission to hospital by ensuring any immediate problems with the family or home are dealt with. RE. Check the patient's facial expression and body posture for reduced muscle tension. Monitor, if, when and for how long the patient sleeps. 4. Provide a sputum pot with lid, and tissues. Explain how to collect sputum in the container. Label it with the patient's name, the date and starting time of collection. RE. Inspect the sputum at least once a day, measure the quantity and assess whether sputum is becoming liquefied in response to rehydration. Check sputum pot is replaced at least once a day. 5. Try to remove any possible causes of bronchospasm from the patient's environment. Fur, feathers, flowers, smoke and house dust may all act as triggers for individual patients. A bed near an open window may be helpful. RE. Check with the patient all the recognised triggers have been removed. Observe for any unexpected causes.

Further action

1. A sputum specimen collected in a labelled sterile container may be requested for culture and antibiotic sensitivity before antibiotic therapy commences.

RE. Observe that the patient does not contaminate the inside of the container when holding it. Check the label gives the correct details. Ensure rapid delivery to the laboratory.

2. Mucolytics (drugs which lessen the tenacity of mucus) such as bromhexine, may be given for short periods. The effect is unproven.

RE. Inspect the sputum every six hours to see if it becomes more liquid. Ask the patient to report any upset of digestion or bowels.

3. Bronchodilating drugs may be prescribed to relax the smooth muscle in the bronchioles. Salbutamol may be given via a nebuliser, using compressed air or oxygen as the carrier gas.

RE. Peak expiratory flow rate (maximum rate of flow of air during forced expiration) measured before and after the use of a nebuliser, indicates the response to the drug. The highest of three readings is recorded for each test. Normal range 400-600L/min.

4. Pocket size aerosols may be prescribed for use by patients with chronic problems. Ask the patient to demonstrate their use. Warn them that it is dangerous to exceed the prescribed dose and frequency. A slow, deep breath taken as the aerosol is released and held for 5 to 10 seconds before breathing out again gives the best effect.

RE. Observe that the anxious patient does not overuse the drug. Check for side effects such as increased pulse rate and shakiness.

5. Aminophylline may be given by intravenous injection, infusion, orally or as a suppository. Check the rectum is empty before giving a suppository so that complete absorption of the drug will occur.

RE. Inspect peri-anal skin for inflammation. Ask the patient to report any rectal tenderness or soreness as proctitis can occur. Intravenously the drug may cause a fall in blood pressure, nausea, vomiting, diarrhoea, rapid pulse, cardiac arrhythmias or fits. It must be given slowly. An ECG may be useful if there is any history of arrhythmia.

6. Physiotherapy can aid expectoration and prevent lung consolidation. Clapping and shaking the chest wall loosens sputum and may be carried out by a nurse.

RE. Observe for exhaustion which can occur quite quickly in an ill patient. Record whether an increased amount of sputum is produced in the hour after treatment.

7. Humidified oxygen may be prescribed, the rate depending on the underlying cause of the bronchospasm. A fresh sterile humidifier and tubing should be used for each patient, and it should be changed daily. Sterile water should be used. Oxygen sustains fire so anyone entering the area should be asked not to smoke tobacco. A 'No smoking' sign may be used.

RE. Check the face mask fits comfortably and does not cause pressure, especially on sweaty skin or behind the ears. Check the level of water at least hourly and top up as necessary. Also check the flow rate remains at the rate prescribed.

8. A skin test may be used to identify an allergic response. Suspect antigens are injected intra-dermally. A course of desensitising injections may be prescribed if allergy is confirmed.

RE. A red wheal occurs at the injection site if the patient is allergic to the antigen. A control injection is used for comparison. A severe reaction may occur during a desensitising injection. Adrenalin and resuscitation equipment should be available in case of severe bronchospasm.

Associated medical diagnoses	Asthma Bronchitis Cardiac asthma Cardiac failure Chronic obstructive airways disease

---

Problem	**Exhausted by rapid respirations.**

Assessment findings	Respiratory rate over 30 per minute Shallow breathing Less movement on one side of the chest than the other Fever Increased metabolic rate (raised BMR) Restless Headache Weakness Blurred vision
Information for the patient	When breathing is an effort, tense muscles use up precious energy and increase the body's need for oxygen. Relaxing the muscles and lying back against a comfortable chair or pillows can reduce the energy needed and help ease breathing.
Nursing action	1. Provide at least five pillows to prop the patient in a comfortable sitting position when in bed. Consider whether sitting in a chair would provide a more comfortable position. Leaning forward on to a pillow placed on a bed table may help. RE. Ask the patient if the position is comfortable. Check respiratory rate after five minutes. Note if facial muscles appear to relax. 2. Plan extra rest periods during the day. Discuss the need for rest with other staff involved with the patient's treatment. RE. Note how much rest the patient is given. Note if any staff ignore a request to allow the patient to rest, so that the need for therapy and the times it is given can be reviewed and the care plan adjusted. 3. Review fluid balance, as the increased loss of water vapour in breath requires replacement. RE. Record fluid intake and output. Observe for loss of skin turgor and dry mouth. Confusion and increased restlessness can occur if dehydration is not treated. 4. Adjust height of bed and be ready to help the patient change position, as a

breathless person is usually a restless one. Examine bed area for possible safety risks. Avoid use of cot-sides as the feeling of being hemmed in may increase distress.

RE. Observe for change in the level of restlessness and check the skin for redness from increased friction from restless movement.

Further action

1. Blood gas analysis results may indicate that oxygen therapy is required.

RE. There is a correct ratio of oxygen to carbon dioxide in arterial blood (the normal values are pCO = 30–40 mm Hg and pO = 90–100 mm Hg per 100 ml arterial blood) and a fall in one and a rise in the other will alter the pressure gradient and inhibit gas exchange in the alveoli, leading to cyanosis and dyspnoea. Blood gas levels may need to be checked at frequent intervals.

2. Avoid giving narcotic drugs unless an antagonist such as Naloxone is available to treat possible respiratory depression.

RE. If a narcotic is given record respiratory rate and depth every 15 minutes following administration by injection. If after 30 minutes the rate has fallen by half, inform the doctor as depression of the respiratory centre may lead to inadequate oxygen levels in the blood. Naloxone by injection acts within 2–3 minutes; the analgesic property of the narcotic is also lost at the same time.

3. Tracheostomy may be considered in extreme cases, as the reduction in the length of the airway through which air must be drawn before reaching the lung tissue, may significantly reduce the effort of breathing. The operation to form the opening below the larynx is usually undertaken in the operating theatre. A plastic tracheostomy tube with a soft cuff inflated with air provides an artificial path for air, while sealing off the lungs from fluid collecting above the tube in the trachea. Record the exact volume of air used to inflate the cuff. Check the pilot balloon is inflated. A nurse should remain with the patient for at least 24 hours after such surgery.

RE. Check the tapes used to tie the tracheostomy tube in place are changed when soiled. Inspect the pilot balloon for signs of deflation at least every half hour.

4. Deflate the cuff at regular intervals and for the length of time prescribed by the doctor to reduce the risk of pressure necrosis on the trachea at the site of the cuff. Record the amount of air needed to reinflate the cuff sufficiently to achieve a seal (no leak of air around the tube).

RE. Report any decrease in the amount needed as this may indicate oedema or other swelling.

5. Suction of the airway may be needed, especially if the patient has become too exhausted to cough effectively. Aseptic technique is essential. Humidified oxygen may be prescribed, using sterile water, to reduce drying of secretions and to replace the moistening effect of the nose and upper trachea. (See page 24).

RE. Check sufficient sterile equipment remains at hand so that the need to re-use suction catheters is avoided. Assess state of secretions at least every four hours. Assess whether tracheostomy lumen remains clear of dried secretions. The tube may need replacement if its lumen narrows and increases the difficulty of breathing.

6. Inspect the tracheostomy site for bleeding and air leakage into the surrounding subcutaneous tissues at least half hourly for the first two hours, and hourly thereafter for 24 hours.

RE. Slight oozing should decrease within two hours of the surgery. Replace the dressing only if heavily soiled otherwise bleeding may be increased by its movement. The risk of infection increases if the surrounding dressing remains moist, especially if humidified oxygen or air is being given. Observe for signs of infection or slough at least daily. Secretions may contain blood even when the edges of the wound have sealed over.

7. Observe blood pressure, respiratory rate, pulse and skin colour every half hour.

RE. An increasing respiratory rate with rising pulse may indicate the need for suction of the airway. Cyanosis and distress may increase if suction is ineffective in clearing the airway. Rapid pulse rate with restlessness may indicate bleeding or hypoxia (low tissue oxygen levels).

8. Provide a means of non-spoken communication, such as a note pad or list of symbols, while the patient cannot talk. Fear is increased if needs cannot readily be made known. The procedures needed to care for the tracheostomy and for suction are uncomfortable and frightening for the patient. Explain each step in simple terms. When the patient can be left unattended provide a hand bell or buzzer within easy reach, so that attention can be attracted quickly if necessary.

RE. Check the patient does not become tired while trying to communicate, pointing at symbols in reply to questions may be less effort than writing. Observe for signs of apprehension or discomfort. Note frequency of use of bell to attract attention, as regular use may indicate fear or feelings of insecurity.

9. Physiotherapy at regular intervals aids the removal of secretions, but must be balanced with the amount of energy the patient has so that the procedure does not exhaust them further. A daily chest X-ray may be requested to monitor lung condition.

RE. Plan treatment at periods when it can be followed by at least half an hour's rest.

Associated medical diagnoses

Anxiety state
Atelectasis
Bacteraemia
Cerebral vascular accident
Chronic obstructive airway disease
Encephalitis
Hyperthyroidism
Interstitial lung disease
Meningitis
Pneumonia
Pontine lesion
Pulmonary embolism
Salicylate poisoning

Problem	Unable to breathe deeply due to pain, muscle weakness or pressure on diaphragm.

Assessment findings

Shallow, rapid respirations
Chest wall moves less than normal
Tense body position, and facial expression indicating pain
Cyanosis (blue lips and fingertips)
Drowsiness
Asymmetrical expansion of chest
Tense, swollen abdomen

Information for the patient

Oxygen from the air is transferred into the body by the lungs. In order to get the right level of oxygen the body has a number of chemical triggers. Shallow breathing becomes more rapid if the body needs to raise the oxygen level. Giving extra oxygen via a mask can relieve rapid shallow breathing.

The diaphragm is a broad sheet of muscle which divides the chest from the stomach, liver and other organs. It will move downwards to help draw air into the chest if the stomach and intestines are not pressing on it, and thus sitting up can make breathing more comfortable and effortless.

Painful spasms when taking a deep breath are part of a vicious circle in which the muscles become tense because of the pain. Controlling the pain will help the muscles relax and aid deep breathing.

Nursing action

1. Relieve pain with regular prescribed analgesia.

RE. Ask the patient about the degree of pain relief half an hour after analgesia. If it remains inadequate discuss medication with the doctor. Consider using a pain chart to record the pain and the effect of the drugs.

2. Support the patient in an upright sitting position to use gravity in moving abdominal organs away from diaphragm.

Position the patient's arms comfortably away from the chest to avoid any restriction of chest movement from their weight. Offer regular bedpans or urinals so that a distended bladder does not add to abdominal volume.

RE. Assess whether the change in position allows an increase in respiratory depth shown by increased movements of the chest wall. Check that respiratory rate decreases.

Further action

1. Humidified oxygen may be given by a Polymask or Venti-mask at 4 litres per minute (60% oxygen) if cyanosis is present.

RE. Assess any change in the patient's colour after 15 minutes. Check that the respiratory rate decreases as the depth increases. Check whether sputum becomes thinner and easier to expectorate.

2. Physiotherapy will help achieve increased chest expansion and loosening of secretions. Gentle slapping and vibrating over the ribs may be required if a coughing spasm fails to produce sputum.

RE. Balance the patient's need for help in expectorating with the need for rest. Adjust care plan to provide time to recover from vigorous physiotherapy before other procedures are carried out.

3. Analgesia may be prescribed for pain. Give the initial doses at the most frequent intervals prescribed. Aim to make the patient pain-free, and ask

them to report as soon as the pain begins to return so that the next dose can be given straight away. Opiates are normally avoided as they depress respirations.

RE. Assess the level of pain and the respiratory rate half an hour after each dose of analgesia. Report the pain level to the doctor if the prescribed dosage and frequency does not control the pain and allow more comfortable respirations.

4. Sputum specimens may be required for culture and sensitivity, or for cytology. If the patient repeatedly swallows sputum, then gastric washings, taken before breakfast, may be required. A naso-gastric tube (12 or 14 FG) is passed into the stomach. Air is injected to confirm that the tube is in the stomach, and 10 ml normal saline is then introduced into the stomach and aspirated back. The specimen obtained is transferred to a sterile container and sent to the laboratory.

RE. Infected sputum may be resistant to some antibiotics. Review the culture results in case isolation of the patient is necessary to prevent cross infection.

5. Gross abdominal distension by ascitic fluid may be relieved by abdominal paracentesis. The cannula is inserted through the abdominal wall so the urinary bladder should be emptied beforehand to prevent accidental puncture. The drainage tubing and bag should be handled using strict aseptic techniques. The drainage rate should be controlled with a clip so that no more than 500 ml drains in an hour. A specimen may be collected for cytology.

RE. Record fluid intake and output. Check the patient's pulse and respiratory rate after the first hour. Check the blood pressure at least twice a day. Protein is lost in ascitic fluid so large volumes drained off will alter the fluid distribution between the circulation and tissues. A high protein diet may be required.

Associated medical diagnoses	Ascites
	Bronchial asthma
	Carcinoma
	Cholecystitis
	Congestive cardiac failure
	Emphysema
	Fractured ribs
	Lymphoma (involving hilar nodes)
	Metastatic deposits in ribs or thoracic spine
	Myasthenia gravis
	Pleurisy
	Pneumonia
	Poliomyelitis
	Tuberculosis

| Problem | Unable to expel thick tenacious sputum. |

Assessment findings	Unproductive cough
	Thick jelly-like sputum plugs
	Exhaustion

Too breathless to drink more than sips of fluid
Dehydration — dry, inelastic skin
Reduced urine output
Fluid loss exceeds fluid intake

Information for the patient

The phlegm is thick and sticky so it is hard to cough up from deep inside the lungs. Drinking a little and often will help make the inhaled air moist and so soften up the phlegm. If possible, cough any phlegm up and spit it into the pot provided, so that it can be checked to see if it is becoming less sticky.

Nursing action

1. Provide a disposable sputum pot labelled with the patient's name, date and time, and paper tissues.

RE. Check the sputum consistency and the amount coughed up at four hourly intervals or at least twice during the daytime. Rehydration should be accompanied by the sputum becoming thinner and less tenacious.

2. Moist, warm inhalation of water vapour ('steam'), with or without tincture of benzoin, can be given two- to three-hourly, depending on the patient's energy level, to encourage the patient to breathe deeply and to temporarily increase moisture level in bronchioles. The presence of tincture of benzoin provides the patient with a reason to breathe deeply.

RE. Supervise the patient during the inhalation and check respirations are deep by placing a hand lightly on each side of the rib cage to detect degree of movement.

3. Provide the patient with small frequent drinks of cool fluids. If necessary agree a 'contract' with the patient for the nurse to provide and the patient to drink an agreed volume of fluid each hour. Encourage the patient by informing them on how close to the target they are getting.

RE. Chart fluid intake and output. The average insensible loss is 500 ml in 24 hours; 1000 ml is required for adequate urinary excretion, therefore fluid intake should exceed output and be at least 1500 ml per day.

4. Supervise deep breathing exercises, teach the patient forced expiration, 'huffing' and coughing. The juice of half a lemon in a glass of very hot water can help the reluctant patient to cough, the sharp taste often causing rapid indrawing of breath which leads to coughing.

RE. Assess the respiratory effort and effect of coughing.

Further action

1. Physiotherapy — clapping the chest and assisting expiration by shaking the rib cage will help in the coughing up of sputum. Postural drainage of the lungs by lowering the head of the patient's bed, will assist drainage of blocked bronchioles.

RE. Measure the amount of sputum coughed up after postural drainage.

2. Bronchodilating drugs may be given orally, by injection or by inhalation. The last route is only effective if the airway is not coated with sticky mucus. Salbutamol may be given by an inhaler, and correct use is essential if the drug is to be effective. Demonstrate the use and supervise the patient until the skill is achieved. A slow deep breath as the aerosol is released should then be held for a count of 5—10 before breathing out.

RE. Check that the bronchodilating drug is given before any planned exertion, to prevent exercise-induced bronchospasm. Activities may need to be replanned to fit in with the prescribed times for the drug. A spirometer may be used to measure peak flow immediately before and 10 minutes after the drug is given. Report any decrease in the effect of the drug, having confirmed that the patient takes it correctly. This may indicate a deterioration in the patient's condition.

3. Nebulised salbutamol may be prescribed for those who cannot use an inhaler. The patient should be helped into an upright sitting position and instructed in the correct use of the nebuliser. It is usually connected to an oxygen supply of 5 litres/min until the bronchodilator (mixed with sterile sodium chloride 0.9%) is used up.

RE. Check the mask fits snugly. Side effects from salbutamol occur less often with the inhalation method of administration. Report any marked increase in pulse rate, nervousness, tremor, dizziness or insomnia.

4. Aminophylline is another bronchodilator which may be prescribed. Like theophylline it enhances the effect of salbutamol, so the dose should only be increased with caution. Both drugs may be given orally, or by rectal suppository. Aminophylline may also be given by slow intravenous injection for severe bronchospasm. Advise the patient to limit their intake of coffee to two cups a day. Smokers should limit themselves to 10 cigarettes a day if they cannot stop smoking, as drug interactions can occur.

RE. Toxic levels can occur, especially in the elderly, and plasma levels may be measured to monitor and adjust the dosage. Side effects to be reported include nausea, vomiting, diarrhoea, rapid or irregular pulse, and with suppositories, rectal irritation, soreness or inflammation. In epileptics, fits may increase in frequency.

5. Corticosteroid drugs decrease the amount of mucus produced and the viscosity of the sputum, easing expectoration. They also aid bronchodilation. They include beclomethasone by inhalation, and prednisolone tablets or intravenous hydrocortisone for acute asthma. Their use requires careful monitoring and dose adjustment, as with any steroid drug.

RE. Observe for signs of low potassium if diuretics are also prescribed (see page 108). Check the blood pressure at least once daily. If large doses are in use, test the urine for glucose at least once a day as blood sugar levels may rise. Prolonged use of steroids can lead to rapid weight gain from fluid retention. Record body weight once a week. Osteoporosis can sometimes occur, increasing the risk of fractures from minor falls, especially in the elderly. Cushing's syndrome may also occur due to the effects of cortisol.

Associated medical diagnoses

Asthma
Bronchial asthma
Bronchitis
Bronchiectasis
Pneumonia

Problem	Unable to expel sputum due to muscle weakness.

Assessment findings

Unable to cough up sputum
Chest sounds wet and gurgling
Bluish colour of lips and nails (cyanosis)
Tires very easily
Restless
Increased pulse rate

Information for the patient

The phlegm (sputum) collects in the main air tubes within the lungs. Coughing it up takes a lot of effort, so instead it can be removed by suction, using long thin sterile tubes called catheters. The suction will also remove some of the oxygen so it will only be done for a very short time. As a guide to how long to suck at any one time, the nurses will hold their own breath while using the suction catheter. The suction machine is very noisy, and the tone changes during the suction. Signals can be agreed to indicate the need for suction, or when it feels uncomfortable. Removing the phlegm can be helped by changes in body position so the different tubes in the lung get emptied into the main one (trachea). Keeping the phlegm loose by drinking extra fluid will also help.

Nursing action

1. Clear secretions from trachea and pharynx via an established airway (see further action) or use a Guedel airway (Fig. 2.1). Choose the smallest size catheter that will collect sputum. Set the suction control to give −5 mmHg. Use a 'Y' connection or a side opening at the catheter connection to avoid suction during insertion. Cover the opening when suction is applied during the withdrawal of the catheter along the airway. Repeat until the airway is clear. Limit length of suction to the time during which you can hold your own breath. Record size of suction catheter used on nursing care plan.

RE. Note any difficulty in aspiration, reflex coughing stimulated by suction and the patient's reaction during suction. Note the colour of the sputum. Look at the patient's colour after suction. Consider giving oxygen for 5−10 minutes prior to future suction application if cyanosis occurs. Record time of suction. Assess whether the frequency with which secretions accumulate changes, by recording the time span between periods of suction.

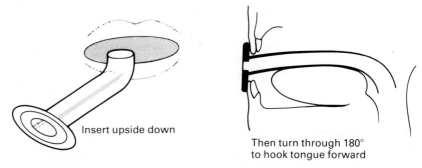

Insert upside down

Then turn through 180°
to hook tongue forward

Fig. 2.1 Insertion of a guedel airway to hold tongue forward and maintain the airway

2. Clear suction tubing of sputum at the end of the procedure by sucking up about 100 ml of sodium bicarbonate solution (1 level 5 ml teaspoon of the powder to 500 ml water) made up in a sterile jug and kept covered between aspirations. Replace with fresh solution at least every 12 hours.

RE. Record volume of solution for later calculation of sputum volume.

3. Wear thin, disposable plastic gloves when aspirating or handling soiled equipment, to limit contamination and the risk of cross-infection. Replace suction tubing at least once in every 24 hours. Empty and measure fluid in suction jar at least once every 6 hours and disinfect jar or replace it with a sterile one at least once every 24 hours. An anti-foaming solution may be added if necessary.

RE. Calculate the amount of sputum aspirated by subtracting the volume of bicarbonate solution from the volume emptied from the suction jar. Record colour and quantity. Report any skin infection of the hands; herpes simplex (cold sores) can occur on the fingers from handling infected catheters.

4. Change patient's position every one to two hours to aid drainage of secretions into the main bronchial tree. Gravity may be used by tipping the head of the bed down by 30—40 degrees from the horizontal if the patient's condition permits. Gentle clapping and shaking of the chest wall may help loosen sputum.

RE. Note whether more sputum can be aspirated after a period in a particular position. Observe patient for increased cyanosis or discomfort while the head of the bed is lowered.

5. Keep sputum loose by maintaining a fluid intake of at least 2 litres in 24 hours, more if fever is present. No fluid should be given by mouth if an endo-trachael or tracheostomy tube is in use. If oxygen is given it should be passed through a humidifier. In a centrally heated room a bowl of clean water by the radiator adds moisture to the air as it evaporates.

RE. Note consistency of sputum. Review fluid balance chart once every 12 hours. Report any bleeding during suction, which may indicate damage to the lining of the airway. Consider reducing the size of the suction catheter lumen as thick sputum loosens.

6. Provide a call system and agree signals to be used if the patient wants sputum cleared from the airway, and so that any discomfort during suction can be made known to the nurse.

RE. Note whether the patient develops confidence in particular nurses, and plan to allocate them to care for the patient if possible. Reducing use of hand signals may indicate growing skill from the nurse or a tiring patient.

7. Consider whether the problem will be a long term one, and if the relatives would wish to and could be taught to undertake the suction. Discuss the idea with the patient and relatives at separate times to avoid emotional pressure on either party. Plan a teaching programme with both patient and relative if both are willing. Home visits may then be possible for the patient with chronic illness, if suction is the main requirement of treatment.

RE. Note if any interest is shown in the use of suction by the relatives, as for some people the idea is too unpleasant to contemplate. Observe for any strain in the relationship between patient and relative. Assess the level of skill and confidence of the patient and relatives before planning any reduction in supervision.

Further action

1. An endo-tracheal tube may be passed into the trachea either through the mouth or the nose. A laryngoscope is used so the tip of the tube can be guided through the vocal cords. Remove any dentures and extend the patient's head back to straighten the airway during insertion. This semi-rigid

25

plastic tube provides a path for air to enter and leave, as well as for the suction catheter. It is left in position, held in place by adhesive tape or bandage. Constant observation by a nurse is necessary to ensure it does not become blocked. The tube prevents swallowing and speech, so fluid replacement may require intravenous therapy. Provide a notepad or other means for the patient to communicate.

RE. This type of tube is normally only used as a temporary measure. If assisted ventilation is required the small cuff around the tube can be inflated with air to provide a loose seal. Note the patient's facial expression for signs of distress or fear. The tube can be very uncomfortable, and loss of speech may add to the discomfort.

2. A tracheostomy may be performed if the muscle weakness is expected to last for several days. The opening is made in the trachea so lessening the distance air and oxygen must be drawn in before reaching the lungs. A cuffed tracheostomy tube will be used to provide an air-tight seal around the tube. This is inflated with air. The tube is kept in place with tapes.

RE. The patient may be able to learn to use the suction themselves if they have the strength. Record the size of the tracheostomy tube used and the volume of air put into the cuff.

3. Sterile saline may be prescribed for instillation into the tube immediately before suction is used. Start with 5 ml or less and observe whether the sputum is easier to remove.

RE. Record the volume of saline used so that it can be included in the calculation of the volume of sputum produced.

4. Sputum samples can be collected during suction by inserting a sterile, disposable sputum trap into the suction tube. Check the specimen obtained is correctly labelled and delivered to the laboratory as quickly as possible.

RE. Infection may indicate poor technique, unsterile equipment, auto-infection or cross-infection.

Associated medical diagnoses	Atelectasis Bronchitis Cerebral vascular accident Disseminated sclerosis Encephalitis Guillain-Barré syndrome Meningitis Multiple sclerosis Myasthenia gravis Pneumonia
Problem	Uncomfortable from dry cough.
Assessment findings	Repeated unproductive cough Fatigue Breathless Patient reports a dry tickle in throat

Information for the patient	A cough is a reflex action designed to clear foreign particles from the lungs. It can be set off by irritation without there being any actual material to be removed (cold or dry air can also cause coughing). If there is no mucus or infection then it is safe to try to stop the cough.
Nursing action	1. Ensure the patient's local environment is warm, smoke free and if necessary increase the humidity by leaving clean water to evaporate near a central heating radiator.
	RE. Check the patient feels comfortable and any known irritants have been removed.
	2. Give the patient warm drinks. The juice of half a lemon mixed with a tablespoon of honey and topped up to a cup of liquid with hot water can be sipped as a soothing drink. Sucking boiled sweets may also help.
	RE. Note if the rate of coughing decreases sufficiently to allow the patient to rest, or if the patient mentions that the throat and cough feel soothed.
Further action	1. Codeine or the synthetic pholcodine may be prescribed as a syrup. These may depress the rate and depth of respirations. They should be given at night to help the patient gain some rest.
	RE. Note the total dose taken by a patient. Observe rate and depth of respirations half an hour after a high dose is given. Pholcodine is less likely to cause constipation than codeine preparations.
	2. In severe cases where malignancy is involved diamorphine linctus may be prescribed. It has a powerful action in stopping coughing, but its considerable depressant effect on the respiratory centre must be taken into account. It is addictive and is therefore used with caution except in terminal illness.
	RE. Note how much rest and relief from coughing follows so that the dose prescribed can be repeated early enough for a coughing bout to be avoided. As tolerance may occur the frequency or dosage may need to be altered in time. Each patient requires individual assessment.
Associated medical diagnoses	Aortic aneurysm Asthma Bronchogenic carcinoma Coryza Croup Emphysema Mitral stenosis Pleurisy Tuberculosis

Problem	Hyperventilation (Overbreathing)
Assessment findings	Feels 'lightheaded' Reports 'pins and needles' or numbness in fingers or toes. Extreme anxiety, 'hysteria' Rapid deep respirations Forced respirations used by patient to overcome pain (as in 'natural childbirth') Salicylate (aspirin) ingestion Muscle twitching

Information for the patient	The breathing pattern has changed from the normal and more carbon dioxide waste is being blown off through the lungs than is usual. This upsets the body's internal chemistry leading to 'pins and needles'. Slowing and calming the breathing rate and resting will help things return to normal.
Nursing action	1. Count respirations. Supervise the patient taking slower breaths. Use a paper bag and instruct the patient to breathe into the bag and then breathe the same air back for two minutes. Breathing the exhaled carbon dioxide trapped in the bag helps to stop further loss of carbon dioxide, allowing the chemical imbalance to be restored.
	RE. Count the respirations after five minutes. Ask the patient if tingling or numbness has decreased. Repeat nursing action once more if there has been no change.
	2. Talk with the patient to identify if there is any emotional problem behind the overbreathing. Acting as a willing listener and providing emotional support may aid the patient to regain self-control.
	RE. Assess how much the patient is willing to open up during such a discussion, and consider whether other professional help may be more effective.
Further action	1. Puffs of 5% carbon dioxide may be prescribed to correct the oxygen/carbon dioxide balance. Close supervision should be given when the gas is administered.
	RE. Compare the respiratory rate before and after the small amounts of carbon dioxide are given. Ask the patient to report any change in numbness or tingling.
	2. Aspirin (salicylate) poisoning may be treated by forced alkaline diuresis, which increases the rate of excretion tenfold if the urine pH is increased from 6.0 to 7.7. Intravenous infusion of alkaline fluid also rehydrates the patient.
	RE. Record the respiratory rate at least half hourly. The rate should drop as the alkaline level of the blood is reduced. Record the pH of the urine hourly.
	3. Analgesics such as the morphine derivatives may be prescribed for pain. They have a direct effect by depressing the respiratory centre in the brain, as well as inducing euphoria.
	RE. Assess the pain relief and respirations half an hour after intramuscular injection of analgesia. Use a pain chart to monitor site(s) and control of pain.
	4. Treatment by a psychotherapist may be prescribed if an emotional cause is suspected.
	RE. Assess the patient's understanding of explanations about psychotherapy. Report to the doctor any comments which indicate misunderstanding and fear of mental illness.
Associated medical diagnoses	Anxiety neurosis Aspirin overdose Cerebral lesion in pons Diabetes Hyperparathyroidism Pulmonary embolism Salicylate poisoning

Problem	Dependent on oxygen therapy

Assessment findings

Anxious
Increased respiratory rate
Feeling of breathlessness
Confusion
Blue colour to lips (cyanosis)
Blue colour to nail beds (cyanosis)
Rapid pulse

Information for the patient

Oxygen can be added to a person's air intake to increase the oxygen reaching the tiny airsacs deep inside the lung. There it can be taken up by the red cells in the blood and carried to the body tissues. The gas is dryer than the air so it will be moistened by bubbling it through water. The face mask is designed to control how much oxygen is mixed with the air breathed, and it must fit snugly on the face. Oxygen increases the rate at which things can burn so extra care must be taken. Smoking is not allowed near oxygen to reduce the risk of fire.

Nursing action

1. Oxygen therapy is normally only given when instructed by a doctor, but in an acute episode of respiratory distress it may be commenced by a nurse. Oxygen of less than 40 per cent concentration may be given provided there is no chronic airway obstruction (4 to 6 litres per minute via a face mask). The doctor should be informed immediately.

RE. Check respiratory rate and colour after 3–5 minutes while awaiting medical aid. Cyanosis should begin to decrease.

2. Humidify compressed oxygen by bubbling it through sterile water in the humidifier at room temperature. Use a sterile humidifier, and refill it every two to four hours while in use. Some types of plastic face mask increase local humidity by mixing expired air with the oxygen.

RE. Check water level in humidifier at frequent intervals to avoid a reduction in the humidity of the gas as the water level drops. Observe whether the sputum becomes looser (more liquid). Ask the patient whether their nose and mouth feel comfortable. If they complain of dryness, keep the water level close to maximum mark by frequent top-ups.

3. Provide a no-smoking notice for patient area. Explain to the patient and visitors that although oxygen is colourless and tasteless, it enables things to burn faster, and so increases the risk of fire.

RE. Be extra careful that the patient and visitors do not smoke cigarettes or pipes while oxygen is being given. Check that staff know where the nearest fire extinguisher is situated.

4. Remove oxygen face mask to wash and dry face at least every two hours. Offer a drink or mouthwash. Apply a little petroleum jelly to the lips to reduce dryness. Adjust the fit of the face mask for comfort, and to ensure the oxygen level is correct.

RE. Inspect skin of face and head for signs of local pressure such as redness. Apply padding beneath face mask straps for comfort if necessary.

Further action

1. A polymask provides a high concentration of oxygen, the MC Mask provides 70–100 per cent and can be administered more accurately. Oxygen given by either type should be humidified.

RE. The thin straps of the polymask may cause discomfort especially over the ears, and the high humidity can increase the damage by producing masceration of the skin. Increase the frequency of removal of the mask for drying the face and adjusting the fit, particularly if the patient needs to use it over a long period of time.

2. Edinburgh mask and Venturi mask provide a precise oxygen level and do not allow rebreathing of expired air, which contains waste carbon dioxide. Use for patients with chronic airway disease with carbon dioxide retention. Select the Venturi mask for the prescribed percentage of oxygen, ie 24/28/35/40 per cent oxygen.

RE. Metal edge can get distorted and dig into the skin. Patients with chronic airway disorders tend to be more restless, therefore frequent adjustment is necessary to maintain a correct fit. Check flow rate of oxygen to ensure the correct percentage is reaching patient.

3. Nasal cannulae provide a high oxygen level and allow freedom of movement. They are less distressing for patients who may feel suffocated by a mask over the face. Rebreathing of expired carbon dioxide is avoided, but the level of oxygen reaching the patient cannot be controlled accurately. Oxygen needs to be humidified.

RE. Inspect nasal mucosa for signs of drying. Petroleum jelly may help to reduce this, but it must be applied as a thin layer or the lumen of the tube may become partially blocked. Check position of cannulae as they can easily be dislodged.

4. Blood gas estimation may be carried out at intervals, and the oxygen flow rate adjusted according to the results.

RE. Record respiratory rate, depth and rhythm at least every two hours. Record pulse rate and observe whether cyanosis is present. A rising pulse and restlessness may indicate that insufficient oxygen is reaching the lungs.

5. An oxygen tent may be used for the very confused and restless patient, but the concentration of oxygen reaching the patient cannot be adjusted, and may be unreliable due to leakage. It is also more difficult to assess the patient.

RE. The risk of fire is increased by the larger volume of oxygen rich air surrounding the patient. Ensure the no-smoking rule is followed.

Associated medical diagnoses

Anaemia
Asthma
Atelectasis
Carcinoma of lung
Carbon monoxide poisoning
Cerebral vascular accident
Congestive cardiac failure
Emphysema
Fibrosing alveolitis
Hyperthyroidism
Lung abscess

Mitral stenosis
Myasthenia gravis
Myocardial infarction
Pleurisy
Pneumoconioses
Pneumonia
Pneumothorax
Pulmonary embolism
Pulmonary oedema
Sarcoidosis
Tuberculosis

Problem	Secreting excessive pleural fluid.

Assessment findings

Increased respiratory rate
Pain especially during inspiration
Sharp stabbing pain over chest
Feels breathless
Unequal chest expansion

Information for the patient

The inside of the chest and lungs are covered by a lining (the pleura) which is lubricated by fluid. This allows the two layers of lining to move slightly and easily with each breath. Extra fluid can collect if the drainage path is partially blocked. If there is an area of inflammation in the lung which irritates the lining, then more fluid may be produced to try to improve the lubrication. Sometimes there is infection, and as the white cells move from the blood to fight the infection, the fluid becomes thicker. As fluid collects it takes up more and more space, squeezing the lung and making breathing more difficult and uncomfortable. The irritation can also produce pain.

Nursing action

1. Provide extra pillows to prop the patient in a comfortable sitting position in bed or on a chair, so that gravity will encourage fluid to collect at the base of the lung.

RE. Record respiratory rate at least twice daily. Ask the patient to report any increase in pain or change in the site of pain. Check that their position is comfortable enough to allow sleep when necessary.

2. Teach the patient deep breathing exercises. Time analgesia administration so that the greatest level of pain relief coincides with the time allotted for exercises.

RE. Note whether the pain level is low enough to allow the patient to breathe deeply. Place hands over their lower ribs to assess how well the lower ribs move during breathing exercises.

Further action

1. Pleural aspiration of the fluid for culture, presence of cells, or to reduce the pressure, may be carried out under local anaesthetic. A sterile needle is inserted through the chest wall using aseptic technique, usually with the patient leaning forward with their head and arms resting on pillows on a bedtable.

RE. Measure the total volume of fluid removed. A specimen in a sterile container may be sent for culture.

31

2. Following the procedure the puncture site is sealed with plastic spray and a firm dressing. A chest X-ray may be performed to check no air has entered the pleural cavity.

RE. Observe the patient's colour and respiratory rate during the procedure, as there is a risk of puncture of the lung and air entering the chest cavity (pneumothorax). Air leakage may also occur in the first few hours after the procedure. Record the rate, rhythm and depth of respiration. Report any increase in cyanosis (blue colour of lips and nails). Observe for increased coughing, or blood appearing in the sputum. Report such changes to the doctor.

4. Inform the physiotherapist that the aspiration has been performed so that lung expansion exercises can be carried out.

RE. Check patient understands and carries out the breathing exercises as frequently as instructed.

Associated medical diagnoses	Ascites
	Carcinoma of lung
	Cirrhosis of liver
	Congestive cardiac failure
	Metastatic carcinoma of breast
	Lung abscess
	Lymphoma
	Pleurisy
	Pneumonia
	Pulmonary infarction
	Rheumatoid arthritis
	Systemic lupus erythematosis
	Tuberculosis

Potential problems

Potential problem	Risk of airway obstruction.
Assessment findings	Falling level of consciousness
	Loss of consciousness
	Absent gag reflex
	Rising pulse rate
	Slow stertorous breathing
	Respiratory rate 8 breaths or less per minute
	Sweating
	Anxiety
	Wheezing breath sounds
	Coughing
	Local swelling of throat or tongue
	Wired jaw
	Broken jaw
	Eating while lying down
	Rapid eating or drinking
	Bleeding in the mouth
	Post-operative breathing eg following tonsillectomy

Information for the patient	The path to the wind pipe is protected by a small leaf like flap, the epiglottis, which normally covers the entrance when a person swallows so no food or drink can get in. If it does, then coughing would normally shift the particles of food out again very quickly. Anything which interferes with swallowing puts that path to the lungs at risk. A suction machine can be used with a thin tube to suck out saliva or particles if necessary. Sometimes it is more important to keep the path clear by leaving a tube in place, which goes down into the top of the wind pipe. That has an added advantage in that the tongue cannot fall back and block off the path of air to the lungs.
Nursing action	1. Place a mobile suction machine or wall suction near the patient while the risk remains high. Provide sterile suction catheters with a side hole or those without and a 'Y' connection.
	RE. Check at least once every 24 hours that the equipment works properly. Record this in the progress notes. Review the level of risk each day. The equipment may be removed from the bedside when the risk is low, as long as it is still easily available if needed.
	2. Provide an adult size Guedel airway or Brook airway, and gauze swabs for clearing the airway of large particles. Note if the patient wears dentures, or has crowned or loose teeth.
	RE. Check the airway is kept close to the patient. Check that the valve on the Brook airway is in place, and that it has not perished.
	3. Make sure there is an oxygen supply, oxygen mask and tubing close to the patient. If an oxygen cylinder is used, check the spanner/key is attached so that it can be turned on readily.
	RE. Check at least once in every 24 hours that the oxygen equipment works.
	4. If the level of consciousness is falling, place patient in the semi-prone position, and tip the head of the bed down by 15–20 degrees from the horizontal to reduce risk of saliva collecting. Observe patient's colour and respiratory rate.
	RE. Assess the patient's neurological state every 15–30 minutes. Report any deterioration or difficulty in breathing to the doctor.
	5. Place wire cutters near the bedside if jaws are wired. Supervise or observe during eating or drinking.
	RE. Check staff know which wires should be cut for fast release and access to the airway, should obstruction occur.
	6. Sudden choking on food may require the use of the Heimlich manoeuvre. Stand behind the patient with arms under his, clenched fists under his diaphragm. Pull the fists up and into the chest with a sharp, jerking movement.
	RE. The increased intra-thoracic pressure should expel the foreign body or food from the airway. If not repeat the manoeuvre. (Fig. 2.2). Request medical aid as abdominal organs may be damaged by the pressure.
Further action	1. Bronchospasm due to asthma may require salbutamol, given by an inhaler in two puffs, 5 minutes apart.
	RE. Observe respirations to see if there is less effort. A peak flow rate may

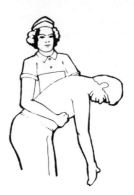

1. Stand or kneel behind the person choking
2. Clench one fist, fingers and thumb against their abdomen between umbilicus and sternum, grasp with other hand
3. Jerk firmly up and back to compress the abdominal organs against the diaphragm to force air out with the obstruction. Repeat until obstructing object appears.

Fig. 2.2   The Heimlich manoeuvre

be recorded immediately before and 10 minutes after the drug is given if the patient is able to control respirations sufficiently to cooperate in using the meter.

2. If bronchospasm is still not relieved, then aminophylline 250 to 500 mg, diluted in 10—20 ml of water for injection, may be given slowly into a vein over a period of at least 5—10 minutes by a doctor. Then an infusion of 200 mg of aminophylline, in 500 ml of 5 per cent dextrose, is given over each 8 hour period for 24 hours.

RE. Record pulse rate at 5 minute intervals during the slow intravenous injection, and at least every 4 hours after that. Changes in the pulse rhythm may occur, and sometimes convulsions. Ask the patient to report any feeling of nausea, and any palpitations.

3. Steroid therapy, either intravenously or orally, may be prescribed to reduce an inflammatory reaction. Hydrocortisone sodium 100 mg in 1 ml may be given by intravenous injection, or methylprednisolone 40 to 80 mg.

RE. If treatment lasts for more than four days, record blood pressure at least daily and report any rise. Test urine for glucose, and weigh patient on alternate days to detect fluid retention. Ask the patient to report any nausea, vomiting or feelings of weakness.

4. Opiate drugs should not be given. Hypnotics such as nitrazepam should be avoided. If sedation is absolutely necessary diazepam 5—10 mg by intramuscular injection may be prescribed.

RE. Elderly people may be more sensitive to diazepam, and its effect is increased by alcohol. Respiratory depression may sometimes occur as a side effect.

Associated medical diagnoses	Asthma Anaphylaxis Alcoholism Bronchial plug or cast Cerebral palsy Cerebral vascular accident (CVA) Diphtheria Epilepsy Head injury Hodgkin's disease Inhaled foreign body Inhaled vomit Lymphoma Poliomyelitis Tumour of larynx

Potential problem	**Risk of pulmonary oedema due to fluid overload.**

Assessment findings	Known heart damage Urine output under 500 ml in 24 hours Patient receiving intravenous fluids Patient receiving blood transfusion Pounding headache Sweating Anxiety Restlessness

Information for the patient	In the lungs fluid can collect between the tiny air sacs if it flows in at a faster rate than it can drain away. Oxygen then takes longer to cross into the blood, and carbon dioxide waste takes longer to leave. The tiny air tubes get squeezed by the collecting fluid, and some may get shut off altogether. The lungs become stiffer, and breathing gets harder. If the left side of the heart ceases to pump the blood around the body efficiently, then the blood collects in the lungs and starts to build up. The kidneys need a good blood flow to remove excess fluid from the body, otherwise they can increase the problems for the heart by not getting rid of enough urine, and the pressure builds up. If the fluid taken into the body is not balanced by the fluid excreted from it, then one of the symptoms may be fluid collecting in the lungs.

Nursing action	1. Monitor the flow rate of intravenous fluids at least half-hourly. If possible use a volumetric pump, burette or special giving set so that the flow rate can be precisely controlled. If a rapid flow rate is administered the urine output should keep pace: provide a urinal or bedpan at frequent intervals and measure each volume or urine passed. RE. Record fluid intake and output by all routes. Review fluid balance at least every four hours, more often if the risk of fluid overload is great, in order to identify any fall in urine production compared with intake. Allow for insensible loss of fluid from the body. 2. Assess respiratory rate and breathing effort every two to four hours, more often if the risk is high, or if a rapid intravenous infusion is in progress. Check

the pulse rate, and, look for any increase in the distension of the veins. Check for increasing blood pressure.

RE. Report to doctor an increase in the respiratory rate, and wheezy or wet sounding respirations. Observe for non-productive coughing. Ask patient to report any increased difficulty in breathing as the onset of symptoms may be rapid. A pounding headache, cold sweating or a feeling of anxiety may precede the onset of more obvious symptoms.

3. If pulmonary oedema is suspected, slow the rate of any intravenous infusion or transfusion. Sit the patient upright in bed or in a chair to use gravity to keep more fluid in the legs and lower trunk. Call the doctor.

RE. A diuretic may be prescribed and given intravenously. Record fluid output and assess response after one hour. Check pulse, respirations and blood pressure at least half hourly during this time.

Further action

1. Chest X-rays may be carried out at intervals to assess the rate of fluid accumulation. Remind the patient that during the X-ray they will have to take a deep breath and hold it for a few seconds. Consider whether oxygen by mask may be needed before and after the X-ray.

RE. If pulmonary oedema is present, for example in left ventricular failure, the chest X-ray report may include engorged lymphatic channels and pulmonary veins, areas of alveolar filling and areas of lung collapse. Bilateral pleural effusions may also be present. When excess fluid is removed, these changes should decrease.

2. Physiotherapy will be needed to ensure the collapsed small airways reopen and secretions are cleared.

RE. Measure sputum volume and observe for changes in colour or consistency indicating infection.

3. Central venous pressure measurement may be decided on for patients at severe risk. The readings may be used to adjust the flow rate of any intravenous infusion or transfusion. Readings may be hourly, or more frequent if the risk is high.

RE. Normal CVP is 4 to 6 mmHg (or 5 to 8 cm water). A rising CVP indicates that fluid intake should be reduced. Electrolyte levels may need more careful monitoring if the CVP falls, as diuretic therapy may need to be adjusted as well as fluid intake.

4. Oxygen may be given by mask at 4 litres a minute if respiratory efficiency decreases.

RE. Observe the patient for restlessness and intolerance of mask, which may occur if oedema is getting worse.

5. Diuretics such as frusemide or bumetanide reduce circulating blood volume and therefore pressure by increasing urine excretion. Digoxin may be given to improve cardiac output. Dopamine also increases cardiac function and renal perfusion. The dose is calculated according to body weight.

RE. Each time the urine is passed, record the time and volume of urine to assess the effect of the diuretic. Both diuretics can cause ringing of the ears or deafness if given in high doses. Bumetanide may cause muscle pains or leg cramps. Both digoxin and dopamine can cause nausea and vomiting, or changes in pulse rate. Blood pressure may fall after dopamine administration.

6. Venesection, haemodialysis or peritoneal dialysis may be considered as emergency measures if renal function is impaired.

RE. One or more pints of blood may be removed to lessen the pressure by reducing the circulating blood volume.

7. Oral diuretics may be prescribed during blood transfusion if there is a high risk of pulmonary oedema. No drug should be added to the unit of blood.

RE. The administration of the diuretic should keep pace with the rate of transfusion, and be related to the volume of blood already given. Record fluid intake and urine output on a fluid chart. Report if the urine/fluid output lags more than 400 ml behind the intake.

Associated medical diagnoses	Congestive cardiac failure Left ventricular failure Myocardial infarction Nephritis Renal failure Septicaemia Shock lung

---

Potential problem	**Risk of cross infection from infected sputum.**

Assessment findings	Productive cough Yellow/green sputum Rusty coloured sputum Foul smelling breath and sputum Weight loss Raised temperature
Information for the patient	The phlegm (sputum) which is coughed up contains germs (bacteria or virus particles) and white blood cells which the body sends to the lungs to fight the infection. Some of these germs will still be alive and could infect other people. As they cannot be seen they may be passed to other people through objects touched by the patient unless the hands are kept clean. A cough can spray out the germs in tiny droplets of moisture as when someone breathes on a cold mirror. Trapping a cough in a thick tissue which can then be burnt will help stop the transfer of germs.
Nursing action	1. Assume any sputum is infected when handling containers or tissues containing sputum, and when supervising coughing exercises. Suggest the patient uses thick, folded tissues rather than thin ones. Provide a disposable sputum container or polythene bag for soiled tissues. Dispose of these by burning. Provide disposable moist tissues to cleanse fingers and face after patient expectorates.

RE. Check that the patient is able to reach and remove the lid of the container easily and always replaces the lid after use. Check soiled tissues are used once and disposed of straight into the polythene bag. Check the polythene bag is sealed with a tie when two thirds full and replaced.

2. Write the time and date that the sputum container is given to the patient so that the volume of sputum expectorated can be measured.

RE. Inspect and record the volume, colour and consistency of the sputum at least daily.

3. Stand beside or behind the patient when supervising coughing exercises. Use disposable oxygen masks. Send oxygen tubing for disinfection after use if it is not disposable.

RE. Ensure the patient directs cough away from the nurse.

4. Review the condition of other patients in the same room to identify any with possible reduced resistance to infection, such as low white blood cell count, or patients receiving drugs which lower their immunity. Consider moving either them or the patient to another room. Explain the risk to the patient.

RE. Observe 'at risk' patients for signs of infection if contact with the patient occurred before the chest infection was suspected.

5. Isolate the infectious patient in a room with the airflow to the outside of the building. Provide face masks for staff and visitors entering the room only if recommended to do so by the microbiologist. If open tuberculosis is suspected, limit staff contact to those who have received BCG immunization or who have a positive tuberculin test.

RE. Note the date and time isolation nursing was commenced. Negative sputum specimens may be required before the microbiologist approves the ending of isolation.

Further action

1. A specimen of sputum for culture and sensitivity to antibiotics may be required before treatment with antibiotics commences, and also during treatment. Remind the patient to expectorate straight into the sterile container. If saliva or sputum soil the outside of the container wear disposable plastic gloves while wiping the area with the locally recommended disinfectant.

RE. Check the specimen is sent to the laboratory as soon as possible after collection. Check the accompanying form includes a warning if tuberculosis is suspected. Laboratory staff are at greater risk of developing the disease than other staff.

2. Erythromycin may be prescribed for gram-positive infections except where liver damage is present.

RE. Report any abdominal discomfort or nausea.

3. Metronidazole may be prescribed: the tablets should be swallowed without chewing and washed down with at least half a tumbler of water during or after a meal. The suspension should be taken at least one hour before a meal. Suppositories may be prescribed. An infusion may be given over 20 to 30 minutes. No alcohol should be taken during treatment with the drug.

RE. Nausea, a furred tongue, drowsiness or dizziness may occur as side effects. If alcohol is taken there may be flushing and a rapid pulse with a low blood pressure. Occasionally loss of sensation or tingling in the fingers or feet may occur with high doses. Observe gait for ataxia.

4. If tuberculosis is suspected, three anti-tubercular drugs may be prescribed for three months, followed by further treatment with two of these drugs. This is because each drug prevents organisms proliferating which are resistant to the other drugs. Isoniazid, rifampicin, ethambutol or streptomycin are most frequently used. The first two are used with caution if liver damage is suspected. Disposable gloves should be worn when preparing and giving streptomycin injections. There is risk of damage to the 8th cranial nerve when streptomycin is given, so an ENT consultation every month is advised.

RE. Observe for skin rashes. Fits may occur with isoniazid as may depression or joint pain. Note the colour of the urine, saliva or tears when rifampicin is being used as the orange-pink colour indicates the drug is being taken. Fever, shock or breathing problems may also occur. Ask the patient to report any change in vision while being treated with ethambutol as loss of red-green colour discrimination or tunnel vision may occur. Gastric upset or loss of sensation in fingers or feet should be reported. Ask the patient to report any change in hearing or sensation about the mouth during treatment with streptomycin. Observe for loss of co-ordination or dizziness.

Associated medical diagnoses

Bronchitis
Diphtheria
Infectious mononucleosis
Influenza
Pertussis (Whooping cough)
Pneumonia
Tuberculosis

References and further reading

Grenville-Mathers, R. (1983). (2nd edn.) *The Respiratory System.* Penguin Library of Nursing/Churchill Livingstone. Edinburgh.
Health Education Council. (1983). *The Facts About Smoking – What Every Nurse Should Know.* Health Education Council. London.
Yates, A.K., Moorhead, P.J., Adams, A.P. (1984). *Intensive Care.* Modern Nursing Series. Hodder & Stoughton. London.

Useful addresses

The Health Education Council, 78 New Oxford Street, London WC1A 1AH

in Scotland:

Scottish Health Education Group, Woodburn House, Canaan Lane, Edinburgh, Scotland EH10 4SG

ASH (Action on Smoking and Health), Margaret Pyke House, 5–11 Mortimer Street, London W1N 7RH

3 Eating

Optimum environment

Mouth

In the adult a full set of teeth consists of two incisors, one canine, two premolar and three molar teeth on each side of the mouth. A healthy tooth has a hard, translucent, insensitive layer of enamel over the crown. This is mainly hydroxyapatite which is made up of calcium and phosphorus. It protects the sensitive, tough, elastic dentine which lies around the pulp with its nerve fibres, blood vessels, lymphatics and connective tissue. The

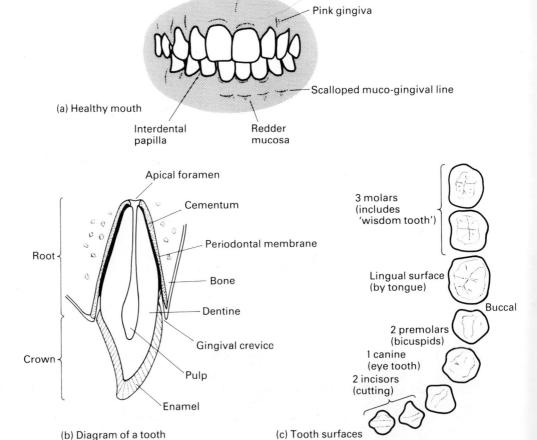

(a) Healthy mouth

(b) Diagram of a tooth

(c) Tooth surfaces

Fig. 3.1 Dentition

cementum covers the root, where the enamel is absent; it acts as a shock absorber and anchors the tooth to the peridontal membrane.

The healthy gum or gingiva is pink in colour and it is in close contact with the tooth up to the epithelial attachment after which it is separated from the tooth surface and forms the gingival crevice. Healthy gums do not bleed when brushed. (Fig. 3.1)

Oral hygiene

Plaque results from food debris, bacteria and mucus. It collects around the necks of teeth and can form tartar. This is composed of calcium and other salts laid down within a network of filaments of bacteria. Calcium is present in saliva, and plaque may be thickest near the salivary ducts. It also collects in the gingival crevice.

When it is first deposited, plaque is soft, porous and whitish yellow. On hardening it will take up stains, including for instance from tobacco smoke. Gingivitis may also occur, leading to receding gums and bleeding.

Bacteria, protected from saliva by plaque, break down carbohydrates into lactic and other acids strong enough to attack enamel. As it decalcifies the enamel looks white, eventually disintegrating and allowing bacteria to invade towards the dentine. Protein dissolving (proteolytic) organisms then speed up the destruction. Dental caries affect a large proportion of the British population.

Removal of plaque by at least twice-daily use of a tooth brush will help maintain healthy teeth and gums. The correct use of dental floss to remove plaque from the gingival crevice is also helpful. The use of disclosing tablets to stain old and new plaque provides a useful check on how efficiently the teeth have been brushed.

Tooth brushing technique

Using a flat, trimmed nylon, multi-tuft brush with rounded strands:
1. Clean the outside (buccal and labial) surface of the upper teeth and gums with short, gentle back and forth strokes.
2. Clean the inside (palatal) surface of all the upper teeth and gums with short, gentle back and forth strokes.
3. Clean the outside (buccal and labial) surface of the lower teeth and gums with the same brush strokes.
4. Clean the inner (lingual) surface by tilting the brush. A child's toothbrush may be more effective if the angle is difficult.
5. Brush the biting surface of upper and lower teeth with horizontal strokes.

Tooth floss technique

Use unwaxed dental floss.
1. Cut a length 12 inches (30 cm) to 18 inches (45 cm) long.
2. Wind an end around the middle finger of each hand until there is a gap of about 2–3 inches between the fingers.
3. Using the thumb and forefingers work the floss *gently* into the space between gum and teeth until resistance is felt.
4. Hold floss tightly against the tooth in a curved 'C' shape.
5. Slide floss down the tooth away from the gum to scrape off the plaque. The fine strands of floss fan out and collect the debris.
6. Repeat steps 3 to 5 for each tooth.

Use of disclosing tablets

1. Clean the teeth by brushing and flossing in the normal manner.
2. Chew one disclosing tablet.
3. Swish round the mouth with a small amount of water.
4. Spit out.
5. Look in the mirror to see if any plaque was left. It will have been stained by the dye.

6. Use toothbrush to remove stained plaque, noting the most effective strokes required for its removal so that they can be incorporated into the normal brushing routine.

7. Repeat after each teeth cleaning session until the technique is so effective plaque is always removed. Make random checks every few weeks to ensure the cleaning technique is still efficient.

As staining of the gums may take time to remove it is best to use disclosing tablets at bedtime.

Most toothbrush manufacturers will provide leaflets for hospital or dental surgeries to give to patients. Health Education Units can also supply a range of dental health leaflets.

Dentures

Thermoplastic materials used as a denture base absorb water and if they dry out the material will contract. Dentures should always be stored in cold water when not in use.

Acrylic resin is not resistant to abrasives so the use of toothpaste or block dentifrice will damage the polish. Cleaning and soaking solutions should be used with gentle brushing to remove particles. Sometimes foods are difficult to chew with dentures.

Diet

Sweet, sticky foods, particularly when eaten between meals, provide a good acid medium and food source for the bacteria which always live in the mouth. The old idea of a crunchy apple to clean teeth, when brushing them is not possible, is now thought to increase the chance of damage. The fruit acids and apple pulp can provide bacteria with extra food. Instead some dentists recommend eating a piece of hard cheese at the end of a meal.

Storage and care of foods to prevent infection

Bacteria and yeasts live on the surface of food, as they do on everything else in the environment. Some are harmful to humans, but most are killed during the preparation and cooking of food. When food poisoning occurs, it can result in vomiting and diarrhoea. Some foods carry a greater risk than others.

The effects of *Salmonella* poisoning appear within 4 to 48 hours. The bacteria comes from animal sources and their excreta may contaminate water. Most types of *Salmonella* are killed by heating to at least 60°C for 15 minutes. Frozen meat and poultry must be completely thawed before cooking so that the heat will cook it right through. Do not use the same surface and cutlery to prepare cooked food as have been used for raw food. Disposable kitchen towels should be used to mop up spills, or use a cloth regularly boiled or soaked in bleach to kill bacteria. Surfaces and equipment should be washed in hot detergent and then dried to kill as many bacteria as possible. (Bacteria thrive in damp surroundings.) Special care should be taken to clean meat slicers and in kitchens catering for large numbers of people.

Foods which carry an increased risk from *Salmonella* include frozen chickens, ducks and duck eggs, sliced cold meats, custards, mayonnaise dressings and cream fillings.

Gastroenteritis occurring within 5 hours of a meal is likely to be caused by *Staphylococcus*. This organism lives on the skin and in the nose. Infected cuts or nose picking can contaminate food. If it then remains in a warm area the staphylococci multiply rapidly, and produce an enterotoxin in the food itself, and this toxin makes the consumer ill. Food should be stored at 4°C or below and covered. Leftover food should be cooled quickly, and when reheated it should be cooked thoroughly. Foods with an increased risk of contamination include cream, mayonnaise, confectioner's cream or custard.

Clostridium welchi is another organism particularly associated with reheated foods, especially those containing meat such as gravy or soup. It is fairly common in communal eating places, such as canteens.

Tinned food should be checked to make sure the can is not 'blown'. Contamination from the soil organism *Clostridium botulinum* (botulism) is a rare danger. The toxin produced by the anaerobic bacteria (able to grow in the absence of air) is very potent and can cause death. Home canning of food must be carefully carried out.

Frozen foods should be carefully prepared. Blanching (scalding in water or steam) stops enzyme activity and may reduce surface bacteria.

Poor handwashing or sanitation can lead to faecal bacteria contaminating food. Dysentery, some *Escherichia coli* (E. coli) and typhoid are risks which face the traveller in certain countries, particularly where sanitation is poor. Rapid air travel can mean the infection does not become apparent until after the journey home.

Some bacteria and yeasts may cause infection in malnourished individuals, and special care should be taken in the preparation of food for those with chronic illness, or a reduced resistance to infection (immunosuppressed).

Eating for health

Food has an important social role as well as being essential for energy and building healthy tissues. There are fashions in food. Travel and new manufacturing processes provide an ever increasing range of combinations of the main constituents. The food industry must provide products which meet specified standards. Prepared foods and meals are often more expensive to buy but save time and effort in the cooking. Frozen foods do lose some vitamins but the nutritional difference between cooked fresh foods and cooked frozen foods is small. Frozen vegetables may have more vitamin C than vegetables bought from the shop or market. The freezing process may follow soon after picking while the 'fresh' vegetables may have to travel to the wholesaler and retailer before reaching the customer. Some would argue that the significant difference is in the flavour.

A single day's diet should provide carbohydrate, fats, proteins, vitamins and minerals. Protein usually forms the smaller proportion of the diet so carbohydrates and fats contribute most to the energy intake, one gram of carbohydrate providing the same Calories as one gram of fat. Most people measure the energy intake in Calories rather than using the SI unit, the Joule. If the energy intake is greater than the energy used, then it may be stored by the body as fat. If the energy intake is less than the energy used, the deficit is made up from the body's stores. This is the basis of most slimming diets which recommend reducing carbhohydrate and fat intake. If more protein is taken in than the body can use, it is broken down and the nitrogen portion is excreted. The remaining part is converted to glucose and used for energy or stored. Substituting the expensive protein foods for the carbohydrates which some 'slimming' diets recommend is a costly way of losing weight. All protein foods also contain some fat so the intake of energy is larger than may at first be realised.

The fibre foods are less easily digested. The body relies on the bacteria in the large bowel to break up the cellulose in vegetables and fruits. Some of the plant cells contain lignin and this takes even longer than cellulose to break down. The material has often left the gut before the final break down is achieved. Wheat bran has a high proportion of lignin and it is this which makes coarse bran useful in 'slimming' diets and for treating constipation. It has the added bonus of being cheap to buy. One problem which dietary fibre brings with it is in the increase in 'wind' (flatus) caused by the gases produced by the bacteria when they break up the fibre. A slow increase in the amount of bran-containing foods and pulse vegetables will help limit the problem. At least 23–30 mg a day is recommended.

A well balanced diet is often talked about as healthy but is difficult to describe as the prepared dishes will vary with cultural and religious beliefs. In

Table 3.1   An example of components of a well-balanced diet, modified from Huskisson (1981)

A. **Milk and Cheese**: 2 portions each day, chosen from:
   1 cup of whole, semi-skimmed or skimmed milk
   1 cup of yoghurt — whole or skimmed milk
   40–50g cheese — low fat, cottage or hard cheese
   Provides:
      protein, calcium, phosphorus
      vitamins A & D, thiamine and riboflavin
      fat in full-fat products

B. **Meat, poultry, fish or eggs**: 1 portion each day, chosen from:
   Meat
   Chicken
   Fish
   Bean sprouts
   Liver, kidney or heart
   4 tablespoons peanut butter
   1 egg
   1 cup peas or beans or lentils
   Provides:
      protein
      iron in meat and eggs
      iodine in fish
      vitamins B complex, D
      fat in meat, dark-fleshed fish, egg yolk

C. **Fruit or vegetables**: 4 portions each day, chosen from:
   Citrus fruits
   Apples, pears
   Tomatoes
   Raw cabbage
   Green salads
   Root vegetables
   Potatoes
   Provides:
      carotene
      vitamin C
      cellulose

D. **Cereals and bread:** 4 portions each day, or more, depending on Calorie requirements chosen from:
   1 slice wholemeal bread
   Half-cup cooked brown rice
   Half-cup cooked wholemeal noodles
   Half-cup cooked cereal
   30g ready-to-eat breakfast cereal or porridge
   Provides:
      carbohydrates
      vitamin B complex
      calcium
      iron
      cellulose

Europe a wider range of ethnic dishes is becoming available. A useful way of describing a well balanced diet is that of Huskisson and is set out in modified form in Table 3.1. (Huskisson, 1981.)

Calcium, iron and vitamins A, B, C and D are all important for healthy body functioning. There has been a growing interest in other minerals and vitamins, notably zinc, magnesium and vitamin E. Vitamin D aids the absorption of calcium, and is important for bone development. The introduction of increased amounts of bran into the diet carries with it the possible reduced absorption of calcium, zinc and iron. Phytic acid in the bran makes calcium insoluble and unavailable to the body. In elderly people the risk of broken bones from minor falls is increased if insufficient calcium is absorbed. The easiest way to ensure calcium intake is to have a daily milk drink, especially at night, when no wholemeal or bran foods are eaten. Spinach and rhubarb also interfere with calcium absorption, but are not normally eaten in sufficient quantities to be a problem.

Vitamin D is produced in the human body when the skin is exposed to sunlight. It is linked to calcium absorption. Asian families are particularly at risk of vitamin D deficiency in the less sunny European climate, especially if their clothing covers most of the body. Margarine then becomes important to their diet, as do eggs and oily fish.

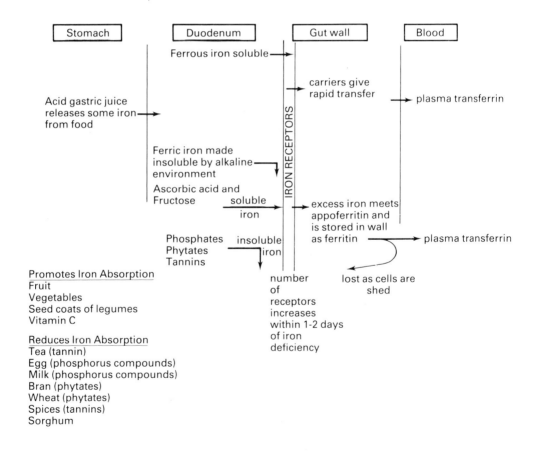

Fig. 3.2   Iron absorption

Iron loss is increased during the menstrual period, so that women have an extra risk of iron deficiency and anaemia, particularly if their periods are heavy. Vitamin C increases the body's ability to absorb iron, but tannin in tea and some Asian spices reduce it. The phosphorous compounds in eggs and milk also reduce it, as do the phytates in bran and wheat. Liver, red meat dark green vegetables and dried fruit provide iron (Fig. 3.2). If heavy periods occur iron intake may be boosted with iron tablets such as ferrous sulphate which can be bought at the chemist. These may be taken for one week starting at the same time as the period. If heavy menstruation is prolonged the doctor should be consulted.

The portions described in Table 3.1 would need to be adjusted for the vegan and vegetarian. The protein that the body needs then has to come from vegetable sources such as nuts, pulses, young plant sprouts and whole grain cereals. The calcium comes from increased amounts of dried figs, currants, raisins and vegetables. The soya bean can contribute protein. As textured vegetable protein it is also used as a 'meat extender' in cheaper tinned and pre-packaged meat dishes.

The energy requirement of the body increases with exercise, and also in cold temperatures when it is needed to keep warm. If a fever occurs the heat production comes first from the sugars, which enter the body from the digestion of carbohydrates, then from the liver stores and later from the body's fat stores. The thyroid gland in the neck controls the rate of heat production. In the winter it increases the rate to balance the heat lost from the body. Those who work in centrally heated offices and live in centrally heated homes will notice the cold more than the person who spends most of the day out of doors in winter, their 'internal thermostats' being set at different levels. Fatty and starchy foods are more palatable when it is cold and the body needs the energy for heat. Salads seem suitable for summer when the weather is warm and internal heat production is not so important. The types of food eaten in Europe therefore tend to vary with the seasons.

Fashion also influences what is an acceptable body weight. Fat people do face physical disadvantages, such as an increased risk of cardio-vascular disease and high blood pressure. In older women there is also an increase in gall-bladder disease. Social pressure can make life unhappy for the 'fatty'. Some people 'eat for comfort' and so risk a vicious circle of eating to excess combined with increasing obesity, disapproval from those around them and increased unhappiness.

The Royal College of Physicians (1983) recommends acceptable weight ranges based on a person's height (Table 3.2). If the weight is 20% above the upper limit of the weight range, then the individual is considered obese.

Eating for recovery from illness

Infection or damage to body tissues increases the need for protein to make more white cells to fight infection, or to repair and replace damaged cells. There is also an increased need for energy. Fever uses more of the body's energy by speeding up the rate at which cells produce heat.

If the food intake is insufficient, the body tissues are broken down to provide the necessary energy and protein (catabolism). The level of insulin produced falls, so blood sugar levels rise and sugar may appear in the urine. Ketones, due to the breakdown of fats, can also be detected. The cells produce less heat. Salt and water are retained while nitrogen is lost into the urine. The body weight falls.

Once cell breakdown is halted, replacement and repair can begin (anabolism). The amount of urine produced by the body increases and more salt is excreted in it. The nutrients from food intake are used first at the site of any cell injury. The amount of nitrogen lost in the blood decreases. The

Table 3.2 Acceptable average adult weight ranges, based on height. (Based on figures from the Royal College of Physicians (1983), Bray (1979) and the Metropolitan Life Insurance Co. (1960).)

Height without shoes			Nude weight Men				Nude weight Women			
Feet	Inches	Centimetres	Stones	Lbs.	Lbs.	Kilograms	Stones	Lbs.	Lbs.	Kilograms
4	10	147.32					7	4	102	46.27
4	11	149.86					7	6	104	47.17
5	0	152.40					7	9	107	48.53
5	1	154.94					7	12	110	48.89
5	2	157.48	8	11	123	55.79	8	1	113	51.25
5	3	160.02	9	1	127	57.61	8	4	116	52.62
5	4	162.56	9	4	130	58.97	8	8	120	54.43
5	5	165.10	9	7	133	60.33	8	11	123	55.79
5	6	167.64	9	10	136	61.69	9	2	128	58.06
5	7	170.18	10	0	140	63.50	9	6	132	59.87
5	8	172.72	10	5	145	65.77	9	10	136	61.69
5	9	175.06	10	9	149	67.58	10	0	140	63.50
5	10	177.80	10	13	153	69.40	10	4	144	65.31
5	11	180.34	11	4	158	71.67	10	8	148	67.13
6	0	182.88	11	8	162	73.48	10	12	152	68.95
6	1	185.42	11	12	166	75.29				
6	2	187.96	12	3	171	77.56				
6	3	190.50	12	8	176	79.83				
6	4	193.04	12	13	181	82.10				

Brushed cotton pyjamas and slippers — add 0.9 kg (2 lbs)
Long cotton nightdress and slippers — add 0.7 kg (1 lb 10 oz)
Note: athletically fit people will be heavier, as muscle weighs more than the same volume of adipose tissue.

appetite returns. Once cell damage is repaired the muscles broken down during the crisis period are gradually rebuilt. The body weight begins to increase once more. When more energy is being taken in than is required for rebuilding the tissues, it is stored as fat until the normal body weight is regained.

The larger the fat stores and muscle bulk the longer the body is able to go on functioning without an adequate food intake. However breaking down body cells to release energy and protein for use elsewhere in the body is inefficient. This process uses energy so it is more efficient to gain energy and protein direct from food.

If possible, eating easily digested food should be encouraged to meet at least some of the requirements and spare the body tissues. Eggs, milk, milk puddings, jelly and ice cream are traditional foods for invalids. However they lack some of the vitamins which may be needed. Fresh fruit juices and thick soups made from meat and/or vegetables should be provided. Extra calories and protein can be added to food by using commercially available supplements based on skimmed milk.

The way in which such food is presented can stimulate a poor appetite. Smaller plates for small portions makes the arrangement of food on the plate look more attractive. Thoughtful touches such as napkins, glass, proper cutlery and table or tray decorations also help. The best restaurants long ago recognised the importance of such details to encourage healthy appetites.

Mealtimes are also social occasions in many cultures. If someone is ill in bed they may welcome the company of a family member bringing two trays to the bedroom to share a meal, rather than being left to eat in splendid isolation.

If the food has to be cut up for the sick person or if they need feeding, the appetite can be better stimulated by cutting the food up in front of them. A mush of all the different parts of the meal mixed together is most offputting. Sitting in an upright position, makes both eating and swallowing easier.

Feeding a sick person should be a relaxed, unhurried activity, with the food being cut up as the meal proceeds rather than all at the start. Unless it is unsafe to do so, a fork should be used for the main course.

Foods causing illness in some sensitive people

Some foods contain vaso-active amines which can trigger a headache in those taking certain drugs, or in migraine sufferers. Monoamine oxidase enzymes break down amines; if they are deficient or inhibited by drugs (monoamine oxidase inhibitors — MAOI) there may be a change in the size of the blood vessels. An intense throbbing headache may occur if foods high in amines have been eaten. Some women become more susceptible before a period or when taking the contraceptive pill. Other people find going without food or stress increases the likelihood of a headache. In classical migraine there may be other symptoms such as a feeling of sickness and blurring of vision.

Trigger foods containing amines include cheese, chocolate, red wine, citrus fruits, raspberries, avocados and yeast extracts. A more detailed list is given in Table 3.3.

Monosodium glutamate (MSG) is increasingly added to soups, meat products, potato crisps and other savoury foods to enhance the flavour. An amine derivative, it is produced by microbiological fermentation and occurs naturally in seaweeds and soya beans. The latter are used in Chinese cooking. In people sensitive to MSG it produces a numbness in the neck extending to the arms and back, general weakness and palpitations. A burning sensation of mouth and lips may also occur.

Gluten is found in wheat, rye, oats and barley. A protein compound of

Table 3.3 Triggers for migraine (based on Wentworth, 1981)

Amines
> Tyramine
> 2-phenylethylamine
> Histamine
> Isoamylamine
> Octopamine
> Synephrine
> 5-hydroxytryptamine

Foods to avoid
Cheeses —
> Blue cheeses
> Cheddar
> Cheshire
> Danish blue
> Derby
> Double Gloucester
> Gruyere
> Irish Cheddar
> Leicester
> Sage Derby
> Scottish Red
> Stilton
> Wensleydale

} tyramine
or
2-phenylethylamine
or
a combination

Foods worth trying, as sensitivity varies
  Brie
  Caerphilly
  Camembert
  Cottage cheese
  Cream cheese
  Edam
  Processed cheese

Fruits to avoid

Grapefruit Lemon Lime Mandarin Oranges Satsumas or tangerines Ugli fruit	synephrine
Raspberries Loganberries Mulberries	tyramine

Other foods to avoid

Avocado pears	tyramine
Chocolate	2-phenylethylamine
Marmite	tyramine
Onions	
Over-ripe bananas	tyramine
Pickled herrings	tyramine
Pork	
Yoghurt	

Foods worth trying
  Bovril
  Carob flour as a substitute for chocolate

Drinks to avoid

Brandy		
Chianti	tyramine	
Cocoa	phenylethylamine	
Cointreau Gran Marnier		synephrine (oranges)
Horlicks		tyramine
Madeira		phenylethylamine
Port Red Wine Sherry Tomato juice		histamine

Drinks worth trying as sensitivity varies

Beer	Vodka
Dry sherry	White wine
Gin	
Lager	

gliadin and glutenin, it is involved in a congenital malabsorption disorder where patches of tiny finger-like villi, which line the small intestine, atrophy. Coeliac disease is an example of malabsorption syndrome. If gluten is removed from the diet these changes are reversed.

Lactose intolerance occurs when the mucosal cells lining the small intestine fail to produce the enzyme lactase. The lactose then passes into the colon where the bacteria ferment it. This results in loose stools which contain lactic acid. Asians and many Africans tend to lose the enzyme as they grow older, and if they are given large quantities of milk, loose stools result.

Shellfish, tomatoes, fish, pork and eggs can all cause an allergic skin rash in susceptible people, for instance eczema or local swelling of the lips and throat. If the symptoms follow very soon after the food is eaten it may be easy to work out the one responsible. In some people the reaction is delayed and it may then be necessary to keep a food diary to work out which food caused the problem. Avoiding the problem food once it is identified is usually easy. However if an allergy to eggs occurs, extra care must be taken to inform the doctor when receiving injections. Immunizing injections for influenza or yellow fever are prepared using eggs and may cause sudden severe illness. Self diagnosis can be difficult and major dietary changes are best made with the expert advice of a doctor and dietitian.

Antacids and indigestion

Indigestion or dyspepsia sometimes follows a meal. It may take the form of nausea, heartburn, abdominal distension or pain and it can follow a large or unusual meal. Self-treatment of occasional dyspepsia is unlikely to cause harm. However regular, frequent use of antacids may delay diagnosis of disease.

The amount of acid produced by the stomach does not have a direct bearing on whether dyspepsia occurs. Overwork or worry may lead to food being eaten rapidly, being poorly chewed, and to swallowing a lot of air. Taking large amounts of alcohol, particulary before food, can irritate the stomach lining causing gastritis and therefore discomfort.

Magnesium hydroxide neutralises acid effectively but may cause diarrhoea, whereas aluminium hydroxide may cause constipation. The tablets contain sugar which may be a problem to diabetics. Tablets should be chewed thoroughly or sucked. The liquid forms are more effective than tablets but are less convenient to carry around. The aluminium hydroxide mixture has a high sodium content, and should be avoided in those with fluid retention or on a low salt diet.

General assessment areas

Amount of food eaten every day
Frequency of eating
Type of food eaten
Religious or cultural beliefs about food
Food likes and dislikes
Hunger and its relationship to eating
Pain associated with eating
Ability to raise hand to mouth
Ability to grip cutlery
Tongue and jaw movements
Difficulties in swallowing
Dentition, crowned teeth, dentures, plaque
Attitudes towards eating
History of abdominal, oral or oesophageal surgery
Weight for height ratio
Food allergy/sensitivity
Special dietary prescription
Loss of taste
Rate of healing of wounds
Halitosis
Vomiting or nausea related to food
Appetite
Colour of oral mucosa
Condition of tongue and gums
Age

Problems

Page

Sore mouth following radiotherapy   53
Sore mouth due to mouth ulcers or local trauma from broken teeth   54
Sore mouth due to oral *Candida* or parotitis   55
Sore throat makes swallowing uncomfortable   58
Frightened to swallow   59
Unable to swallow due to local obstruction   61
Anorexic (lacks desire for food)   63
Unable to feed self   65
Unable to masticate   67
Feels that food 'sticks' in the gullet   71
Nausea and vomiting   72
Pain after eating   74
Feels full after small meals   76
Obese due to overeating   78
Lacks knowledge about what constitutes a healthy diet   80
Lacks understanding of therapeutic diet   82
Impaired sense of taste   83
Unable to tolerate fatty foods   85
Unable to maintain blood sugar within normal limits   86
Protein intake inadequate for current needs   89

Potential problems

Risk of malnutrition (protein and energy intake insufficient for current
    needs)   92
Risk of low body sodium (hyponatremia)   96
Risk that small food intake will not meet protein and calorie require-
    ments   98
Risk of vitamin deficiency   99
Risk of reaction to specific foods   101
Risk of developing low body potassium (hypokalaemia)   108
Risk of developing low body calcium (hypocalcaemia)   110
Risk of developing high blood calcium (hypercalcaemia)   111
Risk of developing low body iron stores   113

Problems

Problem	Sore mouth following radiotherapy

Assessment findings

Mouth feels sore
Mucosa and gums red
Discomfort when talking
Decrease in food intake

Information for the patient

Some cells in the body divide and multiply more rapidly than others. They are found in parts of the body where there is a lot of wear and tear such as in the mouth and lining the gut. Radiotherapy treatment tends to have its greatest effect on these dividing cells. Although great care is taken to aim the radiation beam, these sensitive cells may still be affected. Once the treatments are completed the normal repair rate can return and the soreness should go within four weeks. The white cells of the body which fight infection may also be reduced in number so extra care must be taken to avoid more damage and letting bacteria in to start an infection.

Nursing action

1. Mild alkaline mouth washes such as sodium bicarbonate solution or glycerine of thymol as frequently as the patient desires. (Sodium bicarbonate 1 teaspoon to 2 pints water).

RE. Ask the patient about the degree of discomfort, and whether it is decreasing, inspect the mouth and record the state of mucosa and gums.

2. Bland, soft or liquid foods will reduce mechanical trauma on sore mucous membranes, and will limit further damage to the mouth. Salty or acid foods may sting in the mouth and should be avoided. High protein, high calorie foods will help achieve an adequate intake if anorexia or discomfort limit eating. They will also help aid the replacement of damaged cells.

RE. Record the amount offered and eaten by the patient. If eating tires the patient, plan for small meals every two hours.

3. Ask the patient to clean their mouth after meals with soft swabs soaked in warm water, not a brush. Cells will be shed from the mucous membrane. Gentle cleansing will remove food debris, and reduce the food remnants so depriving bacteria of nutrients and keeping cell loss to a minimum.

RE. Record the amount offered and eaten by the patient. If eating tires the tissue damage.

4. Monitor for ulceration or infection especially if local trauma has exceeded the current rate of repair.

RE. Ask the patient to report any increased local soreness. Inspect the mouth daily for *Candia albicans* infection (thrush).

5. Increase fluid intake by extra 1000 ml to promote elimination of creatinine and uric acid from tissue breakdown. Very hot or cold fluids should be avoided as they can increase discomfort. Fizzy drinks, fruit juices such as orange, but not apple or cranberry, help by making the urine more alkaline which helps keep uric acid in solution. Uric acid and other urates can be deposited in the urinary passages, and lead to stones.

RE. Chart fluid intake and output. Assess pH of urine, aim to keep it between pH 6 and 7.

Further action

1. If infection is suspected a mouth swab may be taken, between mealtimes, for culture and sensitivity. 1% chlorhexidine mouthwash every 4 hours may be prescribed, and dental advice sought if caries are present.

RE. *Candida albicans*, a yeast, may proliferate on damaged mucus membranes, increasing oral discomfort. Check temperature (axilla) at least daily as odontitis or osteomyelitis is a risk from carious teeth.

2. If saliva flow has been reduced by local irradiation, artificial saliva (e.g. Hypromellose solution) may be used to coat and moisten the mouth.

RE. Observe whether speaking and eating are easier. Ask the patient if discomfort is reduced.

3. Aspirin mucilage before meals may provide analgesia and aid eating.

RE. Check the patient is not sensitive to aspirin.

4. Local areas of tissue damage can be coated with anaesthetic gel such as Bonjela before meals and at 2–3 hourly intervals.

RE Inspect the sore areas at least daily for a change in size. Check patient is not sensitive to salicylates.

Associated medical diagnoses

Accidental irradiation
Malignant disease treated by radiation
Receiving radiotherapy especially to head, neck or chest

Problem | **Sore mouth due to mouth ulcers or local trauma from broken teeth**

Assessment findings

Mouth feels sore
Small broken central area which may be surrounded by inflamed mucosa
Less than usual use of lips when talking
Discomfort when talking
Superficial laceration of mucosa adjacent to rough or broken tooth or denture

Information for the patient

A mouth ulcer can form for no obvious reason. Rough or broken teeth can cause small cuts in the mouth. Using a mild mouthwash between meals can ease the discomfort. It also helps to keep the mouth clean and prevents infection. The doctor may prescribe treatment for the ulcer area. The inside surface of the mouth is constantly making new cells so that healing usually takes only 2 to 3 days.

Nursing actions

1. No very hot or very cold food or fluids should be given, to reduce discomfort from extremes of temperature.

RE. Check how much the patient eats. Assess balance of food intake to nutritional requirements.

2. Advise the patient to avoid alcohol, highly spiced food, and tobacco smoke, all of which add to the irritation.

RE. Note if this advice is followed.

3. Warm, normal saline, glycothymol or sodium bicarbonate mouthwashes can be given as frequently as the patient desires. A vacuum flask can be used to provide enough for several hours. Clean teeth with brush as usual but toothpaste may need to be omitted if it causes discomfort or stinging.

RE. Check how frequently the mouthwash is used. Ask the patient whether the discomfort is decreasing. Inspect the mouth and report any change.

4. Encourage an increase in occupations which do not require much talking. Provide books, magazines, handicrafts, television, radio or jigsaw puzzles.

RE. Note which, if any, of the occupations the patient enjoys.

Further action	1. Benzocaine lozenges can provide a local anaesthetic action. Hydrocortisone in pellet form may be prescribed for its anti-inflammatory action if ulcer is very painful. RE. Check the patient keeps the lozenge or pellet over the sore area while it dissolves and does not swallow it whole. 2. Vitamin C and/or B complex may be prescribed if a vitamin deficiency is suspected. RE. Check the patient understands which foods contain high levels of these vitamins. 3. Orabase may be used to protect damaged area. RE. Explain that this is a form of dressing and should not be swallowed. 4. Dental treatment should be sought for a broken tooth, caries or dental disease. RE. Review the tooth cleaning technique with the patient.
Associated medical diagnoses	Agranulocytosis Apthous stomatitis Dental caries Gold therapy Herpes simplex Infectious mononucleosis (glandular fever) Leucoplakia Pernicious anaemia

---

Problem	**Sore mouth due to oral *candida* or parotitis**

Assessment findings	Small white plaques or reddened mucosa or gums Mouth feels sore Discomfort when talking or swallowing Breath smells foul (halitosis) Swollen face – on one or both sides Local inflammation over parotid glands Purulent material visible at duct from parotid Patient complains of an unpleasant taste Thick saliva – decreased volume Badly discoloured teeth, tartar

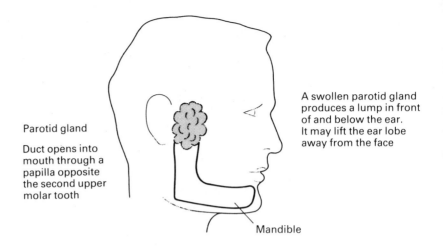

Parotid gland

Duct opens into
mouth through a
papilla opposite
the second upper
molar tooth

A swollen parotid gland
produces a lump in front
of and below the ear.
It may lift the ear lobe
away from the face

Mandible

Fig. 3.3   The location of the parotid gland

Inflamed or receding gums (gingivitis)
Raised body temperature

Information for the patient

When the body's resistance to infection is lowered, infections can occur more easily. Powerful antibiotics can kill bacteria normally present, and so allow other less benevolent organisms to move in and increase. Thrush is caused by a yeast called *Candida albicans*. The *albicans* part of its name is due to the white patches it produces. In hospital other patients may also have a lowered resistance so special precautions are taken to avoid spreading the infection. Bacteria can get into the salivary glands, particularly the parotid gland. This gland gets its name from its position – beside the ear. (Greek para = beside, otos = ear). Infection causes swelling and interferes with the flow of saliva. Pus can pass down the duct from the gland to give a foul taste and bad breath. (Fig. 3.3).

Nursing actions

1. Reduce the risk of cross-infection by providing disposable crockery and cutlery or marking the crockery and cutlery and washing it separately in very hot water and detergent. Sodium hypochlorite solution (Milton) can be used to kill the organisms but it will damage metals and cannot be effective through a residue of food. Soak equipment in a solution of Milton 1:1000. Check that any suction equipment is disposable or is sterilized after use.

2. Provide bland fluids and foods, avoid acidic fruits (e.g. citrus). Acid foods stimulate the secretion of saliva and can also sting when in contact with 'raw' areas. The salivary ducts can be blocked by inflammation and eating, which stimulates saliva flow, increasing the discomfort.

RE. Observe what and how much the patient eats.

3. Increase the patient's intake of protein and carbohydrates to provide at least two portions of milk and/or cheese and two portions of meat or eggs with six portions of cereals or bread. See Table 3.1.

RE. If increased levels of protein are not tolerated, substitute with egg flips or supplementary drinks based on skimmed milk powder.

4. Increase the fluid intake to at least 2.5 to 3 litres in 24 hours, more if temperature is of 38.5°C or higher.

RE. Record fluid intake and output.

5. Cleanse the mouth 2–3 hourly with swabs soaked in mouthwash, water, saline, a sodium bicarbonate solution or hydrogen peroxide. As discomfort decreases toothbrushing should recommence.

RE. Inspect the patient's mouth twice a day and record condition. Increase frequency of cleansing if improvement does not occur after 24 hours of treatment.

6. Record body temperature at axilla or using a rectal thermometer at 6 hourly intervals if temperature is raised to 37.5°C or above. NB: Axillary reading 0.5°C lower than oral readings.

RE. Pyrexia should subside within 48 hours from the commencement of medical treatment. Reduce frequency of recording to twice daily after 48 hours if patient's body temperature has returned to normal.

Further action

1. Antifungal agents such as nystatin suspension, amphotericin lozenges or miconazole gel may be used for *Candida* infection.

RE. Monitor for spread of infection to lungs or gut. Report the production of sputum or loose stools.

2. Paint oral cavity with 1% aqueous gentian violet three times a day for four days to kill *Candida*. Protect pillowcases from saliva as the dye stains permanently.

RE. Monitor for spread of infection. The dye makes the plaques difficult to see.

3. Take a throat or mouth swab for culture and sensitivity so that suitable antibiotic or antifungal therapy can be commenced. No milk should be given with tetracycline as calcium chelates it rendering it unabsorbable.

RE. If infection does not respond to antibiotics within about 48 hours then incision and drainage may be required.

4. If oral hygiene and dental care are generally poor the advice of a dentist or an oral hygienist may be requested on the patient's behalf.

RE. Check how much the patient understands of the advice given. Observe their oral hygiene technique for evidence of improvement.

Associated medical diagnoses

Carcinomatosis
Dental caries
Gingivitis
Leukaemia
Mumps
Periodontitis
Pyorrhoea
Treatment with antibiotics such as tetracycline or chloramphenicol
Alcoholic cirrhosis
Sarcoidosis

Problem	**Sore throat makes swallowing uncomfortable.**
Assessment findings	Swallowing feels uncomfortable Patient swallows with concentration and care Saliva trickles from mouth or is spat out into tissue Pharynx appears red Tonsils enlarged and red Uvula red and swollen Swollen glands (lymph nodes) in neck (Fig. 3.4) Fever

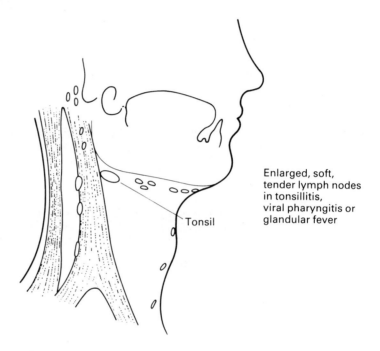

Enlarged, soft, tender lymph nodes in tonsillitis, viral pharyngitis or glandular fever

Tonsil

Fig. 3.4   Glands in the neck which may enlarge

Information for the patient	A sore throat is due to local inflammation. The tissues become red and swollen particularly if there is infection. While the body is fighting off the cause it is important to provide it with enough food to aid recovery. Eating little and often will help. Gargles will be soothing and also help to keep the sore tissues clean.
Nursing action	1. Warm rather than hot food should be given to prevent possible discomfort from increased vasodilatation. Provide frequent small meals. RE. Observe how much is eaten. Increase amount and temperature of food as discomfort decreases. 2. Provide soft, bland food to reduce irritation and possible trauma to inflamed tissues. RE. Observe how much of each meal is eaten. Assess the balance between food intake and nutritional requirement. Provide fluid supplements to increase intake if necessary.

3. Gargles of warm, normal saline should be provided in a vacuum flask at the bedside for frequent use as desired by the patient.

RE. Inspect the mouth and throat, using a torch and tongue depressor, once a day. Record condition. Ask patient about relief of discomfort.

Further action

1. Obtain a throat swab for culture and sensitivity. If infection is present a broad spectrum antibiotic may be prescribed.

RE. Monitor temperature four times a day. An antibiotic course normally lasts for five days.

2. Local analgesia such as aspirin mucilage, or aspirin gargle, which is then swallowed, may be given before meals.

RE. Check for aspirin sensitivity and degree of relief from discomfort.

3. A local anaesthetic may be prescribed for severe discomfort, such as a benzocaine lozenge every six hours.

RE. Check for degree of relief from discomfort.

Associated medical diagnoses

Coryza
Encephalitis
Infectious mononucleosis (glandular fever)
Streptococcal pharyngitis

Problem	Frightened to swallow

Assessment findings

History of past swallowing difficulties
Facial nerve paralysis
Partial oesophageal obstruction
The doctor agrees that the patient may eat
Tongue deviates when protruded (Fig. 3.5)
Anxious facial expression at mealtime
Fear of eating expressed
Asks for clearly impossible foods for meals
Refuses meals
Spits out food

Information for the patient

Normal swallowing involves the use of the tongue and the muscles at the back of the throat. As the food is passed to the back of the tongue the palate rises up to block off the path to the nose. The voice box is closed by a flap (epiglottis) and the entrance to the gullet opens wider. The tongue flips the food backwards into the only open path, the gullet. Once in there, waves of pressure from the gullet walls squeeze the food down towards the stomach. It is easier to swallow solid food than fluids so that eating can start even when the patient still has difficulty swallowing saliva.

Nursing actions

1. Provide tissues and a polythene bag (for their disposal) or a sputum pot or receiver into which the patient can spit saliva. A thick towel or absorbent pad can be used during sleep. (Incontinence pads have a polythene backing and could cause suffocation).

RE. Check amount of saliva being lost by weighing 20 dry tissues in a bag and comparing with the weight of the bag of used tissues. Subtract the dry

(a) No stimulus to left side of the tongue if brain damage on right from cerebral vascular accident

(b) 12th nerve damage (hypoglossal) in lower motor neurone disease causes lack of stimulus to the same side as the damage. The tongue muscle may waste.

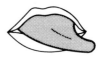

Muscle fibres which are stimulated will extend - the healthy side curves around the affected one.

Fig. 3.5 Damaged control of tongue muscles

weight from the wet weight and calculate volume (5.06 g = 5 ml saliva) or measure volume in pot/receiver. Record on fluid chart.

2. Avoid acid foods and sweets, such as citrus fruits, apple and pineapple juice and lemon drops as these increase saliva production.

RE. Observe saliva production for decrease in volume.

3. Make sure that the suction machine is in good working order and available at the bedside for immediate use if the patient starts to choke.

RE. Record frequency of suction and patient's reaction. Check and clean equipment daily.

4. Vaseline (petroleum jelly) or lip-salve can be gently massaged into lips protect them from repeated contact with saliva.

RE. Ensure that lips do not become sore or cracked.

5. Sit upright, if possible or raise the patient's head for eating or drinking.

RE. Observe that effective swallowing occurs.

6. A high calorie semi-solid or, if there is obstruction, fluid diet should be given to maintain Calorie and protein intake sufficient to maintain body weight.

RE. Weigh patient every 2—3 days to check that the Calorie and fluid intake are sufficient to maintain a stable body weight.

7. Discuss exactly how the fear of swallowing influences the patient's activities. Include activities in the care plan which give the patient a feeling of confidence and control.

RE. Ask the patient how they feel. Increase the texture of their food and gradually withdraw special attention at mealtimes as confidence returns.

8. Provide privacy when eating to reduce embarrassment caused by the presence of other patients. Remain nearby to assist the patient if necessary and give positive reinforcement when food is eaten without difficulties.

RE. Record how often they require a nurse's help at mealtimes.

Further action	1. Essential drugs should be given by intramuscular, subcutaneous or intravenous route through an intravenous cannula. Some drugs can be given by inhalation or suppository.
	RE. Check the hospital rules for the administration of intravenous drugs by a nurse. Monitor how easily the patient can retain a suppository. Insertion — blunt end first may increase surface area in contact with rectal mucosa above anal sphincter.
	2. Intravenous fluids or feeding through a fine-bore naso-gastric tube may be needed for rehydration of the patient if he has not had fluids for some time.
	RE. Observe for increased skin turgor.
Associated medical diagnoses	Bulbar palsy Cerebral vascular accident Lower motor neurone disease Parkinson's disease

---

Problem	**Unable to swallow due to local obstruction.**

Assessment findings	Saliva pools in mouth Coughing from material trickling into larynx Body weight falling Muscle wasting Poor or little control of tongue and palate No swallowing reflex
Information for the patient	Swallowing requires that nerves and muscles work *together* to pass food back from the tongue and into the gullet. There, waves of muscle action push the food along towards the stomach. Damage to the nerves which control swallowing anywhere along their path from brain to gullet can interfere with the process. Any outside pressure on the gullet can also stop food being pushed down by the muscles. The small flap which closes over the windpipe as food is passed into the gullet may also be affected so it 'goes down the wrong way' and causes coughing. The saliva or spit is being made all the time but its flow increases at mealtimes. If it cannot be swallowed it must be collected to prevent coughing or choking. The doctor will decide how food and fluid will be given when swallowing is impossible.
Nursing actions	1. Position the patient so that saliva cannot pool at the back of the mouth, for instance, sitting up with the head forward if the patient is well enough. If the patient is very weak or only semi-conscious, place them in a lateral or semi-prone position, with the foot of the bed tipped up by $15-30°$.
	RE. Check position uses gravity to drain saliva towards lips. Coughing or choking should decrease.
	2. Suction apparatus with a catheter or Yankauer suction tip should be near the patient for immediate use if the patient starts to cough or choke.
	RE. Record frequency of suction and patient's reaction. Check and clean equipment at least once a day.

3. Provide adequate nutrition by the prescribed route.

RE. Weigh patient every 2 days to check Calorie and fluid intake is sufficient to maintain a steady body weight.

4. Check all visitors understand they must not give the patient food (or fluid). An interpreter should be used when English is not the first language as a precaution against misunderstanding.

RE. Observe visitors frequently if there is any doubt that they may fail to comply with the request not to feed the patient.

5. Apply petroleum jelly or 'lip salve' to lips and skin around the mouth to prevent excoriation from constant wetting by saliva.

RE. Check the patient's lips and skin for redness or early excoriation.

6. Provide soft tissues and a polythene bag for their disposal or make a wick of ribbon gauze to drain saliva into small receiver. A thick towel or pad of absorbent material under the chin can be used during sleep. (Incontinence pads have a polythene backing and could cause suffocation).

RE. Check amount of saliva lost by weighing 20 dry tissues and polythene bag, reweigh bag of used tissues, subtract dry weight from wet weight to calculate volume (5.06 g = 5 ml saliva) or measure volume in receiver. Record on fluid chart.

7. Discuss with the patient how it feels to be unable to swallow. Check if there are any activities which cause them discomfort or if they have any other problems or fears.

RE. Observe for increased tension or distress.

Further action

1. Insertion of a plastic or reinforced tube along the oesophagus through the obstruction and anchored to the stomach wall may be undertaken to provide an open channel. Drugs should be given in syrup form.

RE. A weekly X-ray should be taken to check tube remains correctly placed.

2. The fluid diet can be replaced by thicker purées and well masticated solid food. Avoid pulpy foods such as fresh oranges.

RE. Observe for discomfort.

3. In severe cases a gastrostomy tube may be inserted through the abdominal wall into the stomach. A fluid diet may be given ideally as a continuous drip or in 100–200 ml feeds. Wide bore tubes may allow puréed meals to be used. Drugs in syrup form may be given by this route.

RE. Check skin for damage from gastric acid splashes when the tube is aspirated and also for leakage. Use 'Stomahesive' or 'Rediseal' for protection.

4. Parenteral feeding involves hypertonic (concentrated) nutrients which irritate small veins. The intravenous cannula is usually inserted so its tip lies in a wide central vein where dilution by blood flow reduces the damage. The sub-clavian route to the superior vena cava is a popular route. Insertion is carried out with strict asepsis as infection is a major risk. Change the administration set each day. Attach a note to the prescription chart that no drugs are to be given via the line.

RE. Mark the insertion point on catheter. Check there is no strain on catheter or kinking and that it is covered by a clean dressing. Monitor vital signs for infection; a rigor may indicate septicaemia.

5. The prescription of fluid volume, electrolytes, vitamins, fats and minerals will vary according to the patient's condition. A volumetric infusion pump should be used to control the rate of flow to reduce the risk of entry of air into the giving set. The more viscous the solution, the smaller the drop size will be.

RE. Weigh the patient at the same time each day in the same clothes. Fluid intake and output should be strictly monitored. Test urine for glucose at least daily, up to six hourly in severely ill patients.

6. Salivation may be suppressed by giving atrophine.

RE. Drying of eyes and other mucuous membranes may occur. Urinary retention is possible.

7. Drugs should *not* be given through the parenteral feeding line. The intramuscular, subcutaneous or rectal routes should be used. This should be specified on the prescription chart.

RE. Check new staff understand the policy.

Associated medical diagnoses	Aortic aneurysm Cerebral vascular accident Carcinoma Cerebral palsy Enlarged mediastinal lymph nodes Foreign body in oesophagus Goitre Motor neurone disease Myesthenia gravis Pharyngeal paralysis from glossopharyngeal damage (to 9th cranial nerve) Poliomyelitis Post-oesophagectomy Vagal nerve damage
Problem	**Anorexic (lacks desire for food)**
Assessment findings	Onset of loss of appetite Food refused Toys with food Eats no more than 2–3 mouthfuls at a meal No sensation of hunger Digitalis therapy Low serum potassium Weight loss Elderly Unconcerned about poor appetite Ketones in urine

Information for the patient

In illness the appetite may be lost at a time when the body's need for food is actually increased. It is important to try and eat even though it seems a big effort. The body's continuing need for energy, protein and other nutrients means the tissues will be used as a temporary measure to provide these if the diet is inadequate. This is an ineffective source and leads to weight loss and a reduced ability to fight illness.

Nursing actions

1. Provide frequent small, attractively presented meals on small plates. The visual presentation of food plays an important role in stimulating appetite and salivation.

RE. Record food intake and calculate calorie requirement and daily intake. Weigh patient every two days to check that their food intake is sufficient to maintain the body weight or increase it.

2. Provide milk based supplements midway between meals. A variety of flavours are available which can be served hot or chilled.

RE. Record intake on fluid chart, add nutritional intake to calculation for food. Report if intake is less than calculated requirement after 48 hours.

3. Discuss with the patient whether worries about illness, problems at home or any upsetting sights and sounds in the hospital ward are reducing appetite.

RE. Observe for non-verbal signs of tension. Consider if another member of the team has a good rapport with the patient and could act as a counsellor or confidant.

4. A small glass of dry sherry 20–30 minutes before meals may be given to stimulate the appetite. In hospital, if drug therapy is in use the doctor's permission must be obtained to avoid possible interference with other treatments.

RE. Observe patient's response to being offered sherry and effect on their subsequent meal. The alcohol provides extra calories so include in estimate of intake.

5. Ask relatives and/or visitors to bring in small quantities of the patient's favourite foods. If they are willing and the patient agrees, relatives may help by coaxing the patient at mealtimes.

RE. Check that food does not become a disruptive factor in the relationship between family and patient. For some people food becomes the vehicle for emotional communication.

6. Low potassium levels — encourage high potassium foods, including orange, pineapple and tomato juice, bananas, Bovril, Marmite, soups, meat, fish and milk. See potential problems section.

RE. Check any subsequent electrolyte results for increase in serum potassium.

7. Tobacco smoking decreases appetite. It should be discouraged.

RE. Observe whether smoking decreases, give positive reinforcement if this is achieved.

Further action

1. Anabolic steroids such as nandrolene increase the appetite. The effect of the drug lasts for three weeks.

RE. Observe for side effects of masculinization in women such as deepening of voice, increasing body hair and increased libido. Weigh weekly to identify increase in body tissues. Rapid weight gain may indicate salt and water retention. Uterine bleeding may occur with some compounds when treatment is stopped.

2. Alcohol before meals is not prescribed if liver disease is present or for a 'dry' alcoholic. It may also interfere with antibiotic activity.

RE. Check that alcohol does not conflict with the patient's cultural or religious beliefs. Observe how much food is taken during the meal.

3. Nitrogen excretion may be measured from a 24 hour urine collection. Serum albumin measurement may also be used to review the need for enteral feeding.

RE. The volume of urine collected should include that excreted after the start time (i.e. throw away the first urine passed and write the time of its passing on the bottle). The urine passed up to the end of the following 24 hours should go into the bottle. If a sample has to be taken for other purposes note the volume as 'aliquot of . . . ml removed'. If the patient cannot empty the bladder at the close of 24 hours add the urine passed after the usual finishing time together with the actual time this last quantity was produced.

4. Thiamine (Vitamin B_1) may be useful in deficiency disease as it plays an important role in carbohydrate metabolism.

RE. The oral route of administration is preferred as anaphylactic reaction may occur if it is given intravenously.

Associated medical diagnoses	Bacterial endocarditis Beri beri Carcinomatosis Gastritis Glomerulonephritis Hepatitis Hypothyroidism Kwashiorkor Leukaemia Pernicious anaemia Radiotherapy for malignant disease Sprue Vitamin deficiency
Problem	**Unable to feed self**
Assessment findings	Muscle weakness affecting arms Poor neuromuscular co-ordination Loss of use of arm Deformity of joints Poor concentration Stiff elbow or shoulder joints Weak grip Loss of positional sense

Lying flat in bed
Deformity of fingers
Loss of sense of touch
Contracture of fingers
Muscle spasm
Incoordinate muscle activity
Cog-wheel rigidity in arms
Receiving phenothiazine drugs

Information for the patient

When a patient is unable to feed unaided the nurses or relatives may help. It is not easy to find the rhythm and food mixtures on the fork that another person like to use while eating. It helps if the patient explains how they like to eat their meals and feels free to ask for changes if it isn't quite right. It takes a while to sort out all the details but once they are clear they can be added to the care plan so that other staff don't have to start right from the beginning at each mealtime. If a patient feels able to start feeding themselves they should tell the staff.

Nursing actions

Ask the patient if they prefer to eat in the relative privacy of their bed area or at the table with other patients. Adult patients may feel embarrassed by their dependence on others.

RE. Observe how comfortable the patient appears in the chosen meal setting.

2. Position the patient comfortably before a meal; if possible sitting upright and well supported by pillows. Lower the height of adjustable beds so the patient is within a comfortable distance of the meal tray and the nurse. Patients who have to be fed lying down may find chewing and swallowing easier if the bed head can be tilted upwards. Insert the patient's dentures if necessary.

RE. Observe the most comfortable feeding position for the patient. Incorporate information in care plan. Modify texture of food if mastication or swallowing proves difficult.

3. Use absorbent cellulose wadding or tissues beneath a napkin for fluid meals or if saliva tends to dribble from mouth.

RE. Make sure clothing does not become damp or soiled during the meal.

4. Feed patient by sitting on patient's righthand side if nurse is righthanded, patient's left if lefthanded. Cut up food and load the fork or spoon as if eating the meal. Place the food in the patient's mouth or if the patient prefers hold the food an inch or so away from their mouth so that they can move their head to reach it. If the patient has facial paralysis on one side place the food in the opposite side of the mouth to aid swallowing.

RE. Note how much of the meal the patient eats and when, or if, fatigue sets in. Weigh the patient at least once a week to check food and fluid intake is sufficient to maintain steady body weight.

5. Keep hot food hot and cold food cold, so that it remains palatable however long the patient needs for eating. Meals served on plates with a heated pellet in the base remain hot for 10–15 minutes once the lid is removed.

RE. Check temperature of food by asking patient or using a clean teaspoon to taste it.

6. Take time to feed the patient. If possible the same nurse should feed the patient for the whole meal. Talk with the patient to make it a more normal social occasion and to provide natural pauses in the feeding rhythm so the patient can 'get his breath'.

RE. Observe patient for fatigue or tension. Adjust the rhythm of feeding according to the verbal and non-verbal cues.

7. Make full use of any feeding skills the patient is still able to use. Independence is a valued possession for most adults. A polythene tube may allow thin soup to be sucked from a cup unaided.

RE. Note any movements which could, with aids, allow the patient to begin feeding himself once more. Consider further action.

Further action	1. Seek occupational therapist advice in the selection of feeding aids such as:-

Lightweight cutlery with shaped or padded handles to aid a weak grip.
High friction mats to hold plates steady.
A plate shaped to provide a pushing area.

RE. Check aids are kept in good repair and made available for every meal.

2. Arrange speech therapy advice for the patient on regaining or strengthening muscle control in lips or tongue. Photographs or diagrams may convey exercises or facial positions better than words.

RE. Check exercises or feeding methods are used as prescribed. Results may be slow so the patient or helper may give up the effort, if not encouraged.

Associated medical diagnoses	Alzheimer's Disease Bone fracture in arm or hand Burns Cerebral palsy Cerebral vascular accident Extrapyramidal disorder Intracranial tumours Myasthenia gravis Parkinson's disease Pre-senile dementia Rheumatoid arthritis Schizophrenia Senila dementia Spinal cord injury

Problem	**Unable to masticate**

Assessment findings	Edentulous Unable to clench teeth Wired or broken jaw Reluctant to wear dentures Lost or broken dentures or dental bridge Loss of muscle bulk of masseter muscle (which assists in elevating the lower jaw) (Fig. 3.6) Involuntary tongue movements Loss of sensation (Fig. 3.7) Weakness of one side of the face

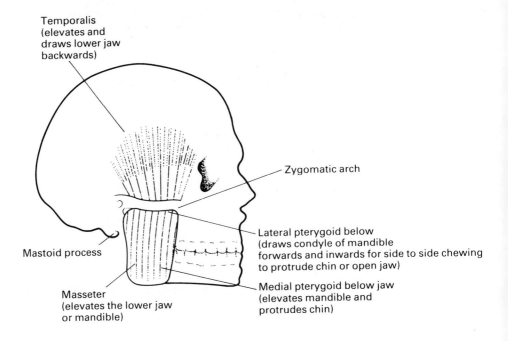

Fig. 3.6 Muscles used in mastication

Poor chewing movements
Able to suck and swallow
Dry mouth (xerostomia)
Mouthbreathing

Information for the patient

Chewing helps to stimulate the flow of saliva and appetite. Soft or liquidized food can provide as much energy and protein as the more solid form but it is digested more quickly. Eating little and often helps to stop the hollow feeling between meals.

Nursing actions

1. Provide a mechanically soft diet (Table 3.4) or liquidized foods such as those listed. Select food for texture, colour, variety and add garnishes. Puréed foods should be served in small containers on a plate.

RE. Observe how much is eaten and calculate intake and nutritional requirements.

2. Help the patient to feed slowly and give small amounts. Small frequent meals may prove less tiring and will prevent hunger pangs if fluid foods are given. Fluids pass through the digestive tract more quickly.

RE. Observe for signs of tiredness, and increase proportion of high calorie, low bulk foods if tiredness occurs.

Table 3.4   Mechanically soft diet

Breakfast
  Fruit juice
  Porridge — with sugar, butter or syrup
  Cornflakes — with sugar, milk or cream
  Bran flakes
  Wheat flakes
  Bread, butter, honey or jelly or thin-shred marmalade
  Scrambled or soft boiled eggs
  Poached or coddled eggs
  Minced bacon and tinned tomato
  Omelettes with herbs or fine chopped fillings

Midmorning snack or tea
  Sponge cake
  Madeira cake
  Bread and butter with grated cheese or mashed bananas
  Drinking chocolate
  Milk shake

Lunch or dinner
  Chilled melon
  Strained vegetable or meat soups
  Puréed vegetables
  Consommé — hot or cold
  Tomato mould
  Savoury mousse
  Avocado pear — ripe
  Minced chicken, beef, ham, pork, rabbit, with mayonnaise, curry, herbs or
    as a mould
  Cottage pie with grated onion
  Omelettes with fine-chopped fillings
  Savoury mince with grated vegetables
  Poached or baked fish
  Chopped spaghetti or small pasta shapes in sauce
  Tinned fish
  Baked beans
  Mashed potatoes, swede, turnip
  Leaf spinach
  Tinned sweetcorn
  Cauliflower florets
  Marrow
  Young carrots or peas
  Jelly
  Milk puddings
  Fruit mousse or fool
  Yoghurt
  Mashed banana
  Black, red or white currants
  Tinned grapefruit or mandarin oranges chopped up with juice
  Melon
  Tinned peaches, pears, raspberries, strawberries — chopped up with juice
  Stewed apples, pears without skins
  Trifle
  Ice cream with sauce
  Egg custard
  Cream caramel
  Sponge pudding with custard or sauce
  Water ices (granita)

3. Improve the muscle tone of the weak side of the patient's face by holding their jaw closed and briskly stroking the affected cheek down towards the lip.

RE. Improvement may take weeks to achieve; increasing ability to close the lips heralds increasing muscle activity.

4. Improve muscle tone by holding jaw up gently and mimic chewing movements by moving lower jaw from side to side with rotating movements.

RE. Improvement will take weeks to become obvious.

5. Cleanse mouth after food with mouthwashes or gentle brushing. Check food has not collected between cheek and gums.

RE. Inspect mouth after cleansing to confirm food has been removed.

6. Observe for mouth breathing leading to the patient having dry mouth.

RE. Check oral temperature for fever. Inform doctor so that the cause can be investigated.

Further action

1. Speech therapy advice should be sought when the 7th cranial nerve has been damaged and mouth movement is limited. Photographs or diagrams of exercises are often easier for the patient to understand than words.

RE. Check exercises are continued as frequently as advised as progress may be slow with the patient or helpers losing interest and enthusiasm.

2. Dental advice may be helpful if the bite or occlusion is inadequate.

RE. Orthodontic treatment can be lengthy, the patient needs to understand the treatment and to co-operate in maintaining good oral hygiene.

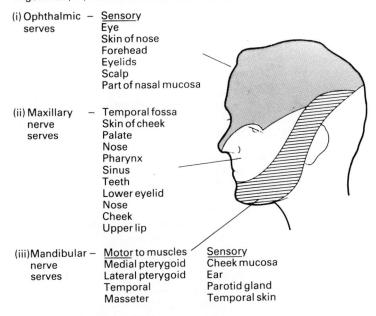

Trigeminal (5th) nerve divides into three branches:-

(i) Ophthalmic –   <u>Sensory</u>
serves   Eye
                Skin of nose
                Forehead
                Eyelids
                Scalp
                Part of nasal mucosa

(ii) Maxillary   –   Temporal fossa
nerve   Skin of cheek
serves   Palate
                Nose
                Pharynx
                Sinus
                Teeth
                Lower eyelid
                Nose
                Cheek
                Upper lip

(iii) Mandibular –   <u>Motor</u> to muscles   <u>Sensory</u>
nerve   Medial pterygoid   Cheek mucosa
serves   Lateral pterygoid   Ear
                Temporal   Parotid gland
                Masseter   Temporal skin

Fig. 3.7   Areas of the face where sensation is influenced by the trigeminal nerve.

Associated medical diagnoses	Cerebrovascular accident
	Dehydration
	Diabetes mellitus
	Fractured mandible
	Myasthenia gravis
	Trigeminal (5th) nerve paralysis (Fig. 3.7)
	Vincent's angina (Trench mouth)

Problem	**Feels that food 'sticks' in the gullet**

Assessment findings

Poor food intake
Avoids all hard foods
Vomiting after small food intake
Localised discomfort in chest
Pain radiating into back and neck
Chest infection
Reducing body weight

Information for the patient

Swallowing requires the nerves and muscles to work together to pass food back off the tongue and into the gullet. These waves of muscle action push the food down towards the valve (sphincter) which opens to let it enter the stomach. Outside pressure on the gullet or stiff inelastic tissue can interfere with this muscle action. If acid from the stomach has been able to pass back through the valve it can burn the gullet and leave scars. Sometimes the valve is slow to open. If any of these problems occur it feels as if the food has got stuck. The muscles above the food keep on pushing and that increases the discomfort. A soft or liquid diet can usually reach the stomach but it will be passed on down the gut more quickly. So to stop feelings of hunger food must be taken 'little and often'.

Nursing actions

1. Semi-solid or liquid diet providing at least 3500 Calories in 24 hours. See list of foods in Table 3.6.

RE. Weigh the patient at least once a week and at the same time each day to check their calorie and fluid intake is sufficient to maintain a stable body weight.

2. Small frequent meals or drinks prevent the hollow feeling that follows the more rapid digestion of liquid food. Tiredness may also be prevented.

RE. Observe how much food is taken at each meal and for any signs of tiredness.

3. Sit the patient upright, if possible, or raise the head of the bed for eating or drinking and leave it raised for up to an hour afterwards.

RE. Observe if effective swallowing occurs. Record occurrence of discomfort or pain and any particular food involved.

4. Keep suction equipment and a receiver in case of vomiting or choking. However, avoid having them within the patient's sight to reduce the suggestion that trouble is anticipated.

RE. Record the amount and type of vomitus if the patient vomits and the relation to meal time.

5. Provide carbonated (fizzy) drinks or water after a meal to cleanse oeso-hagus.

RE. Check for distension or abdominal discomfort from carbonated drinks. Record the patient's fluid intake.

6. Offer privacy for meals to reduce embarrassment caused by vomiting. Remain nearby to assist the patient if necessary.

RE. Observe for reduced tension at mealtimes. Record the amount of assist-ance required by the patient.

Further action

1. Oral drugs should be given as an elixir, syrup or suspension. Suggest that the patient sits upright to swallow and washes medicine down with at least half a glass of water.

RE. Observe for nausea or vomiting after medication.

2. Investigations of the cause of the difficulty may include a chest X-ray, barium swallow, oesophagoscopy or gastroscopy, ultrasound, radio-isotope scan or angiography.

RE. Check the patient understands what the doctor tells them about these investigations. Explain in simple terms if necessary.

Associated medical diagnoses

Aortic aneurysm
Carcinoma of oesophagus
Enlarged mediastinal lymph node
Goitre
Oesophageal stricture
Oesophagitis with hiatus hernia
Oesophageal pouch
Plummer-Vinson Syndrome (or Paterson-Brown-Kelly Syndrome)

Problem **Nausea and vomiting**

Assessment findings

Pale
Sweating
Increased salivation
Careful body movements
Nausea preceding vomiting or vomit regurgitated without effort
Vomit – amount, colour, type of odour, presence of recognisable food
        particles
      – presence of blood
      – presence of tablets
      – frequency
Abdominal discomfort or tenderness.
Retching (involuntary spasmodic muscular activity).
Nausea following food or drug ingestion.

Information for the patient

Vomiting happens when the vomiting centre in the brain is triggered from the stomach. Fright, unpleasant sights, smells or severe pain can also act as triggers. Being sick can be a safety measure for the body but if it goes on too long it upsets the body's salt and water balance. Noting the amount and frequency of vomiting can help the doctor to decide on the cause and the best treatment to try. A vomit bowl or receiver should be used so the nurses can measure how much is being brought up.

Once the sickness stops, fluids then food can be taken. Until that time nothing should be eaten or drunk.

Nursing actions

1. Nothing should be given by mouth until there has been no vomiting for 2 hours.

RE. Chart volume and type of vomitus each time it occus so that frequency and any change in content can be identified. Electrolyte replacement may be required for prolonged or severe vomiting. Exhaustion can occur due to the extra effort.

2. A clean receiver should be provided covered with a paper towel or cloth to reduce suggestion. Empty and rinse after each emesis. Odour and sight of vomitus may increase the vomiting. Stay with the patient during vomiting bouts. Taking deep breaths may help the patient's nausea.

RE. Record if taking deep breaths reduces nausea.

3. Clear liquids, warm or cool, should be offered, or carbonated (fizzy) drinks, e.g. soda water, or soda-water and milk in equal proportions.

RE. Chart fluid intake. No further vomiting and increasing hunger pangs indicate more solid food may be tried if not contra-indicated.

4. Dry cream crackers or plain biscuits can be given once nausea abates.

RE. No further vomiting and a returning appetite indicate other foods can be tried.

5. Mouthwashes of cold water or glycothymol after each bout of vomiting should be given to cleanse the mouth and remove the unpleasant taste.

RE. Check the taste of glycothymol does not increase the sense of nausea.

6. A change of the patient's position should be carried out slowly especially if the inner ear is affected.

RE. Observe for any relationship between movement and the onset of nausea or vomiting.

7. Discuss what is being done with the patient and check they understand the treatment planned. Worry and fear can increase gastric motility (remember pre-exam butterflies?)

RE. Observe for signs of anxiety. Ask the patient to repeat your explanation in his own words.

8. Report the presence of blood to the doctor. Haematemesis (vomiting blood) from a gastric ulcer may occur if a blood vessel breaks in the base of a gastric ulcer. Comfort the patient who will be distressed at the sight of blood.

RE. Check pulse rate and blood pressure at frequent intervals to estimate the effect of blood loss.

Further action	1. Anti-emetics reduce gastric motility and can depress the vomiting centre in the brain. Intramuscular or intravenous routes may be used if vomiting is present. Examples include metoclopramide, prochlorperazine, domperidone, chlorpromazine. Ask patient to remain supine for half an hour after the injection.

RE. Ask the patient if their symptoms are relieved or reduced. Compare the time of vomiting with the time the drug was given to identify how long the drug remains effective. Record frequency of bowel actions and compare with patient's usual pattern as constipation may occur.

2. Loss of the electrolytes sodium and potassium may be monitored by blood samples. Replacement is usually by intravenous infusion.

RE. In frequent vomiting there is a marked risk of hyponatremia (low sodium) and hypokalaemia (low potassium). See problems under these headings.

3. Investigations for the cause may include barium studies, gastroscopy, ultrasound, X-rays and brain scan.

RE. Check the patient understands what the doctor has said about these investigations. To reduce anxiety, ensure the patient takes a vomit bowl and tissues with them when visiting other departments.

4. Drug toxicity may occur in sensitive individuals or where excretion routes are diseased. Drug therapy should be reviewed for the possible cause. The blood level can be compared with the usual therapeutic level for some drugs.

RE. Digitalis and cytotoxic drugs require careful monitoring for side effects such as nausea. |
| **Associated medical diagnoses** | Carcinoma of stomach
Cholecystitis
Drug toxicity especially cytotoxic drugs and digitalis
Gallstones
Gastric ulcer
Gastroenteritis
Hepatitis
Hiatus hernia
Meningioma
Menière's disease
Myocardial infarction
Pancreatitis
Pyloric stenosis
Radiotherapy |

Problem	Pain after eating

Assessment findings	The time pain occurs in relation to food
Burning or ache
Site of pain — epigastric, or radiating towards the back
Relief of pain by food
Pain at night — duodenal ulcer
Steady body weight or weight loss
Vomiting frequency and presence of bile

Haematemesis
Melaena
Pain ½–1 hour after food – gastric ulcer
Pain 2–4 hours after food – duodenal ulcer
Smoking habits

Information for the patient

The inside of the stomach is lined with cells which produce acid to help digest food. Hormones stimulate the cells to do this, especially at mealtimes. Irritation of the stomach lining in gastritis or ulcer formation can produce pain. Not everyone who has pain has an ulcer, and not everyone who has an ulcer has pain.

The treatment is intended to lower the level of stimulation and allow the lining to heal. The diet may need to be adjusted. The milk and fish bland diet is considered old-fashioned and a much wider range of foods can be eaten. Rest and relaxation are still considered important. Meals should be regular, unhurried and chewed well. A rest or gentle activity after a meal is helpful. Antacids neutralize the stomach acids and need to be taken between meals to give extra protection to the lining.

Nursing actions

1. An antacid (usually magnesium trisilicate) can be given as required or as prescribed for epigastric pain. Aluminium hydroxide and calcium carbonate tend to cause constipation.

RE. Monitor pain frequently as the dose can be adjusted to control it. Review pain management at least once a day. Sudden intense abdominal pain with shock and a rigid abdomen indicate perforation of an ulcer and the need for immediate medical aid.

2. Discuss which, if any, foods precipitate or increase discomfort. Plan the diet to omit these, together with meat stock or beef extracts (Oxo is used in gastric research to stimulate gastric production of acid).

RE. Observe for signs of pain or discomfort after meals. As pain decreases with ulcer healing, broaden the range of foods offered.

3. Provide milk, preferably in a vacuum flask by the bed, at bedtime.

RE. Ask the patient how many times he needed to take the milk during the night. Nocturnal pain from a duodenal ulcer should decrease with healing.

4. Observe for signs of bleeding from an ulcer or gastritis. Ask the patient to report if faeces become darker or tarry.

RE. Bleeding from the base of an ulcer may be sudden and severe. Haematemesis or melaena may accompany the signs of shock, and will need immediate medical assistance.

5. Discuss with patient his normal use of alcohol and smoking, as these should be avoided if possible or taken only after a meal. Cigarette smoking in particular increases gastric motility and secretion. Plan a programme of education and support to reduce, and if possible, eliminate smoking. Incorporate any alternative support mechanisms the patient has found useful in times of stress. Enlist the help of relatives, visitors or other patients to provide alternative activities.

RE. Chart the number of cigarettes or cigars smoked each day. Ask the patient to explain in their own words the new knowledge about smoking and alcohol to assess recall and understanding.

6. Help the patient to learn to relax by identifying with them activities which produce or increase feelings of stress. Suggest that work is forgotten about for a while. Plan the resumption of work with increased meal breaks, periods of relaxation and delegation of activities so that the patient can readjust their lifestyle if necessary.

RE. Assess the patient's activities and their co-operation in trying to relax and plan.

Further action

1. Cimetidine at adequate blood levels inhibits the secretion of acid by the parietal cells when stimulated by histamine, gastrin or acetylcholine.

RE. Observe for side effects such as diarrhoea or gynaecomastia in men.

2. Haemoglobin levels may be estimated regularly, or if sudden, acute pain occurs.

RE. Normal level of haemoglobin is 11—15 g per 100 ml. Women of menstrual age may be at the lower end of the range.

3. If bleeding is suspected, a small sample of stool may be sent for occult blood level. A specimen from each of the next three stools may be requested. The rate of transfer of faeces along the colon varies among individuals, and it may take 48 hours or more for faeces containing the blood to leave the body.

RE. Inspect each stool for malaena (partly digested blood) which is dark in colour and sticky. Iron preparations give a dull black colour to the stool.

4. Investigations into the cause of the pain after eating include an abdominal X-ray, barium studies, gastroscopy and ultrasound.

RE. Check that the patient understands what the doctor has told them about the tests.

Associated medical diagnoses

Duodenal ulcer
Duodenitis
Extensive burns
Gastric ulcer
Hyperparathyroidism
Renal transplant
Rheumatoid arthritis
Zollinger-Ellison syndrome (gastrinoma)

Problem | **Feels full after small meals**

Assessment findings

Sensation of fullness
Distended abdomen — ascites, loaded colon
Belching
Post-gastrectomy
Body weight falling
Recent change to high fibre diet with extra pulses

Information for the patient

The stomach has waves of contraction passing along it to churn up the food and juices during digestion. When food first enters the stomach it relaxes and dilates to make more room. If it cannot expand properly because of pressure from the organs around it, or after surgery, then it feels full after only a small amount of food. Gas in the stomach, especially from fizzy drinks, or lower in the gut from peas or beans, causes pressure. Fatty foods stay inside the stomach longer than others before they are passed out through the sphincter valve into the gut for digestion. Liquids only spend a short while in the stomach. Altering the diet can help reduce the discomfort.

Nursing actions

1. A semi-solid or liquid diet with high Calorie content to low volume should be given if local obstruction is suspected. Meat is sometimes not tolerated. Avoid carbonated drinks as these increase distension, although small quantities may help the patient burp and release swallowed air.

RE. Weigh patient every 4 to 5 days at the same time of day, to assess Calorie and fluid intake are sufficient to maintain body weight. Take account of fluid loss from paracentesis or from passing of faeces.

2. Small meals should be given every 2 hours. Remind the patient to eat slowly and chew well. Clear fluids leave the stomach more rapidly than solid or fatty foods. Small quantities may reduce the feeling of fullness and make eating less tiring.

RE. Record the amount left to identify likely deficiencies in nutrition.

3. Peppermint water, tea or peppermints can be offered after meals to relieve flatulence.

RE. Ask the patient whether discomfort decreases within 30 minutes.

4. Deep breathing exercises before meals should be encouraged to maintain aeration of lower lobes of lungs. Shallow breathing is more comfortable when the abdomen feels full or distended, and atelectasis or chest infection may occur.

RE. Supervise exercises until the patient demonstrates that they can perform them effectively. Check oral temperature and pulse twice daily for indications of infection.

5. Observe for signs of dumping in post-gastrectomy patients. Nausea, crampy abdominal pains, dizziness, muscular weakness, sweating, palpitations, fainting or diarrhoea may occur during or after a meal. Refined carbohydrates such as sugar, salty foods or a large meal are usually involved.

RE. If symptoms do occur adjust the diet and provide smaller dry meals with fluids between meals to slow gastric emptying. Reduce refined carbohydrate content. Suggest the patient eats slowly and rests for half an hour afterwards. Artificial sweeteners may be used to replace sugar.

Further action

1. Investigations of the cause include abdominal ultrasound, barium studies and gastroscopy.

RE. Check the patient understands what the doctor has said about any tests proposed.

2. Tip the head of the bed by 30–45° if a hiatus hernia is present. Advise the patient not to bend over to reach things but to bend the knees, keeping the back straight.

RE. Ask the patient to demonstrate the correct technique for picking up low items.

77

3. If the patient has marked ascites, paracentesis may be needed to relieve the pressure on the diaphragm and abdominal discomfort. A rigid catheter is inserted through a small incision in the abdominal wall under a local anaesthetic. The fluid is drained through sterile tubing into a bag, the rate of flow being controlled by a gate clip to no more than 100 ml an hour. Ascitic fluid may be sent for cytology or culture.

RE. Record the volume of fluid drained each hour and the total each 24 hours. Record oral temperature, pulse, respiration and blood pressure to monitor how patient adapts to changes in pressure and fluid compartments. The risk of peritonitis increases with the frequency of paracentesis and the length of time the cannula is in place.

4. Regular laxatives or enemas may be required to relieve constipation and re-establish normal bowel activity.

RE. Record frequency, consistency and amount of stool for comparison with normal bowel activity.

Associated medical diagnoses	Ascites Carcinoma of stomach Cholelithiasis Hepatomegaly Hiatus hernia Post-gastrectomy Pregnancy — during third trimester Severe constipation Splenomagaly

---

Problem	**Obese due to overeating**

Assessment findings	Body weight 20% in excess of that recommended for height (Table 3.2) Single skin fold thickness of more than 1 inch. Dyspnoea on exertion Excessive food intake High carbohydrate intake Abnormal eating pattern Eating snacks or sweets between meals
Information for the patient	Obesity carries an increased risk of ill-health, especially if other members of the family have diabetes, high blood pressure (hypertension) or ischaemic heart disease. People in their twenties who are already fat run a particular risk of illness. Fat is stored in the body when more energy is taken in than is burnt up during metabolism. Food is used to keep the body warm, provide energy for movement, for healing of tissues and for growth. Hormones can affect the rate at which energy is used. Smoking cigarettes also increases the rate, and can also blunt the taste of food, so smokers tend to weigh less than non-smokers taking in the same energy. The proportion of fat in the body increases with age. Reducing diets should be adjusted to ensure that fewer Calories are taken in than the body requires. Then the fat in the body is converted to energy to make up the amount. A slow steady rate of weight loss is safer than a drastic diet. A change in eating habits is given the chance to develop, so that the excess weight stays off!

Nursing actions

1. Discuss with the patient their Calorie requirements and eating pattern. A diary of time of eating, and the type and amount of food taken could be kept by a patient well enough to do so. The doctor and dietitian will advise on the appropriate Calorie intake for the individual. Pace the discussion according to the patient's level of interest and apparent understanding.

RE. During discussions assess how much the patient remembers and accepts. Some people seem to resist all attempts to help them face the fact that excessive Calorie intake over output leads to fat storage. Food can be used to replace love — 'eating for comfort'.

2. Reduce Calorie intake to 1000–1500 Calories (4.2–6.3 MJ) per day. A reducing diet should encourage healthy eating habits. High fibre foods increase the feeling of satiety. Fat, fried foods and sugar should be kept to a small proportion of the diet.

RE. Observe how much of the meal gets eaten, check for eating between meals and increased consumption of 'diabetic' sweets and drinks.

3. Weigh the patient at the same time once a week, preferably before breakfast and with bladder empty.

RE. An initial phase of weight loss should be followed by a steady loss of 0.5 – 1 kg (1–2 lb) per week.

4. Provide high fibre foods and increase intake of water to reduce risk of constipation. Note patient's normal elimination pattern.

RE. Monitor frequency and consistency of stools for decreased frequency of dryer, hard faeces.

5. Discuss whether the patient uses food as a comforter. Some people eat when bored, upset or angry. Plan for non-edible rewards as substitutes. Suggest the patient talk about their feelings when tempted to break the diet.

6. Substitute raw vegetables or fruit high in fibre in place of sweets.

RE. Check how well the patient complies with these substitutions.

7. Help the patient stop smoking as it carries a greater risk than obesity.

RE. Check use of food to substitute for smoking. Note number of cigarettes smoked each day.

Further action

1. Severe reducing diets of under 1000 Calories per day should be undertaken with extreme caution, as deaths have occurred in some circumstances. Liquid protein diets may occasionally induce cardiac arrythmia.

It is difficult to teach sensible eating habits during this type of diet, and it needs to be planned together with supervision of meal choice, once the severe diet is stopped.

RE. Record the patient's pulse rate and rhythm at least 6 hourly. Monitor meal plans once the teaching phase starts.

2. Anorectic drugs include amphetamines which stimulate the sympathetic system, and may also cause insomnia. The feeling of wellbeing which they create can help a patient persevere with an unwelcome dietary regime. However they may produce tolerance and dependence, and because of the risks involved are only used in extreme cases.

RE. Record how much the patient sleeps each night. Monitor level of mental and physical activity. Monoamine oxidase inhibitors should not be given if amphetamines are in use or if there is history of migraine. If there is a history of migraine any headache should be reported to the doctor.

3. Bulk producing products such as methylcellulose provide a feeling of fullness but are not digested. The recommended volume of fluid should be taken with each dose so that the optimum bulk is produced before the meal is eaten.

RE. These products should be given at least 30 minutes before the mealtime. Bowel action may be more frequent than normal as the undigested bulk stimulates the colon. NB: Bulk producing products are sometimes used to treat constipation.

4. In severe obesity the opinion of a gastroenterologist may be sought on the advisability of jejunal bypass. Dental advice on limiting eating by splinting the jaws together may be sought as an alternative.

RE. The patient's co-operation and consent are essential if either of these methods is to be effective in the long term. If the patient expressed doubt or misunderstanding this should be reported to the doctor.

Associated medical diagnoses	Diabetes mellitus
	Hypertension
	Hypothyroidism
	Hypopituitarism
	Myocardial infarction
	Rheumatoid arthritis

Problem   **Lacks knowledge about what constitutes a healthy diet**

Assessment findings

Diary of day's usual food intake records mainly 'junk foods' (e.g. crisps, cola drinks, chips, chocolates)
Refuses a wide range of foods
Adheres to diet possibly deficient in proteins, vitamins, calcium or iron
Educational attainment – type of school
Patient's assessment of own learning ability
Unable to describe why the body needs a balanced diet

Information for the patient

The human body needs different types of food to keep it working properly. Different foods give mixtures of the important nutrients, carbohydrates such as starch, fats, proteins, vitamins, other minerals and trace elements and roughage or fibre. Clear healthy skin, shiny healthy hair and a good body shape can be helped by eating a healthy diet.

To help in learning about what it is best to eat, the information is planned into small steps; once one step is learnt, the next can begin, and plans made to try different foods and select a healthy diet. There are are leaflets to take home as reminders.

Nursing actions

1. Use the knowledge of the patient's educational attainment and learning ability to plan a step by step programme with the patient to explain how the body used:
– carbohydrates – for energy, storing temporary excess in the liver and long term excess as fat.

- fats for energy, storing excess in the fatty tissues.
- proteins – for rebuilding cells, excess excreted in the urine
- iron – for red blood cells, to carry oxygen
- vitamins – for healthy cells, excess excreted in urine or faeces, except for vitamins A and D which are stored.
- calcium – for bones, excess excreted in urine
- roughage – indigestible fibre in the gut, helps the stomach feel full after a meal, helps prevent constipation.

RE. When the patient's attention slackens, stop. Before starting on the next step ask the patient to explain what was discussed in the previous session. Revise what was forgotten, then move on to the next step.

2. Describe the four main food groups and the number of portions needed each day for a normal adult. Ask the patient to sort out which group, if any, their favourite foods fit into.

RE. Assess how much the patient has understood by their decisions about their favourite foods. Explain what was incorrect. Record how much has been learnt.

3. Ask the patient to list all the activities usually undertaken on a normal working day and on a day off. Discuss the typical energy requirement and which foods, if any, should be added to the normal adult diet.

RE. Assess whether current intake matches energy expenditure. Discuss and plan any necessary adjustment.

4. Tell the patient what is on the menu for the day. Ask the patient to plan the day's meals. If possible let the patient serve up the food. Fit some snack food into plan. Discuss any unsuitable choice. Praise good plans and selections.

RE. Assess how well patient can use information from previous sessions. Plan to recap items forgotten or misunderstood.

5. Introduce different foods slowly. Explain what food groups they belong to. Praise patient for tasting and eating them.

RE. Observe how willing patient is to try new foods. Record those which have been found acceptable. Include new foods in weekly menus.

Further advice

1. Supervision by a dietitian may be needed if the diet is markedly deficient in one or more components.

RE. Strongly held beliefs may not be changed by advice. Observe for compliance at meal times.

2. Iron and/or vitamin supplements may be given. Iron absorption is promoted by fruit, vegetables and vitamin C in the diet.

RE. Warn the patient that iron will make the stools black in colour.

Associated medical diagnoses

Iron deficiency anaemia
Obesity
Scurvy

Problem	Lacks understanding of therapeutic diet

| Assessment findings | Eats food prohibited in diet
Asks visitors to bring in prohibited foods
Uses prohibited condiments (salt, pepper, etc)
Calorie intake exceeds prescribed amount
Unable to explain rationale for prohibition of specific foods |

Information for the patient

The healthy body can balance the amount of the food absorbed that it requires to repair cells and provide energy. If disease alters its ability to do this then the balancing must be thought out and done before eating. Special diets do this and if they are not followed very carefully there is a risk of damaging the tissues. It is easy to believe that cheating on a special diet will not matter because the damage to the tissue may build up slowly. By the time the damage is noticed it is usually too late to do anything more than slow the rate of further damage.

Nursing actions

1. Ask the patient to record what is eaten each day. Observe and record what the patient eats. Compare the two records with the diet prescribed, and involve the patient in the discussion. Identify the discrepancies.

RE. Monitor how keen the patient is to co-operate. Some patients may not be able to write. If the patient fails to keep a record offer to do the writing but ensure the patient describes each meal.

2. Discuss with the patient whether they find it easiest to learn using diagrams, pictures, repetition or making notes. Identify the learning pattern the patient feels will best suit him.

RE. Assess how the patient has learnt other things and whether this relates to their choice of learning pattern.

3. Plan the teaching sessions to suit patient's learning pattern, the time available and the information the patient *must* learn to be able to control the food intake within the prescribed diet. Ask them about the information learnt at the start of each session.

RE. Assess what new information has been absorbed, adjust the planned pace in the light of achievements.

4. Check the patient's choice of food at mealtimes. Ask the patient to explain the reasons behind their choice. Do this at a time and in a place which will not embarrass the patient.

RE. Note any discrepancies between what the patient can describe and the actual choice of food. Praise suitable choices for the contribution they make to the patient's recovery and health.

Further action

1. Supervision by the dietitian may be required by the patient as an outpatient after discharge from hospital.

RE. If the patient does not accept and follow the advice given, they cannot be made to do so. Eating the prescribed diet in hospital indicates a positive approach, but enthusiasm may wane without regular reinforcement.

2. Relatives, or those who share the patient's home, may need and appreciate a discussion with the doctor and dietitian to understand the reasons for adhering to the therapeutic diet.

RE. Discuss with the patient and relatives where special foods or cookery books can be obtained locally.

Associated medical diagnoses	Arteriosclerosis Cirrhosis Congestive cardiac failure Diabetes mellitus Gout Hypertension Myocardial infarction Renal failure

---

Problem	**Impaired sense of taste**

Assessment findings	All food tastes the same History of head injury involving front of face Poor appetite Low body weight Uses salt or other seasonings heavily Unable to recognise bitter, sour, sweet and salty solutions dropped onto tongue Difficulty in smiling or frowning Tongue or oral mucosa inflamed Runny or blocked nose Decreased perception of odours Heavy use of tobacco
Information for the patient	Food is tasted in two ways. The tongue has tiny taste buds on its surface arranged in groups. These pick out bitter, sour, sweet and salty foods. At the back of the nose are lots of tiny cells with hairs on their surface. The tiny molecules of odour dissolve in the moisture around the hairs. If they fit the surface shape then a nerve cell is triggered and a message goes to the brain. These nerves run through a tiny plate filled with holes like a colander. If the hairs get clogged up with mucus, for instance from a cold, then the odour molecules can't get through. A head injury which affects the base of the skull can tear the nerves where they pass through the tiny plate (cribiform plate) (Fig. 3.8). If that happens it is unlikely that the person's sense of smell will return. Smell and the specific taste of food are linked, so taste is also lost. To make up for the reduced sense of taste other senses need extra stimulation. Temperature, strong flavours and the look of a meal need extra attention.
Nursing actions	1. Increase the amount of flavour-intensified foods offered to the patient. Monosodium glutamate can be used for most people, but as it is a salt it should not be used in sodium-restricted diets, or if there is a sensitivity to it. It can be bought in jars as 'seasoning salt' and sprinkled over savoury dishes. RE. Observe if food enjoyment or intake increases. 2. Increase the use of seasonings and herbs. Alter the proportions of bitter, sour, sweet and salty dishes to provide variety. Vary the textures.

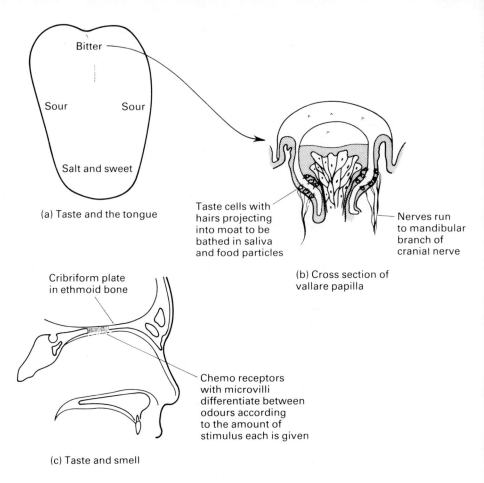

Bitter

Sour   Sour

Salt and sweet

(a) Taste and the tongue

Taste cells with
hairs projecting
into moat to be
bathed in saliva
and food particles

Nerves run
to mandibular
branch of
cranial nerve

(b) Cross section of
vallare papilla

Cribriform plate
in ethmoid bone

Chemo receptors
with microvilli
differentiate between
odours according
to the amount of
stimulus each is given

(c) Taste and smell

Fig. 3.8   The link between the senses of taste and smell

RE. Ask the patient if they find the food tastes better. Check with the doctor at what level the increased use of salt or acid foods would affect the patient's electroyte balance, and adjust diet accordingly.

3. Ensure hot foods are hot, and cold foods cold to accentuate temperature stimulation. Provide hot and cold courses for contrast.

RE. Observe if food enjoyment or intake increases. Note how much of a meal the patient eats. Weigh them at least once a week to check that their food intake is sufficient to maintain a stable body weight.

4. Set out meals attractively and colourfully using extra garnishes such as parsley on savoury foods, and glacé cherries on sweet. Vision plays an important part in the enjoyment of food.

RE. Observe if the patient starts to look forward to mealtimes.

5. Advise the patient to reduce the use of tobacco if they are a smoker. If the patient agrees, plan a step by step programme to replace its use with other pleasurable, distracting activities. Give positive reinforcement when the patient goes without a cigarette/cigar/pipe.

RE. Ask if the food tastes better. Check how many cigarettes/cigars/pipes are smoked each day.

Further action	1. If loss of taste is due to 7th cranial nerve damage a quiet room may be necessary for eating as the patient may be sensitive to noise.
	RE. Check which noises cause the patient distress so that the appropriate action can be taken to reduce or eliminate them.
	2. If an infection is suspected, a mouth and throat swab for culture and sensitivity should be taken between meal times.
Associated medical diagnoses	Allergic rhinitis Basal skull fracture Bell's Palsy Brain or nerve damage — such as facial, glossopharyngeal, or vagus nerve Fracture of cribiform plate Temporal lobe lesion

---

Problem	**Unable to tolerate fatty foods**

Assessment findings	Anorexia Nausea Pale, foul-smelling stools Flatulence Jaundice Abdominal pain Tendency to bruise easily Spontaneous bleeding Rising urobilinogen levels Dislike of fatty foods
Information for the patient	The liver produces bile which is needed to digest fats. If the flow of bile is blocked, or the liver cells no longer make enough, then the undigested fats make the stools smell foul; they are also pale because of the absence of bile pigments. The intestines may also be irritated so that 'wind' (flatulence) occurs. If the liver cannot cope with fats then it must rely first on its store of sugar and then on the body cells for proteins. It is far better to avoid having to use the internal supplies of body tissue for energy by trying to provide a steady flow of foods the body can digest, by eating little and often.
Nursing actions	1. Small, frequent, low fat, high carbohydrate and protein meals should be given, served attractively on small plates. The dietitian will advise on the provision of skimmed milk and fats.
	RE. Record how much the patient is eating so that the Calorie intake can be maintained at above 2000 Calories, unless the patient is obese when 1000 to 1500 Calories should be sufficient. Observe for apathy and forgetfulness which may reduce the amount eaten. Record body weight at least twice a week.
	2. High Calorie powders which dissolve easily in water may be prescribed. Vary the flavours to give variety, diluted to taste with water. No alcohol should be taken. A fluid intake of at least 2 litres per day should be maintained, in small frequent amounts to prevent nausea.
	RE. Record the patient's fluid intake and output. Add the Calorie content to the day's total Calorie intake.

3. Provide private lavatory facilities if possible. A sanichair visit to the lavatory is preferable to a commode by the bed. 'Fresh air' sprays and other deodorisers may be necessary. Ask the patient to report the stool colour.

RE. Observe for embarrassment when bowels have moved. Check toilet area is adequately ventilated.

4. Advise the male patient to use an electric razor and a soft toothbrush to reduce the risk of damage and bleeding. Avoid giving injections if possible.

RE. Observe for signs of bruising or bleeding into the skin (purpura or small purple spots). Record the site and extent if they occur so any increase can be recognised.

Further action

1. Intramuscular or intravenous injections of vitamin K may be prescribed if blood clotting times are abnormal due to liver disorder. Apply firm pressure over the puncture site for at least 3 minutes after injection to reduce risk of bruising.

RE. Bruising from intramuscular injections may interfere with the patient's mobility and increase the risk of skin damage. Record site and size of any new bruises.

2. Fat soluble vitamins A, D, E and K may need to be given by injection if fat intolerance is marked and prolonged. Impaired fat absorption can be worsened if mineral oil (liquid paraffin) is taken regularly as a laxative.

RE. Check patient is not continuing the habit of taking mineral oil.

3. Cholestyramine powder may be mixed with fruit juice or sprinkled on food to reduce the absorption of bile salts and prevent itching. It can decrease the absorption of other drugs and these should be given at least one hour before or after the meal.

RE. Monitor how much food the patient eats. The powder may blunt an already small appetite. Ask the patient to report nausea, heartburn or a rash.

Associated medical diagnoses

Alcoholic cirrhosis
Biliary colic
Carcinoma of head of pancreas
Carcinoma of the liver
Cholecystitis
Cholelithiasis
Cirrhosis
Hepatocellular jaundice
Infectious hepatitis
Obstructive jaundice
Serum hepatitis
Viral hepatitis – infectious hepatitis

Problem

Unable to maintain blood sugar within normal limits

Assessment findings

Age
Blood sugar
Glucose present in urine
Ketone bodies present in urine

Thirst
Recent weight loss in young people
Obesity in middle aged or elderly
Fungal infections of skin or vulva
Parenteral nutrition
Receiving steroid therapy
Receiving total parenteral nutrition
Intravenous dextrose or dextrose/saline
Low blood sugar — under 3 mmol/litre

Information for the patient

A large gland called the pancreas lies below the stomach. It releases the hormone insulin into the bloodstream. This helps the body cells to take up sugar or glucose from the blood to provide energy. Together with another hormone from the pancreas called glucagon it helps to regulate the level of sugars in the blood. If something goes wrong and the blood sugar rises then glucose may cross into the urine. The levels rise and fall after meals especially if a lot of carbohydrate is eaten. If the blood sugar falls to a low level or the cells cannot take in sugar because the insulin is missing, then the body tries to provide energy by using body fat. The waste products from this use of fats are called ketones and they can start to poison the body.

The level of the blood sugar must be balanced so that there is always enough for the cells to use, but not so much that the body tissues are damaged. If the pancreas is still making some insulin it may be possible to take tablets to slow the normal rate of insulin breakdown, stimulate the production of insulin and help the sugar to enter the cells. Then the diet can be adjusted to provide as much unrefined carbohydrate as is necessary to provide the sugars to balance the available insulin. Some people can manage by carefully controlling their diet; others need both a diet and tablets or insulin.

Insulin can be given by injection if the pancreas is not capable of producing any. As it is a protein, it would be digested if it were taken by mouth. Various chemicals can be added to allow for different rates of absorption of injected insulin.

The body cells require different amounts of energy according to how much work they do. Run for a bus and the energy need goes up. If insulin has to be given by injection it also becomes important to balance sugar and insulin to the energy required. Sport, illness and pregnancy, all influence energy and so affect insulin requirements. Too little sugar available leads to headache, dizziness and if these are ignored, to loss of consciousness.

Treatment must be planned to fit each person's particular life style and it will need adjustment with later changes. It takes a while to get the balance exactly right.

Nursing actions

1. When explaining their condition to the patient assess how much information they are able to understand and remember. Explain in simple terms each step of the proposed treatment.

RE. Observe whether the patient takes an interest in learning about their condition, and whether they ask questions. Note how long they are able to concentrate without tiring.

2. Discuss which method of learning the patient finds easiest to understand; diagrams, discussion, drawing, games or models. Schooling history may help identify learning abilities. Plan teaching to help the patient establish the link between what is eaten and the blood sugar.

RE. Assess how much the patient is learning and adjust the pace accordingly. Observe what they eat and drink. Any cheating on the prescribed diet indicates that they have not accepted the link between food and blood sugar. It may then be helpful to use blood sugar estimations before and after a meal to demonstrate the link.

3. Test the urine 15 to 30 minutes before meals. Ask the patient to also empty their bladder 15–30 minutes before the required urine sample time, so that when the collected urine is tested it is freshly made by the kidneys, rather than a mixture of old and new. Use the test strips for ketones and a clinitest tablet for glucose.

RE. Record the result of urinalysis on a urinalysis chart. The level of glucose should decrease as the treatment takes effect. The presence of ketones indicates insufficient sugar is being made available to the cells.

4. Explain the urinalysis result to the patient and when they are fit enough to do so teach the patient how to test their own urine and record the result.

RE. Assess the level of interest shown. Double check the urine result when the patient undertakes the urinalysis, until the patient and nurses agree the patient can take responsibility for this.

5. Discuss with the patient their normal pattern of activities. Plan out with the patient an increase in physical activities, so that the balance between food intake with insulin/drugs and the energy requirement is attained before discharge.

RE. Observe and record the increase in activity and look for any signs of hypoglycaemia — sweating, trembling, hunger, weakness, fast pulse, palpitations and a sense of fear. More severe symptoms include faintness, giddiness, blurred or double vision, confusion and loss of co-ordination, with eventual loss of consciousness. Sometimes the confusion can lead to aggression. Hypoglycaemia can occur:
After soluble insulin — after 2 to 6 hours
Intermediate delay insulin in the morning — symptoms in the afternoon/evening
Slow-acting-insulin — overnight or early morning.

Further action

1. Estimate blood glucose level using finger prick method and a reagent strip at intervals. Use a large drop of blood, time accurately and follow instructions exactly for reliable readings.

RE. Record exact time of sample and time of food intake. Readings should remain between 7 and 10 mmol. Results outside that range should be reported to the doctor unless other instructions are given.

2. Hypoglycaemia (low blood sugar) may be treated by 15 g glucose/sugar in fruit juice or a tablespoonful of honey if the patient can swallow. Intravenous injection of 50 ml 50% dextrose may be needed if blood sugar falls to under 2 mmol. Unstable blood sugar levels may require intravenous therapy to allow easy, frequent re-adjustment of Calorie intake.

RE. Symptoms such as sweating, rapid pulse, faintness or blurred vision should subside within 10 minutes of oral glucose/sugar. Record the symptoms of a newly diagnosed diabetic, as each person usually has a personal pattern and the earliest warning symptoms need to be learnt. Protein, such as a glass of milk or piece of cheese, may be given after a mild reaction to help stabilize blood sugar. Blood glucose levels should be monitored.

3. Hyperglycaemia (high blood sugar) may occur in insulin dependent diabetics, or those receiving parenteral nutrition. If the insulin level is not sufficient for cells to use glucose, then fat is broken down and ketone bodies are produced. Acidosis develops, and urine output increases leading to dehydration and electrolyte imbalance. Test the urine for ketones. Blood samples are taken for electrolyte estimation and pH. Intravenous fluids and insulin will be prescribed according to the results.

RE. Monitor fluid intake and output to identify reduced urine output as ketosis decreases. Measure glycosuria and ketone level in urine at least four hourly. Assess skin turgor for change in hydration. Record patient's pulse and blood pressure quarter-hourly during crisis period, reducing frequency as electrolyte results return to within normal limits. Falling blood pressure may indicate loss of consciousness is near.

4. A glucose tolerance test may be undertaken to asses the ability to stabilize the blood sugar level after a known glucose load. The patient should not eat and should only drink water for six hours before the test, resting on the bed during it. A urine sample is collected together with blood for the fasting blood levels. A glucose load of 50 g dissolved in 200 ml of water is then given as a drink. Blood and urine samples are collected every half hour for two hours. The patient can then eat and drink normally.

RE. In normal people the highest reading should be within the normal range of $2.8 - 8.9$ mmol per litre, occurring within the first hour, and the level should then fall. In diabetics the level rises above the normal range and remains raised. Such a patient may feel thirsty during or at the end of the test.

Associated medical diagnoses	Acromegaly
	Cushing's syndrome
	Diabetes mellitus
	Gastrectomy
	Hyperinsulinism
	Nephritis
	Pancreatitis
	Thyroxicosis

Problem	**Protein intake inadequate for current needs**

Assessment findings	Fever
	Infection
	Increased metabolic rate
	Large area of skin loss
	Shiny legs — early oedema
	Skin wrinkled
	Body fat present
	Dermatitis
	Tissue destruction
	Neoplasm
	Muscle wasting
	Proteins in urine
	Ketones in urine

Weight loss
Wound healing slow
Low serum protein
Low lymphocyte count
Prone to chest infection/poor lung ventilation when intercostal muscles are wasted
Damage to gut mucosa due to toxogenic candida and bacterial species
Diarrhoea

Information for the patient

Proteins make up about 20 per cent of the body weight, they are found in all tissues, antibodies and blood clots (fibrin), they act as carriers for drugs and other materials and they can influence swelling and healing of wounds. Illness can lead to either too little protein being eaten and absorbed by the body, or to an increased rate of protein loss. It is very important that each day's intake of protein meets the body's needs as extra protein from one day cannot be stored for future use. If the body runs short of protein for the day's needs then more body cells are broken down to release it. The body still needs carbohydrates such as starch to help it make the best use of the protein. Adequate protein intake can be achieved by adjusting the diet. Sometimes the body needs more protein than can be taken orally, and when this occurs other ways to increase the intake will be prescribed by the doctor.

Nursing actions

1. Record the food actually eaten by the patient so that the protein intake can be estimated. Include foods supplied by visitors and relatives. Discuss the minimum desirable intake with the doctor and the dietitian.

RE. Compare actual intake with desirable intake to identify any shortfall.

2. Discuss which high protein foods the patient likes and plan how to include these in the day's menu. Meat, fish, cheese, eggs and milk can be increased in proportion to the other components. Add high protein powder to some foods such as puddings (Casilan).

RE. Check the high protein foods are eaten first and that the patient does not get full on carbohydrate first. Both protein and carbohydrate are needed for the most effective use of protein. Calculate daily protein intake. Monitor appetite, when anabolism occurs the appetite returns before the muscle bulk increases.
Review protein requirement every 4 to 5 days to ensure that intake and loss are balanced. Increase intake to help the body replace tissue loss once the patient is able to eat and absorb more than a maintenance protein intake. Test urine daily for ketones. Weigh on alternate days. Monitor serum protein levels. Record regression of symptoms every 3 days.

3. Substitute high protein drinks for some of the patient's fluid intake, e.g. egg flip, skim milk powder drinks, milk shakes, Ovaltine.

RE. Record the volume and type of fluid to include in the calculation of protein intake.

4. Assess whether the patient tires easily when eating. Consider including easily eaten foods which do not need a lot of chewing. Energy can be conserved by feeding the patient if necessary.

RE. Review meal times and eating aids to identify possible reasons for low food intake related to the patient's ability to feed himself.

Further action

1. A 24 hour urine collection can be carried out for urea estimation to indicate the number of grams of nitrogen being excreted

RE. Typical values —

		urea		nitrogen
Starving	=	108–114 mmol	=	3–4 g per day
Normal	=	324–360 mmol	=	9–10 g
Post-gastrectomy	=	540–576 mmol	=	15–16 g
Major trauma	=	1080+ mmol	=	30+ g

1 gram of nitrogen equates with 30 grams of muscle mass lost.

2. Enteral feeding, via a fine bore tube passed through the naso-pharynx and down into the duodenum, may be used when intestinal absorption is normal. The site should be checked by an X-ray. Air can be insufflated to confirm the tube's position. Slow continuous feeding is preferred to reduce the risk of diarrhoea, and a volumetric pump may be used to control the rate of flow. Mark the site where the tube enters the nostril. Store opened containers of feed in a refrigerator until half an hour before use, then remove so that it slowly reaches room temperature. Check from the mark on the tube that its position remains unchanged.

RE. Fluid intake and output should be monitored. Record the frequency and consistency of bowel actions. Diarrhoea may be due to concurrent antibiotic therapy, infected foods, malabsorption or, rarely, to lactose intolerance.

3. Parenteral feeding involves hypertonic (concentrated) nutrients which irritate small veins. The intravenous cannula is therefore inserted with its tip in a wide central vein so that the blood flow dilutes the solution. The subclavian route to the superior vena cava is popular. Insertion is carried out with strict asepsis as infection is a major risk. X-ray confirmation of the position is usual. The patient's giving set is changed each day. Attach a note to the prescription chart indicating that no drugs are to be given via the line.

RE. Mark the insertion point on the catheter. Check there is no strain or kinking of the catheter and that it is covered by a clean dressing. Observe for leakage from the hub as cracking can occur. Monitor the patient's vital signs for infection — a rigor may indicate septicaemia. Pain, difficulty breathing, and cyanosis indicate a pneumothorax, which requires immediate medical aid.

4. The prescription of fluid volume, electrolytes, vitamins, fats and minerals will vary according to the patient's condition. A volumetric infusion pump should be used to control the rate of flow to reduce the risk of air entry into the giving set. The more viscous the solution, the smaller the drop size.

RE. Weigh the patient at the same time each day in the same clothes. Fluid intake and output should be strictly monitored. Test urine for glucose at least daily, or six hourly in severely ill patients. If over ½% of glucose is found, check regulation of the infusion in case a bolus of feed is given which would be high in glucose and lead to a temporary high blood glucose with renal overspill. Serum electrolytes should be checked at least daily by the doctor.

Associated medical diagnoses

Chromium deficiency
Crohn's disease
Cirrhosis
Gastric carcinoma
Decubitus ulcers
Hepatitis
Phosphorus deficiency
Potassium deficiency
Ulcerative colitis
Uraemia
Zinc deficiency (acrodermatitis enteropathica)

Potential problems

Potential problem	Risk of malnutrition (protein and energy intake insufficient for current needs)

Assessment findings

Refuses to eat
Anorexia
Prolonged vomiting
Severe diarrhoea
Intravenous therapy provides little or no protein
Fluid diet of milk, jelly, juices and soups is taken
Prolonged excessive alcohol intake
Self neglect
Low resistance to infection
Loss of body fat
Weight loss
Lowered basal metabolic rate
Ketones in urine
Lowered resistance to chest infection
Wasting of intercostal muscles
Low blood sugar
Lethargy
Fatigue

Information for the patient

The body requires protein to build new cells, and it is not capable of storing extra protein. If the day's protein intake is not enough to meet the body's needs, then cells are broken down to release it. Energy from carbohydrates is also necessary. Excess carbohydrates can be stored as fat, but if this needs to be used in large amounts, byproducts are produced which can act like a poison to the body. These show up in urine tests. Sometimes the body's need for protein and energy is increased by illness. To prevent weight loss and the increased risk of infection, it is important that the body's dietary needs are met.

Nursing actions

1. Weigh the patient daily at the same time of day and in the same clothing. Test urine for ketones.

RE. Monitor for weight loss. If weight begins to fall and ketones are detected, food intake is insufficient for needs.

2. Record the amount of food being taken each day. The dietitian may be willing to help calculate the daily Calorie intake. Observe for possible eating problems.

RE. Identify preferred foods and record calorie intake (see Table 3.6 for selected food values).

3. Assess the daily energy requirement for the current activities of the patient. (See Table 3.5 for sex, age and activity levels).

RE. Estimate energy requirement and compare with intake. Consider any likely cause of shortfall (See Table 3.6 for selected food values).

4. Increase the patient's Calorie intake when indicated by providing supplements containing Caloreen (glucose polymer – 400 Kcal in 100 g), sandwiches between meals, fats such as butter, bananas and cream, chocolate, glucose-

Table 3.5 Energy and protein requirements during illness. (From Buss and Robertson, 1981. By permission of the Controller of HMSO.)

| | Energy | | |
Adult activity levels *	Kilocalories (Kcal)	Megajoules (MJ)	Protein g
Male			
13–34 Low	2510	10.5	62
Moderate	2900	12.0	72
High	3350	14.0	84
35–64 Low	2400	10.0	60
Moderate	2750	11.5	69
High	3350	14.0	84
65–74	2400	10.0	60
75+	2150	9.0	54
Female			
18–54 Moderate	2150	9.0	54
High	2500	10.5	62
55–74	1900	8.0	47
75+	1680	7.0	42

Examples of energy requirements during illness

Low level of activity	— spends most of the day sitting or walking around the room — no fever or infection
Moderate level of activity	— restless, walking about, climbing stairs, resting only 8 hours — fever, some infection, tumour
High level of activity	— hyperactive, getting little rest in 24 hours — high fever, severe infection

Table 3.6 Selected foods for energy and protein intake calculations. (From Buss and Robertson, 1981. By permission of the Controller of HMSO.)

Portion of 100 g	Kilocalories (Kcal)	Kilojoules (kJ)	Protein (g)
Whole milk	447	1841	3.3
Dried, skimmed milk	355	1821	36.4
Yoghurt: natural (low fat)	52	216	5.0
Yoghurt: fruit (low fat)	95	405	4.8
Cheddar cheese	406	1682	26.0
Bacon — cooked rashers	447	1851	24.5
Beef — corner	217	905	26.9
Beef — stewing steak	223	932	30.9
Chicken — roast	142	599	26.5
Ham — cooked	269	1119	24.7
Lamb — roast	291	1209	23.0
Liver — fried	243	1016	24.9
Pork chop	332	1380	28.5
Sausage, pork	367	1520	10.6
Sausage, beef	299	1242	9.6
Steak and kidney pie	286	1195	15.2

Table 3.6 (cont'd.) _Portion of 100 g_	_Kilocalories_ _(kcal)_	_Kilojoules_ _(kJ)_	_Protein_ _(g)_
White fish — filleted	76	322	17.4
Cod fried in batter	199	834	19.6
Fish fingers	178	749	12.6
Herring	234	970	16.8
Kipper fillets	184	770	19.8
Eggs	147	612	12.3
Butter	740	3041	0.4
Margarine	730	3000	0.1
Milk chocolate	529	2214	8.4
Honey	288	1229	0.4
Jam	262	1116	0.5
Marmalade	261	1114	0.1
White sugar	394	1680	0
Beans — canned in tomato sauce	64	270	5.1
Beans — broad	69	293	7.2
— runner	24	102	2.3
Brussels sprouts	18	75	2.8
Cabbage, green	15	66	1.7
Carrots, old raw	23	98	0.7
Cauliflower	13	56	1.9
Crisps, potato	533	2224	6.3
Lettuce	9	36	1.0
Parsnips	49	210	1.7
Peas, frozen, boiled	38	161	5.4
Potatoes, boiled	79	339	1.4
Potatoes, chipped	253	1065	3.8
Potatoes, roast	157	662	2.8
Tomatoes, fresh	14	60	0.9
Apples	46	196	0.3
Apricots, canned with syrup	106	452	0.5
Apricots, dried	182	772	4.8
Bananas	76	326	1.1
Blackcurrants	28	121	0.9
Cherries	47	201	0.6
Gooseberries, green	17	73	1.1
Grapefruit	22	95	0.6
Lemon juice	7	31	0.3
Melon	23	97	0.8
Oranges	35	150	0.8
Orange juice — canned	33	143	0.4
Peaches, fresh	37	156	0.6
Peaches, canned	87	373	0.4
Pears, fresh	41	175	0.3
Pineapple, canned with syrup	77	328	0.3
Plums	32	137	0.6
Prunes, dried	161	686	2.4
Rhubarb	6	26	0.6
Biscuits, chocolate	524	2197	5.7
Biscuits, cream crackers	440	1857	9.5
Biscuits, plain semi-sweet	457	1925	6.7

Bread, brown	223	948	8.9
white	233	991	7.8
wholemeal	216	918	8.8
Corn flakes	368	1567	8.6
Rice	361	1536	6.5
Spaghetti	378	1612	13.6
Apple pie	281	1179	3.2
Currant bun	328	1385	7.8
Custard	118	496	3.8
Rice pudding	131	552	4.1
Soup, canned tomato	55	230	0.8
Trifle	160	674	3.5
Ice cream, vanilla	166	698	3.5

based sweets and drinks such as Hycal (a protein-free, flavoured glucose drink — 415 Kcal in 171 ml bottle).

RE. Record the quantity and type of food eaten each day to calculate calorie intake. Test urine for glucose.

5. Increase the patient's protein intake when indicated by providing meat, eggs, fish, cheese and milk-based foods. Add protein powder such as Casilan to some foods, for instance puddings. Supervise mealtimes.

RE. Calculate daily protein intake. Test urine for ketones.

6. Conserve body stores of energy by keeping both room and patient warm, limiting daily activity and encouraging rest. Consider whether a nurse or relative should feed the patient.

RE. Observe for signs of fatigue. Record oral temperature daily.

7. Supervise deep breathing and chest exercises if muscle wasting occurs, to prevent chest infection. Check that visitors and other patients with upper respiratory tract infections do not visit.

RE. Observe the patient for coughing with sputum production. Report any sign of chest infection to the doctor.

Further action

1. Enteral feeding may be recommended via a fine bore tube passed through the naso-pharynx and down through the stomach to the jejunum. The site of the tip should be checked by an X-ray. The tube is then marked where it enters the nostril.

RE. Check that the mark on the tube remains in the same place each time that a fresh feed is set up. Check the tube is securely taped in place with no strain or kinking.

2. Air can be insufflated to confirm the tube's position, but fluid cannot be aspirated from the gut by suction with a fine-bore tube. Store the opened feed in a refrigerator until half an hour before use, then remove it so it slowly reaches room temperature. Slow continuous feeding is preferred as it reduces the risk of diarrhoea, and increases the amount of nutrition which

can be given in 24 hours. A volumetric pump should be used to control the rate of flow.

RE. Weigh the patient in the same clothes at the same time each day. Ask them if there is discomfort due to the temperature of the feed following a fresh container being set up. Monitor fluid intake and output. Record the frequency and consistency of bowel actions. Diarrhoea may be due to concurrent antibiotic therapy, infected feed, malabsorption or, rarely, to lactose intolerance.

Associated medical diagnoses	Anorexia nervosa Carcinoma Cerebral vascular accident Coeliac disease Malabsorption Meningitis Multiple injuries Peptic ulcer Ulcerative colitis Wired jaw

---

Potential problem · **Risk of low body sodium (hyponatremia)**

Assessment findings

Severe or prolonged vomiting (1000 ml gastric juice contains about 55 mEq sodium ions)
Copious gastric drainage
Copious drainage from a fistula or paracentesis
Profuse sweating (1000 ml perspiration contains about 82 mEq sodium ions)
Prolonged use of salt-losing diuretics
Low salt diet
Adrenal steroid therapy
Falling blood sodium levels (normal = 135–150 mmol per litre).

Information for the patient

Salt in the body tends to attract water to it. The kidneys normally adjust the amount of salt in the body. However the salt and water balance can get out of control, for instance salt can be lost in sweat or vomit. Some drugs may be prescribed to make the body pass more urine, and so more salt than normal may be lost with the urine. The doctor will make regular checks on the salt balance through blood tests. The patient can help their body keep that balance right by watching what kinds and amounts of food are taken each day.

Nursing actions

1. Increase the salt content of the diet to maintain the balance of intake with loss. (Table 3.7). Advise the patient about which foods to include in the daily diet. Tinned tomato juice provides a palatable source of sodium if there is no vomiting. Bacon, kippers, salted butter, margarine, Marmite or milk puddings can be given. Check the salt cellar is available at mealtimes.

RE. Check how much of the advice the patient can remember. Record the amount and type of high sodium foods eaten each day. Monitor blood electrolyte results.

Table 3.7   Body fluids

1000 ml	Sodium Na+/mEq	Ions lost Potassium K+/mEq	Chlorine C1-/mEq
Gastric juice	55	10	90
Perspiration	82	—	12

Normal loss. Urine 60 mmol K+   Average diet 65 mmol K+ (50–150 mmol)
　　　　　　　Faeces 7 mmol K+
　　　　　　　Sweat   3 mmol K+

Replacement	Sodium mg	Potassium mEq
Medium size orange	0.3	4.4
banana	0.85	9.4
pear	2.35	4.0
Orange juice – 250 ml	1.25	6.4
Tomato juice – 250 ml	568.70	14.5
Apple juice – 250 ml	5.0	11.4
100 g cheddar cheese	610	120
100 g bacon	1480	233
kipper	990	520
butter	870	15
margarine	800	5
canned processed peas	330	170
corn flakes	1160	99
marmite	4500	2600

2. Explain the symptoms which may indicate low sodium levels. Ask the patient to alert the nurse if they should occur.
(i)   Headache
(ii)   Vertigo
(iii)   Fatigue
(iv)   Abdominal and muscle cramps
(v)   Falling blood pressure
(vi)   Muscle weakness
(vii)   Poor skin turgor
(viii) Lethargy
(ix)   Confusion

RE. Check how many symptoms the patient can remember. Observe for signs of low sodium. Check blood pressure daily. See p. 149 for 'Risk of sodium imbalance'.

Further action

1. Intravenous sodium replacement using 1.8% saline with close biochemical monitoring of blood sodium levels.

RE. Monitor the flow rate carefully, consider using a volumetric pump for a more accurate control.

2. Sodium tablets may be used but rate of absorption cannot be controlled. Some patients find the large tablets difficult to swallow.

RE. Observe for nausea or discomfort because tablets 'stick' in the gullet.

3. Excessive water intake may cause low sodium by rapid dilution. Water restriction and/or intravenous sodium replacement may be used.

RE. Record the patient's fluid intake carefully. In severe cases epiliptiform fits may occur, so good observation and knowledge of safety precautions are required.

Associated medical diagnoses	Abrupt withdrawal of steroids Addison's disease Anorexia nervosa Ascites Cushing's syndrome Fistulae — ileum, colon, rectum or vagina Dilutional hyponatraemia Gastric ulcer Hypertension Paracentesis Peptic ulcer Myocardial infarction Vomiting

---

Potential problem	**Risk that small food intake will not meet protein and calorie requirements.**

Assessment findings	Hypothermia — need for extra Calories in winter Prone to infections Loss of body fat Weight loss Ketones in urine Fall in metabolic rate Age — elderly Memory impairment Tires easily Food fads Embarrassed by needing help with feeding Loss of appetite Loss of interest in food Grief or bereavement Multiple investigations which involve periods of fasting Fever Increased metabolic rate Ethnic diet requirements Limited menu choice Low blood sugar
Information for the patient	The body needs protein and energy for health. If the appetite is blunted it is possible to eat less than required, but not to notice the change or to feel hungry. Sometimes just being in hospital and not liking the food served, or being too tired to eat can lead to an inadequate food intake especially if the body actually needs more than normal because of illness. While there is a risk from not eating enough, a careful watch must be kept so that steps can be taken if a problem occurs.
Nursing actions	1. Weigh the patient daily, at the same time each day, in the same type of clothing. Test urine for ketones which indicate that the body is using up its own fat supply.

RE. Monitor for weight loss. If weight loss begins and ketones are detected in the urine, then the food intake is insufficient for the patient's needs.

2. Assess the energy and protein requirements needed for the day's activities.

RE. Monitor the temperature of the patient's environment, as a cold room will lead to the body requiring increased energy requirements to keep warm.

3. Assess the daily food intake to calculate its Calorie and protein content.

RE. Check that the food placed before the patient is actually eaten. Monitor interest in food. Confirm that the food served meets any ethnic or other requirements. Check that food, not given while investigations are performed, is later served in a palatable form.

4. Observe the patient at mealtimes to identify any feeding difficulties.

RE. Monitor for increases in the time taken to finish a meal, and for fatigue or toying with food.

5. Discuss their food intake with the patient, and agree on adjustments where required. Compare the meals available in hospital to the normal eating pattern of the patient at home. Assess the need for additional support on transfer home.

RE. Check how much of discussion patient can remember 24 and 48 hours later. Review proposals for additional support if the patient has forgotten. Consider the availability and need for facilities such as meals on wheels, a home help to do the shopping, luncheon clubs, bereavement counselling, extra financial help or social work support. Refer to appropriate bodies for help.

Further action	1. Measure serum albumin levels to assess if the protein intake is sufficient for patient's needs.
	RE. Serum albumin is not an accurate indicator.
	2. Measure triceps skinfold to assess the amount of muscle wasting.
	RE. A decrease indicates loss of muscle mass and therefore a protein deficit.
Associated medical diagnoses	Carcinoma Chronic bronchitis Depression Hypothermia Pneumonia Senile dementia

---

Potential problem	**Risk of vitamin deficiency**

		Vitamin particularly at risk
Assessment findings	Rarely eats citrus or other fruits	A, C
	Rarely eats green vegetables	C
	Heavy smoker	C and B vitamins
	Excessive alcohol intake	B_{12}, folic acid
	Excessive use of liquid paraffin as a laxative	A, nicotinic acid (water soluble), D_2, E,K may also affect water-soluble vitamins

Avoids meat, milk and eggs	A, B_{12}
Eats institutionally cooked food	C
Repeated pregnancies and lactation	D, folic acid
Food fads limit variety of foods eaten e.g. macrobiotic diet	B_{12}
Fed by naso-gastric tube	C
Fat intolerance	A, D, K
Drug therapy with:	
Antibiotics	B complex
Anticonvulsants	B_6, folic acic, D, K
Oral contraceptives	B_6
Oestrogens	C, B_{12}, folic acid
Isoniazide and antituberculosis therapy	Nicotinic acid
Chemotherapy for cancer	B_{12}, folic acid
Antimalarials	B_{12}, folic acid
Neomycin	Carotene, B_{12}

Information for the patient

The body cells need very small amounts of chemicals, found in both animal and vegetable foods, for normal functioning. These are known as vitamins (= vital for life). If a vitamin is not contained in the foods eaten, or it cannot be used by the body cells because drugs interfere with its absorption, then a deficiency disease can occur. Those vitamins which are soluble in fats can be stored, so that the body can make up the amount missing from the diet until its store is used up. The water soluble vitamins are not stored, they are passed out of the body in the urine. Each day enough of these vitamins must be taken in to meet the body's needs. Some illnesses require extra amounts of vitamins for damaged cells to be repaired.

Nursing actions

1. Provide a diet with increased amounts of the potentially deficient vitamin (Table 3.8 gives examples of foods and the vitamins they contain).

RE. Assess how much of the vitamin(s) at risk the patient is taking. Observe for any signs of deficiency. (See Table 3.9.)

2. Discuss the increased vitamin requirement with the patient.

RE. Check how much of the discussion the patient remembers. Plan further teaching if necessary.

3. Suggest which foods relatives or friends may be able to supply to help boost the patient's intake of vitamins.

RE. Observe whether the relatives provide additional foods and if the patient eats them.

4. Discuss the cost of a revised diet, and how to budget for it. Offer to contact a social worker to discuss supplementary benefits for the elderly or unemployed.

RE. Assess the patient's attitude to changing their diet, and possibly having to spend more on it.

Further action

1. Parenteral vitamins can be given intramuscularly or intravenously. High potency vitamins should be given initially, and if a deficiency is developing. Observe the patient carefully for an anaphylactic reaction to thiamine during the first few minutes of intravenous injection.

RE. Ask the patient how they feel. Observe their respiratory rate and their colour for a sudden change.

2. Multiple vitamin tables can be taken as a supplement when institutional cooking cannot be avoided or improved. Vitamin B_{12}, serum folate and Vitamin C levels indicate the absorption of the vitamins.

RE. Check the patient can swallow the tablets easily. Vitamin drops can be added to food or drink as an alternative.

Associated medical diagnoses	Alcoholism Anorexia nervosa Carcinoma Carcinoma of prostate Cerebral vascular accident Epilepsy Gastrectomy Hepatitis Infection Jaundice Oesophageal stricture Tuberculosis Wernicke's encephalopathy

---

Potential problem	**Risk of reaction to specific foods**

Assessment findings	Past reaction to shellfish, strawberries, milk, gluten, lactose Food sensitive migraine Food additive sensitivity; such as to monosodium glutamate Taking monoamine oxidase inhibitors (MAOI)(an antidepressent) History of skin rash Hives Blocked or runny nose Swollen lips or mouth Nausea Vomiting Diarrhoea Headache Flashing lights Temporary numbness
Information for the patient	All foods are made up of a variety of different substances. Sometimes one or more of the ingredients can upset the body. It may be because one of the pathways by which the body makes new cells or other substances is blocked or upset. There are food groups which all contain the same or very similar substances. If the food that causes the upset is known it should be possible to adjust the diet to avoid foods containing it. When the body is also having to cope with illness it can become more prone to food sensitivity.
Nursing actions	1. Identify the food constituent which is involved in the allergic reaction. Write out a list of foods which contain it. Plan out a daily diet with the patient to avoid these foods. Discuss patient's normal diet. Seek advice from dietitian if necessary.

Table 3.8 Vitamins and examples of foods containing them

Vitamin	Recommended intake per day	Precursor	Solubility	Foods: 100 mg of each, raw*		
A Retinol	5000 IU or 750 μg retinol equivalent = 1μg retinol	Carotene	Partially soluble in water	*μg* Raw, old carrots 2000 Spinach 1000 Dried apricots 600		
			Fat soluble	Halibut liver oil 900 000 Cod liver oil 18 000 Ox liver 16 760	Butter 985 Margarine 900 Cheddar cheese 410	
B_1 Thiamine	Related to carbohydrate intake		Water soluble unstable in cooking	*mg per 100 kcal* Marmite 1.80 Corn flakes 0.49 Fresh peas 0.48	Oranges 0.29 Pork 0.18 Potatoes 0.13 Wholemeal bread 0.12	
B_2 Riboflavine	1.6 mg		Slightly soluble in water, unstable in light	*mg* Marmite 11.00 Liver 3.10 Kidney 1.90	Corn flakes 1.60 Cheddar cheese 0.50 Eggs 0.47	
Nicotinic acid Nicotinamide (niacin)	18 mg nicotinic acid equivalent	Tryptophan (if pyridoxine available)	Fat soluble, slightly soluble in water	*mg* Instant coffee (dry) 25.1 Chicken 9.3 Beef 7.3	Pork 7.0 Cheddar cheese 6.2 White fish 4.9	
B_6 Pyridoxine	Related to protein intake		Water soluble	Wholemeal cereals Yeast Liver		

Vitamin	Amount	Properties	Rich sources		Other sources	
B₁₂ Cyanocobalamin	3 µg	Water soluble unstable in light, alkali or strong acid	Ox liver Lambs liver Pigs liver	*µg* 110.0 84.0 25.0	White fish Eggs Cheddar cheese	2.0 1.7 1.5
Folic acid	281 µg	Water soluble, lost in cooking water, unstable in light	Offal Raw green leafy vegetables Pulses		Bread Oranges Bananas	
C Ascorbic acid	300 mg	Water soluble, unstable in light or heat	'Ribena' 264/100 ml Blackcurrants Brussels sprouts Cauliflower	*mg* 200 87 64	Strawberries Oranges Lemon juice	60 50 50
D₂ Calciferol D₃	0-10 µg	Cholecalciferol from sunlight on skin Fat soluble	Cod liver oil Dry Ovaltine Herring or kipper	*µg* 212.5 30.6 22.4	Canned salmon Margarine Canned sardines	12.5 7.94 7.5
E Tocopherol	15 IU	Fat soluble	Vegetable oils Wheatgerm Eggs		Peas Beans	
K Phytomenadione	10 mg	Synthesised by gut flora Fat soluble	Spinach Cabbage Cauliflower		Peas Cereals	

Table 3.9 Vitamin deficiency and excess: early signs and severe symptoms

Vitamin	Deficiency		Excess	
	Early signs	Severe	Early signs	Severe
A Retinol	'Nightblindness' Keratinization of mucous membranes (eyes, nose, throat, gastro-intestinal tract) dry with decreasing mucus production	*Xerophthalmia* (conjunctivitis and corneal atrophy) Dry, scaly skin Slow growth	Fatigue Abdominal discomfort Headache Joint pain	Hair loss Vomiting
B$_1$ Thiamine	Loss of appetite Weight loss Depression Fatigue Irritability	*Beri-beri* Tachycardia Enlarged heart Oedema ECG changes Epigastric pain Peripheral neuritis Tender muscles Muscle atrophy Confusion *Wernicke's encephalopathy* Vomiting Ataxia Dementia	Anaphylaxis occurs (rarely) if administered parenterally	
B$_2$ Riboflavine	Slow wound healing Poor protein utilization Sores in corners of mouth (cheilosis)	Slow growth		

Vitamin			
Nicotinic acid	Anorexia Weight loss Weakness Lassitude	*Pellagra* Itching skin Dermatitis Diarrhoea Confusion Nervousness	Vasodilation
B6 Pyridoxine	Nervousness Skin changes	Peripheral nerve defects Convulsions Anaemia	
B12 Cyanocobal- amine	*Megaloblastic anaemia* Sore, smooth tone Anorexia	Jaundice *Sub-acute combined degeneration of the cord* 'Pins and needles') Fingers cold and numb) and toes Muscular weakness Loss of co-ordination Staggering walk, paralysis	
Folic acid	Megaloblastic anaemia		
C Ascorbic acid	Bleeding gums Delayed wound healing Petechiae after local pressure (e.g. from sphygmomanometer cuff)	*Scurvy* *Anaemia*	
D Calciferol	Tetany	*Rickets* Crooked, bowed long bones muscle pain *Osteomalacia*	Diarrhoea Weight loss Nausea Renal stones Calcification of soft tissues
E Tocopherol K Phytomena- dione	Bleeding tendency Purpura Nose bleeds (epistaxis) Melaena		

RE. Check the food at mealtimes to ensure only those not on the list are eaten. Check that the list is available to those serving the meals.

2. Review the list of foods implicated in a food reaction with the patient. Assess their level of understanding and plan a teaching programme to fill in knowledge of gaps if necessary.

RE. Check how much the patient can remember.

3. Review the drugs prescribed to identify any which contain the offending substance, e.g. lactose in laxatives, tartrazine (yellow colouring agent). Seek advice from a pharmacist if necessary.

RE. Observe the patient's response to drugs, especially where the full list of constituents is unknown.

Further action

1. Elimination diets may be useful if the specific allergy is unknown. Medical and dietetic supervision is required. Start with a total fast for five days, with only bottled mineral water to drink (chlorine free).
List all foods usually eaten more than once in three days.

RE. Foods taken daily or more often are particularly suspect. Check the patient's urine daily for the ketone level. Weigh at beginning and end of five day period to assess weight loss.

2. On each day following the five day fast give a large helping of one suspect food in the evening with mineral water.

RE. Observe for flushing, nausea or usual symptoms of food reaction occuring within two hours after meals. If symptoms occur put the food on a 'black list'. Ask the patient to report if any new symptoms occur, and how long they last.

3. If the patient has recovered, repeat with a new suspect food the next evening.

RE. If there is no reaction add the food to the 'safe list'. Such foods can be given at breakfast and lunchtimes, preferably in rotation.

4. Testing is repeated until all the suspect foods have been listed and the patient understands how to avoid them. Many commercial foods contain a mixture of substances. If food additives are suspected use a pure version of the food first.

RE. If there is no reaction to the food without additives, then in the next test give the version that does contain them.

5. Provocative sub-lingual testing may be tried after a five day fast. Uncontaminated small samples of the suspect foods are liquidized in a clean blender with enough distilled water to make a thin solution. Record the patient's pulse rate and pupil size. Each solution is put in a sterile cup with a disposable 10 ml syringe, together with distilled water, paper towels and a receiver on a tray. Ask the patient to tip their head back with the tongue on the roof of the mouth. Draw up 1 ml of solution. Two drops of solution are put under the tongue.

RE. Observe for any of the main symptoms and a rise in pulse rate. If none occur within two minutes, the patient can bring their head forward and rinse out the mouth with distilled water, ready for the next text solution. Score for first test solution is 0 = no symptoms. If the symptoms occur, write 1 for slight, 2 for moderate, or 3 for severe reaction on a chart against the test solution. Count the pulse rate at 2 minutes and record. Use a 'turn-off solution' to reduce the moderate or severe reaction.

6. Make up first turn-off solution by drawing up distilled water to dilute the first solution to 1 in 10. Place one drop under patient's tongue and leave for 2 minutes. If necessary serial dilutions can be made up by ejecting 9 ml and drawing up a fresh 9 ml of distilled water to give 1 in 100, and the process repeated for 1 in 1000.

RE. Observe for signs that the reaction is decreasing and the patient feels that they are returning to normal. Check their pulse at 2 minutes and record. If pulse is normal, patient should rinse their mouth with distilled water and try the next solution. If the reaction continues, give 1 drop of 1 in 100 solution. Repeat the procedure using serial dilutions until the reaction is over. Record the final dilution used. If the symptoms are severe, oxygen therapy may be required.

7. Modified elimination diets may be used, but results are not so accurate. A whole range of suspect foods would be removed from the diet for one week, then reintroduced to see if any symptoms recur.

RE. Check the patient uses plain foods, and avoids sauces and processed foods. The common offenders to be tested include cane sugar, cereals, instant coffee, tea, chocolate, eggs and milk. Check the patient is aware of which foods in the group are to be omitted. For example in grain-sensitive people beer and whisky must be avoided as well as cakes, bread, breakfast cereals and sauces.

8. A jejunal biopsy may be undertaken using a crosby capsule attached to a semi-rigid radio-opaque catheter, to obtain a specimen of the small bowel tissue which may be sent for microscopy to detect changes in the villi, culture, or biochemical analysis. The patient must fast overnight for biopsy in the morning. Provide mouth washes to ease the discomfort of a dry mouth. The patient swallows the capsule. The position of the capsule, normally in the duodeno-jejunal flexure, is confirmed by X-ray before biopsy. Suction on the catheter draws the mucosa into a side port, the resulting negative pressure fires a small blade which severs the mucosa. The capsule is then withdrawn.

RE. Record the patient's temperature, pulse and blood pressure every half hour for 4 hours following the biopsy and keep the patient fasting. Observe for signs of bleeding or perforation of the bowel wall, such as abdominal pain.

9. A lactose tolerance test may be undertaken if malabsorption of milk is suspected. Fast the patient overnight for a morning test. Provide mouth washes to ease the discomfort of a dry mouth. Give 50 grams of lactose dissolved in 200 ml water as a drink. Blood samples are taken every half hour for two hours for glucose estimation.

RE. The patient can eat and drink again after 2 hours. A gradual increase in blood glucose levels indicates absorption. No rise in the levels of glucose indicates intolerance. Warn the patient they may have loose stools after the test.

Associated medical diagnoses	Asthma Chinese restaurant syndrome (Kwok's disease) Coeliac disease Gluten enteropathy Eczema Hay fever Lactose intolerance Migraine

---

Potential problem	**Risk of developing low body potassium (hypokalaemia)**

Assessment findings	Age 70+ Severe diarrhoea Prolonged use of potassium-losing diuretics — e.g. thiazide Potassium supplements not being taken Potassium supplement 'Slow K' not being absorbed (passed in faeces) Carbenoxolone therapy Corticosteroid therapy Diet low in fresh fruit, meat, fish, cheese, eggs, milk or vegetables High blood urea Falling blood potassium levels
Information for the patient	Most of the body's potassium is found within the cells. Old people have less body potassium and seem less able to absorb it from the gut. Some drugs such as those to make the kidneys produce more urine can cause potassium loss from the body. The digestive juices which mix with food to break it down are high in potassium. If food is hurried through the gut, it cannot be reabsorbed, and it is lost in diarrhoea. To make up for the lower levels of potassium in the blood, it is moved out of the body cells. The muscles cannot work properly and feel weak. The heart can also be affected. To prevent these unpleasant effects it is important to take foods rich in potassium each day, as the body does not store any extra taken on one day to use in future. Fruit and vegetables are good sources of potassium.
Nursing actions	1. Increase the potassium content of the patient's diet to maintain level, by giving cups of instant coffee, potatoes, peas, brussels sprouts, mushrooms, cauliflower, meat, oranges, prunes, bananas, and tomato and other fruit juices. If anorexia is present, start by giving fruit juices at 250 ml per hour. 250 ml tomato juice provides 14.5 mEq potassium 250 ml apple juice provides 11.4 mEq potassium 250 ml orange juice provides 6.0 mEq potassium

RE. Record the intake of potassium-containing fluids. Check any serum electrolyte results for changes in level. Observe for signs and symptoms of low potassium such as the following
(i) weakness
(ii) apathy or depression
(iii) constipation
(iv) abdominal distension
(v) soft flabby muscles
(vi) cardiac arrhythmias or bradycardia, especially if digoxin is also being administered.
(vii) mental confusion (if loss of potassium is severe)

2. Avoid the use of laxatives or enemas which speed the passage of food through the gut. Increase the dietary fibre if possible. Use glycerine suppositories to stimulate the rectum if bowel action is less frequent than normal.

RE. Record the frequency of bowel actions. Constipation is one symptom of falling body potassium. Measuring the volume of diarrhoea aids assessment of potassium lost.

Further action

1. Potassium supplements can be given by intravenous infusion, up to a maximum rate of 20 mEq per hour and 200 mEq in 24 hours. If potassium is added to an intravenous solution ensure that it is mixed thoroughly or a concentrated solution may be given for part of the administration period. Consider using a mechanical pump to give greater control of the flow rate.

RE. Check the patient's pulse rate and rhythm during administration. Excessive blood potassium levels may produce muscle weakness, lethargy or confusion.

2. Oral potassium supplements in effervescent or slow release form can be used. Advise the patient to sit upright to swallow the tablets, and to take at least one full glass of water with them.

RE. Ask the patient to report any discomfort or feeling that tablets 'stick' in the gullet. Oesophageal ulceration may occur if the tablet does not reach stomach readily. Observe the stools if bowels are opened frequently, as tablets may not remain in the gut long enough for absorption to take place. An alternative form of supplement may be needed.

3. If a cardiac monitor is in use, the pattern of the tracing may change as potassium levels alter.

RE. Low potassium – flattening T waves, large U complexes, and depressed ST segments may be seen, and they could lead to cardiac arrest.
High potassium – tall peaked T waves, and depressed ST segments may occur, and progress to ventricular fibrillation with rapid, irregular, weak contractions of the heart, or broad, slow QRS complexes.

Associated medical diagnoses

Alcoholism
Cirrhosis
Congestive cardiac failure
Diverticulitis
Diarrhoea
Diabetes
Glomerulonephritis
Hypertension
Ileitis
Malnutrition
Potassium losing nephropathy
Pulmonary oedema
Renal failure
Ulcerative colitis
Vomiting

Potential problem	Risk of developing low body calcium (hypocalcaemia)

Assessment findings

Age
Large blood transfusion
Rapid spurt of growth
Pregnancy
Lactation
Spends all day indoors
Diuretic therapy for hypercalcaemia, or in the elderly — frusemide not thiazole
Prolonged tetracycline therapy
Falling blood calcium, rising blood phosphate

Information for the patient

Calcium is needed mainly for bones and teeth. It also plays an important part in the clotting of blood following a cut, and is needed for nerves and muscles to work properly. Calcium balance in the body is controlled by hormones. If the balance is disturbed and the level falls, it can bring on feelings of numbness or pins and needles in the hands and feet. Severe muscle spasms can occur over a longer time. Low calcium levels lead to brittle bones, which are more easily broken during a fall. Older people, especially women after the menopause, and those taking a lot of bran in the diet, are especially prone to low calcium and risk breaking a hip bone if they fall.

Some drugs may also interfere with the body's ability to absorb calcium from the food. Calcium is found in milk, cheese, tinned whole fish (because the bones are eaten), eggs and white bread. Vitamin D, which aids the absorption of calcium, is found in fatty fish, eggs and butter. It is also added to margarine. More important still is the vitamin D made by the skin in the presence of sunlight.

Nursing actions

1. Increase the amount of calcium and vitamins C and D in the diet. Plan bran-containing foods for different times to limit the action of phytic acid. A late night milky drink is a useful addition to the diet. Ovaltine provides a useful combination of milk (120 mg calcium per 100 g; vitamin D — winter 0.01 ug to summer 0.03 ug vitamin D per 100 g) and dry Ovaltine (30.60 ug vitamin D per 100g). Cheese, eggs, canned whole fish, white bread and yoghurt are all helpful. A sardine sandwich made with white bread and margarine is a calcium-rich combination.

RE. Note amount of supplementary food tolerated.

2. Increase the exposure to direct sunlight by providing opportunities for sunbathing to promote vitamin D production. Patients in hospital for long periods of time will need to gradually increase their periods of exposure to prevent sunburn. Skin creams and oils should be avoided before, and for a few hours after, exposure to sunlight.

RE. Observe for development of a tan or sunburn in fairskinned people.

3. Regulate blood transfusions as prescribed by the doctor.

RE. Observe for signs and symptoms of low calcium
(i)   numbness and/or tingling
(ii)   muscle twitching or cramp
(iii)   palpitations
(iv)   change to positive for Trousseau's and Chvostek's signs (these demonstrate increased neuromuscular excitability)

(v) irritability

(vi) bleeding from minor trauma to mucous membranes or skin

(Trousseau's sign is the spasmodic contraction of the muscles of the forearm producing a claw-like flexure of the hand which occurs when a sphygmomanometer cuff is inflated around the arm.

Chvostek's sign is positive when on tapping the facial nerve in front of the ear, the upper lip twitches and the facial muscles contract.)

Further action

1. Oral effervescent calcium or calcium with vitamin D tablets may be prescribed. The latter form is chalky and may be easier to chew with a biscuit.

RE. Do not give bran-containing foods at the same time.

2. Symptoms occurring during blood transfusion can be treated with a solution containing calcium gluconate, administered slowly.

RE. Observe the patient's site during and after the transfusion, as the intravenous compound is an irritant and may induce phlebitis.

Hypercalcaemia is indicated by excessive thirst, polyuria, headache, nausea, fatigue, muscle weakness or anorexia.

Associated medical diagnoses

Hypoparathyroidism
Haemophilia, peptic ulcer or trauma requiring blood transfusions
Osteoporosis
Osteomalacia
Parathyroid tumour
Renal osteo-dystrophy
Rickets
Thyroidectomy

Potential problem | **Risk of developing high blood calcium (hypercalcaemia)**

Assessment findings

Age
Vitamin D therapy
Prolonged bed rest
Drinks large amounts of milk
Impaired renal function
Balance when standing and walking
Increased urinary excretion of calcium

Information for the patient

Calcium is needed in the body for bones and teeth, and it plays an important part in the clotting of blood following a cut, and for nerves and muscles to work properly. Calcium is taken into the body from foods such as milk, cheese, tinned whole fish, eggs and white bread. The kidneys get rid of any excess in the urine. Calcium balance is controlled by a hormone produced by the parathyroid glands in the neck. This can encourage calcium to move from the bones into the blood. Weightlessness, such as in space travel, or lack of exercise due to long periods in bed can lead to so much calcium being moved out of the bones that they become weakened and break more easily. Sometimes so much calcium leaves by the kidneys that kidney stones can form.

It is important not to put too much strain on the bones until the calcium balance is improved. Falls could obviously be harmful. The acids in the bran of cereals help to stop the body absorbing calcium from the food, so milk and cheese can still be eaten but with bran in cereals, bread and cakes.

Nursing actions

1. Provide an adjustable height bed, and if necessary assistance to get into and out of it, to reduce the risk of falls for the mobile patient. Keep the bed height low for a restless patient. Supervise the patient if they have a poor sense of balance.

RE. Check the patient understands the need for care to prevent falls. If a fall occurs, request that the doctor examines the patient. Report the incident fully.

2. Instruct the patient not to lift heavy weights, to avoid straining their weakened bone structure.

RE. Check that the patient can explain why he should not lift heavy weights. Observe for evidence that the patient complies with the instruction.

3. Increase the amount of bran and wholemeal bread in the diet to increase the proportion of insoluble calcium passing through the gut.

RE. Check on the amount of bran and wholemeal bread consumed each day.

4. Monitor the patient's fluid intake and output and bowel activity.

RE. Observe for signs and symptoms of high calcium levels, such as:
(i)   muscle weakness
(ii)   local or generalized bone pain
(iii)   headache
(iv)   polyuria
(v)   excessive thirst
(vi)   nausea
(vii)   fatigue
(viii)   anorexia
(ix)   constipation
(x)   stuperose
(xi)   coma (rare)
(xii)   rising blood calcium with falling blood phosphate

Further action

1. Intravenous saline in large volumes (1 litre in 4 hours) to force a diuresis may be combined with a diuretic such as frusemide. Ensure the commode or toilet is within easy reach. Record intake and output.

RE. Compare the volume of fluid infused with the patient's urine output. Check their pulse rate and strength for signs of cardiac failure.

2. Steroids may be used in the treatment of sarcoidosis to reduce serum calcium. Regular blood testing is needed for calcium and phosphorus levels.

RE. Observe for signs of salt and water retention. Weigh the patient twice a week. The normal calcium level is 2.25 to 2.6 mmol per litre.

3. A cytotoxic drug such as mithramycin may be give intravenously to reduce calcium level.

RE. A 24 hour urine sample can be collected to measure the calcium level.

Associated medical diagnoses

Bladder calculi
Bone neoplasm
Duodenal ulcer
Excessive administration of vitamin D (calciferol)

112

Hyperparathyroidism
Peptic ulcer
Renal calculi
Sarcoidosis
Thyrotoxicosis

Potential problem	**Risk of developing low body iron stores**

Assessment findings	Pale colour
	Lethargy
	Breathless on moderate exertion
	Poor intake of iron-containing foods
	Rarely eats fresh fruit or vegetables
	Recent heavy blood loss
	Heavy menstrual periods
	Headaches
	Dizziness or fainting
	Feels the cold easily
	'Pins and needles' in fingers or toes
	Increased pulse rate
	Angina in the elderly
	Pale (hypochromic) red cells
	Small (microcytic) red cells
	Low haemoglobin count, normal range being
	13—15 G in men
	12—14 G in women

Information for the patient	The body uses and stores iron to make the red blood cells which it needs to carry oxygen around the body. Iron is absorbed from foods such as liver, red meat, eggs, raisins and apricots. The rate at which it is absorbed depends on the body's need for iron. The presence of chemicals which bind to the iron may prevent its absorption. Iron in excess of that needed to make red blood cells is stored in the liver — which is why animal liver is useful in the diet.

Nursing actions	1. Increase the amount of iron-containing foods which the patient likes in the diet. Dried fruit should be given instead of snacks. Liver, liver pate, liver sausage or red meat should be eaten as the main meal of the day if possible. Warn the patient that their stools will look dark or black if they are taking iron tablets.
	RE. Assess the daily intake of iron, only a small proportion is absorbed.
	2. Increase the amount of citrus fruit or other vitamin C-containing foods to promote iron absorption. Limit the amount of tea, spices, eggs, milk and bran taken at the same time as the iron foods.
	RE. Assess the daily intake of vitamin C foods.
	3. Suggest extra rest in or on the bed, and limit the amount of even moderate exertion in a day to reduce the strain on the cardio-vascular system.
	RE. Check the pulse rate. If anaemia is present the pulse rate will increase, breathlessness, palpitations or angina may be noticed by the patient. A sore, smooth red tongue sometimes occurs.

4. Advise the patient to avoid standing for long periods, and to rise from a chair or bed slowly to reduce the risk of dizzy spells or fainting.

RE. Check whether the patient follows the advice. Report if they complain of any symptoms.

Further action

1. Oral iron preparations such as ferrous sulphate 200 mg to be taken three times a day; vitamin C may also be recommended to increase absorption. Warn the patient this will cause dark black stools and a change in bowel habit.

RE. Record the frequency of bowel actions.

2. An intramuscular injection such as Imferon or Jectofer is sometimes prescribed. Use a long needle and zig-zag technique into the upper outer quadrant of buttock to prevent leakage and skin staining after intramuscular injection.

RE. Observe for rash, raised temperature, painful joints or swollen glands and report so that iron therapy can be reviewed.

3. A total dose infusion is only used with great caution because of the risk of anaphylactic reaction, irritation of the vein around the infusion site, and occasionally allergic reactions. The infusion is started slowly under the supervision of a doctor. If after 10 minutes no untoward reaction occurs then the infusion rate can be increased.

RE. Monitor the patient's respiratory rate, pulse and blood pressure during first 10 minutes of infusion. Side effects appearing later than this are similar to those occurring with administration by the intramuscular route.

4. A blood transfusion may be used if iron therapy is ineffectual or if the patient's haemoglobin level requires urgent action. Packed cells may be used to avoid large volumes of fluid being transfused. Follow the hospital procedure for checking that the correct, cross-match blood is administered. Check the patient's blood pressure at the start of each unit, and their temperature half an hour after commencement. If there is risk of circulatory overload check the pulse rate at least half hourly during transfusion.

RE. Compare the blood pressure readings, pulse rate and volume, for early signs of circulatory overload. Ask the patient to report any discomfort, particularly around the kidney area. Assess their urine output to identify any decrease in relation to the volume transfused.

Associated medical diagnoses

Anaemia
Carcinoma
Duodenal ulcer
Gastric ulcer
Microcytic hypochromic anaemia
Menorrhagia
Plummer-Vinson syndrome (associated with certain cases of hypochromic anaemia)

References and further reading

Bray, G.A. (ed). (1979). *Obesity in America.* Proceedings of the 2nd Fogarty International Centre Conference on Obesity, No. 79, Washington: US DHEW.

Buss, D., Robertson, J. (1981). *Manual of Nutrition.* HMSO. London.

Davidson, S., Passmore, R. Brock, J.F., Truswell, A.S. (1979). (7th edn.) *Human Nutrition and Dietetics.* Churchill Livingstone. Edinburgh.

Hassan, M., Marsden, J. (1984). *E for Additives.* Thorsons Publishers Ltd, Wellingborough, Northamptonshire.

Health Education Council. (1983). *A Discussion Paper on Proposals for Nutritional Guidelines for Health Education in Britain.* NACNE (National Advisory Committee on Nutrition Education). September.

Huskisson, J.M. (1981). *Nutrition and Dietetics in Health and Disease.* Baillière Tindall Ltd. London.

Metropolitan Life Insurance Co., New York. (1960). Mortality among overweight men and women. *Statistical Bulletin,* **41**. February.

Ministry of Agriculture, Fisheries and Food (MAFF). (1984). *Look at the Label.* MAFF Publications Unit, Alnwick, Northumberland.

Moore, F.D. (1959). *Metabolic Care of the Surgical Patient.* pp. 24–45. W.B. Saunders, Philadelphia.

Royal College of Physicians of London. (1983). Obesity: A Report of the Royal College of Physicians. Reprinted from the RCP *Journal,* **17/1**, p. 7. January.

Tiffany, R. (ed). (1978). *Cancer Nursing – Medical.* Faber & Faber Ltd. London.

Tiffany, R. (ed). (1979). *Cancer Nursing – Radiotherapy.* Faber & Faber Ltd. London.

Waterlow, J.C. (1981). *Nutrition of Man.* British Medical Bulletin, Vol. 37. No. 1. Published for The British Council by Churchill Livingstone, London.

Wentworth, J.A. (1981). *The Migraine Guide and Cook Book.* Sidgwick and Jackson. London.

4   **Drinking**

Optimum environment

Swallowing fluid

Saliva is produced in small quantities all the time. It starts to flow freely when food is anticipated, and for half an hour after eating. This mouthwatering can be stimulated by the thought, sight or smell of food. The three pairs of glands which produce saliva are controlled by the sympathetic and parasympathetic nerves. If parasympathetic activity is blocked then saliva flow decreases and the mouth feels uncomfortably dry. When the body is short of water, saliva flow will decrease from the normal amount of 1 to 1.5 litres in 24 hours. It becomes stickier, as the lubricating mucin is carried in less fluid.

Lubrication of the tongue, teeth and lining of the mouth makes speech easier and protects the tissues from the friction of movement. Saliva also dilutes acids and other irritants, and the enzyme lysozyme is also present, which has an anti-bacterial action. When there is foreign material in the mouth, saliva flow increases.

The lips must close for swallowing to be effective. If there is poor closure, then dribbling occurs. If there is muscle weakness, for example, after a stroke, muscle tone can be improved by holding the jaw closed and stroking the affected side briskly with a finger. Stroke the face in an upwards direction.

The tongue is involved in swallowing by pushing the food bolus or collection of fluid upwards and backwards into the pharynx. This part of the sequence is under voluntary control. Reflex then takes over. The soft palate moves upwards to close off the back of the nose. The larynx moves upwards, closing the entry to the lungs with the epiglottis. The vocal cords come together and breathing stops. The muscle at the upper end of the oesophagus relaxes, providing a funnel into which the fluid drops. Gravity helps this process, so sitting upright makes swallowing easier.

The oesophagus (or gullet) provides a tube of about 25 cm long to guide fluid into the stomach. The cardiac sphincter at the entrance opens to allow it through. A wave of muscular contraction (peristalsis) follows, massaging down any last drops into the stomach.

If the larynx is not closed properly fluid can enter and a bout of reflex coughing follows. If the patient's swallowing is impaired, it is important not to talk to them while they are drinking. Solid food may cause fewer problems than fluid.

In the stomach, at rest about 30 ml of gastric juice is secreted in each hour. The presence of a foreign body, such as a naso-gastric tube, or fear, increases this rate. The stomach of a healthy person may contain 200 ml of gastric juice during a fasting period.

The rate of emptying from the stomach will depend on the constituents of the liquidized meal or fluid. As with solid food, the carbohydrates tend to leave the stomach first, then the proteins and later the fats. The peristaltic action of the stomach will be slowed by anxiety, fear and pain, or by morphine-related drugs and some anaesthetics. Hunt and Knox (1972) report that acid inhibits gastric emptying. Some drugs increase the rate of emptying, such as Metoclopramide, which alters upper gut motility. According to Forrest *et al* (1978), cimetidine, a drug used to treat gastric ulcers, increases the rate for solid food only.

Fluids leave the stomach faster than solid food, so if a person is on a diet of liquids only, hunger pangs may occur two hours after a meal. The intake should therefore be little and often in order to prevent this discomfort.

Thirst

The body contains a lot of water, about 40 litres for a 65 kg man. The cells contain about 25 litres, the rest is found in body fluids such as tissue fluid, blood, intestinal secretions and saliva. Fatty tissue contains little water, so that fat people have relatively less water for their weight. Water is produced by the chemical changes inside the cells (metabolism), it is also obtained from food. These two sources are not sufficient to replace that lost in urine, sweat, faeces and evaporation from the lungs.

The kidneys regulate the amount of water lost from the body. If the sodium concentration in the blood rises it triggers a feeling of thirst through the hypothalamus in the brain. For this reason wetting the mouth with water does not relieve thirst. If salt is lost as well as water, for example through sweat in a hot, dry climate, then this warning is not given. Such dehydration and salt depletion can also occur due to a high fever, or after heavy manual work, athletics and sports. Salt can be added to water to replace this loss. Some sportsmen, especially those competing in hot countries, also take salt tablets before a game.

Urine contains about 96 per cent water, together with urea and sodium chloride (NaCl), and a large number of other substances in tiny amounts. The amount of urea and sodium chloride depends on the dietary intake. Urea is the chief waste product excreted and the quantity produced increases greatly with the amount of protein eaten. A daily diet containing 100 grams of protein produces about 30 grams of urea for excretion.

The kidneys cannot produce urine more concentrated than 1400 mosmol/kg^3 so they are obliged to excrete enough water to excrete this waste. Most people drink more water than that needed to remove waste. If the blood plasma is diluted by this excess water absorbed from the gut, it is sensed by nerve cells in the pituitary gland of the brain. The posterior part of the gland secretes antidiuretic-hormone (ADH), which acts on the renal tubules to increase the amount of water they absorb. If dilution is detected this secretion is reduced. This reduces the water reabsorbed from the filtrate in the kidneys and the urine is diluted by the extra water.

Rix (1983) reports that elderly people may not feel as thirsty or drink as much water as a young person with the same changes in body fluids. This may increase their risk of dehydration in hot weather or illness. Damage to the brain in the area of the hypothalamus may also reduce the feeling of thirst. In other conditions such as diabetes mellitus, excessive thirst occurs.

Feelings of thirst usually cease once the stomach is full. This may be caused by distension of the stomach or dilution of its contents.

Fluid balance

The average amount of water lost in the urine, in sweat from the skin, in faeces and water vapour from the lungs, totals about 2250 ml in 24 hours. The minimum fluid intake required (actually taken as fluid) when a normal diet is being eaten is 1300 ml. The food will provide about 1000 ml and its metabolism a further 250 ml. Urine output is normally about 1500 ml but as little as 400 ml is required by normal kidneys to excrete metabolic waste.

About 900 ml is lost as sweat and from the lungs so it is essential that 1300 ml of fluid is taken as food and fluid each day to balance this loss. If the rate of fluid loss is increased, then the intake must also be increased to balance it. The body can compensate for a while by water movement out of the cells. The urine becomes concentrated and the skin loses its elasticity and can be pinched into folds. The mouth and tongue feel dry, and there may be a headache.

Potassium is found mainly within the body cells (intracellular) and sodium in the body fluids (extracellular). If insufficient water is available potassium moves out of the cells and into the bloodstream. It is then removed from the blood by the kidneys and lost from the body in urine. Water follows the potassium out of the cells but it is not excreted into the urine. The anti-diuretic hormone acts to ensure it is reabsorbed from the filtrate. The rising level of potassium in the blood eventually causes a variety of symptoms.

If the loss of water lags behind intake, the excess water collects in the tissues. At first it may not be noticed, except as an unexpected increase in body weight. Changes in sodium levels can also lead to water retention. Some women become familiar with the bloated feeling and weight gain in the days before a menstrual period. The water tends to collect in the lowest part of the body. The ankles swell, and pressing firmly with the fingers produces small indentations. This is known as pitting oedema.

If the overload of water becomes severe, fluid may collect in the airways. Diuretic drugs may be used to encourage the kidneys to excrete more urine. Mild diuretics are now available over the chemists counter for women who suffer from pre-menstrual water retention. They should not be taken for long periods as electrolyte imbalance can occur.

Fluids

Plain tap water may taste of the salts which are dissolved in it, such as calcium in hard water areas. Some natural waters contain high levels of fluoride. In foreign countries, if there is poor sanitation, cholera and typhoid are water-borne diseases against which the traveller must take precautions.

Bottled waters are becoming popular. Their sharp taste makes them re-freshing and many are also naturally aerated with carbon dioxide. Soda and tonic waters are traditionally mixed with alcoholic drinks such as whisky and gin.

A 150 ml cup of tea contains tannin, 60 to 280 mg, fluoride and caffeine 50–80 mg. The latter acts as a stimulant on the nervous system, it is also a weak diuretic. A cup of tea may contain more caffeine than a cup of coffee. Adding milk and sugar give it some nutritional value.

Instant coffee contains 20 to 40 mg caffeine in a gram of powder and about 0.6 mg nicotinic acid. Freshly ground coffee may contain more caffeine and tannins. Large quantities of coffee or tea may cause sleeplessness. In some people coffee can increase the incidence of cardiac arrhythmias, such as extra (ectopic) beats. It is also a diuretic. Cola drinks also contain caffeine in amounts between 50 and 200 mg per litre. Colas and drinking chocolate/cocoa contain theobromine and tannin.

Fruit juices provide vitamin C in varying quantities. The citrus fruits provide more than pineapple or tomato juice (see Table 3.8). They also contain high levels of potassium, and apart from tomato juice, little sodium.

Fruit squashes and crushes may have vitamin C added, but in general they provide only sugar, and have less than 9 mmol/litre of potassium. Their main value is in adding taste to water. Fizzy (aerated) drinks may cause belching because of the gas they contain. This may provide relief from nausea or indigestion.

Alcohol

Drinking is a word sometimes associated in western minds with alcohol. It is an important part of some cultures, and the pattern of drinking may vary between women and men. Social drinking may be normal behaviour in some countries, but in certain cultures abstinence from alcohol is a religious requirement. (See Table 7.1, Section 7.)

Alcohol provides Calories (1 gram yields 7.1 Calories (29.7 kJ). Some forms provide nutrients such as iron in wine and riboflavin in beer. Alcohol can also increase the effects of some drugs, for instance diazepam. It is also under suspicion as adversely affecting the early stages of embryonic development. Pre-natal preparation should include avoiding alcohol, as well as avoiding it during the first three months of pregnancy.

Alcohol, when taken orally, is completely absorbed, partly by the stomach, but mostly by the small intestine. The brain's function is affected by alcohol. It dulls the perception and impairs fine movement, and can induce sleep or even unconsciousness. It therefore makes it dangerous to drive a vehicle or use machinery after drinking alcohol. Surprisingly, few people have a clear idea of the alcohol content of common alcoholic drinks. (Table 4.1.) Some people are more sensitive to the effects of alcohol than others. The variation in this respect appears as great within races as between them.

Ethyl alcohol or ethanol (C_2H_5OH) is clear and colourless, it has a weak smell and a strong burning taste. Vodka is the drink which most closely resembles pure alcohol. All the other alcoholic drinks contain congeners which add flavour and colour and increase the chance of a hangover. The level varies from 3 g per 100 litres in vodka to 285 g per 100 litres in Bourbon.

Table 4.1   Alcohol content of common alcoholic drinks (adapted from the *AA Book of Driving* (1980) by permission of The Automobile Association).

Alcoholic drink	Amount	Blood alcohol mg of alcohol per 100 ml of blood	Breath alcohol μg per 100 ml
Sweet vermouth	1 glass 4 fl. oz.	20	9
Dry vermouth	1 glass 4 fl. oz.	20	9
Sherry	2 fl. oz	20	9
Sherry	4 fl. oz	40	17
Liqueur	1/8 gill	12	5
Port	2 fl. oz	20	9
Whisky	1/6 gill	15	7
Gin & tonic	1/6 gill	15	7
Brandy	1/6 gill	15	7
Rum	1/6 gill	15	7
Vodka & lime	1/6 gill	15	7
Red table wine	4 fl. oz	15	7
White table wine	4 fl. oz	15	7
Sparkling wine	4 fl. oz	16	7
Sparkling wine	6 fl. oz	24	10
Cider	½ pint	20	9
Stout	½ pint	20	9
Export lager	½ pint	20	9
Light ale	½ pint	15	7
Draught bitter	1 pint	30	13
Draught mild	1 pint	25	11

To convert blood alcohol to breath alcohol divide by 2.3 (figure rounded to nearest whole number)

Some wines (e.g. Chianti) contain high levels of tyramine which can trigger a headache in migraine sufferers and those taking monoamine oxidase inhibiting drugs. (MAOIs).

The rate of absorption of alcohol from the stomach and gut varies. It is soluble in both water and lipids, so a fatty meal may slow it down. The presence of carbon dioxide and bicarbonate increase the rate of absorption and sparkling wines like champagne 'go to the head' faster.

Once absorbed, alcohol soon appears on the breath and in the urine, a fact used by the law to decide whether an individual is drunk when driving. Less than 10 per cent is excreted by these routes. The remainder is metabolised by the liver. It is oxidised to acetaldehyde by an enzyme, alcohol dehydrogenase inside the liver cells. In heavy, regular drinkers a second system may be present which can use the acetaldehyde as a source of energy which can pass into the blood for use by the muscles.

The level of alcohol in the blood therefore depends on the liver metabolism, the body weight, the amount of alcohol in the drinks and the time which has elapsed since they were drunk. Table 4.2 illustrates the change over

Table 4.2 Changing levels of alcohol in the blood over different periods of time (adapted from the *AA Book of Driving* (1980) by permission of The Automobile Association).

Total consumed (mg/ml blood)	1 hour	2 hours	3 hours	4 hours	5 hours	6 hours	7 hours	8 hours	
15	0	0	0	0	0	0	0	0	
30	15	0	0	0	0	0	0	0	90 mg = 3 pints draught bitter
45	45	30	15	0	0	0	0	0	
60	60	45	30	15	0	0	0	0	90 mg = 6 glasses of wine
75	75	75	60	45	30	15	0	0	90 mg = 6 gin & tonic
90	90	90	75	60	45	30	15	0	90 mg = 6 vodka & lime
105	105	105	90	75	60	45	30	15	80 mg = 2 schooners of sherry
120	120	120	105	90	75	60	45	30	
135	135	135	135	120	105	90	75	60	
150	150	150	150	135	120	105	90	75	
165	165	165	165	165	150	135	120	105	
180	180	180	180	180	165	150	135	120	
195	195	195	195	195	180	165	150	135	
210	210	210	210	210	210	195	180	165	

Driving affected

OVER LEGAL LIMIT

80 mg/ml

Note:
For 8–10 stone (51–63.5 kg) body weight
Adjust for weight: Above 8–10 stone, deduct 1 hour; below, add 1 hour.

time for a man of 51–63.5 kg (8–10 stone) body weight.

If planning to drive after drinking, it is important to stop drinking in sufficient time for the liver to deal with the alcohol before leaving. The legal limit in the blood is 80 mg per 100 ml blood. The new breath alcohol limit as measured in a police station is 34 μg per 100 ml. As even small amounts of alcohol impair judgement, the driving organisations advise people not to drive at all after taking alcohol.

Several anti-diabetic drugs e.g. chlorpropamide inhibit alcohol breakdown and cause an accumulation of acetaldehyde which leads to nausea, vomiting, headache and a fall in blood pressure.

Effects of alcohol

The blood vessels dilate at the skin surface increasing the rate of heat loss and reducing the body temperature. People have died of exposure after staying out in the open overnight while very drunk.

Some drinks such as brandy, gin, whisky, rum and liqueurs contain high levels of alcohol (up to 40 per cent) and this can cause gastric irritation with an increase in gastric juice production. If severe, any vomit may contain traces of blood.

At blood alcohol levels over 50 mg per 100 ml blood there is euphoria, increased self confidence and decreased inhibitions. Attention is easily lost and judgement decreases as co-ordination decreases. Driving skills are affected at 30 mg per 100 ml blood and by the time the legal limit of 80 mg is reached the impairment is serious. The mood can change very quickly, reaction time lengthens and co-ordination may be poor so that staggering occurs. Nausea or a strong desire to lie down may occur.

Confusion sets in with blood alcohol levels of about 100 mg per 100 ml blood. There may be dizziness and exaggerated emotions such as fear or anger. Pain sensation decreases. Perception changes, balance is impaired and the speech slurred. At levels over 250 mg apathy occurs, there is a marked lack of response to stimuli. The individual cannot stand or walk. There may be vomiting, incontinence and deep sleep or stupor. Alcohol levels over 500 mg can lead to death from respiratory paralysis or inhalation of vomit while unconscious. Sadly, each year young men die after a stag night's drinking.

Hangovers

The congeners which add flavour to alcoholic drinks seem to be connected with the severity of the headache and nausea which constitute the hangover. Brandy produces the worst type of hangover, followed by red wine, rum, whisky, white wine and gin. Vodka produces the least effect.

Pure alcohol is used in preparing tissues for staining as it draws out water from the cells. Not surprisingly, alcohol produces thirst. Part of the dull headache of a hangover may be due to dehydration. Drinking one or two glasses of water after the evening's alcohol may reduce the severity of the next morning's symptoms.

Fructose has been claimed as a beneficial pick-me-up in the morning. Fruit such as apples and pears contain more than apricots and peaches. Several large glasses of fruit juice may help, they will also aid rehydration.

Alcoholism

According to Reed (1983) response to alcohol varies between individuals. Regular drinking of alcohol produces a reduced response to the same quantity, or tolerance. Larger quantities are then needed to produce the same effect. The liver cells also increase the level of enzymes available to break down the ethanol. Heavy drinkers acquire tolerance. People in some occupations may tend to drink more than others for instance, printers, journalists, barmen and publicans.

In alcoholism, there is a compulsion or craving for alcohol, and the pattern of daily drinking becomes established. The nightly drinking session may be reinforced by lunchtime alcohol. Drinking takes a high priority over other activities, and may feature frequently in conversation. The typical intake would be 8 pints beer, a bottle of wine or 4 doubles of spirits each day.

The effect of alcohol on the nervous system becomes apparent when the blood alcohol level drops. There may be shakiness, sweating and nausea. Then the 'hair of the dog' is required before normal activities are possible. Drinking may be hidden and great ingenuity may be used to avoid detection at home or at work. Sexual impotence may increase marital strain.

Some people confine their drinking to binges, which may last for several days. There may be periods of amnesia or 'blackouts' afterwards. The blood alcohol may take two or more days to drop. If food has not been taken, there may be hypoglycaemia or acute gastritis. Regular weekend bingers risk inflammation of the pancreas. They may draw attention to a problem by Monday morning absenteeism from their job.

Large intakes of alcohol blunt the appetite, as does the resultant gastritis. Vitamin deficiences may occur, protein intake may be inadequate and infections may take longer to fight off. Strong (1983) claims that one in five men admitted to medical wards has problems related to drink. The incoordination of a person when drunk increases the accident rate. The loss of self control may lead to fights and subsequent cuts, bruises and head injuries. It may also result in petty crime.

The alcoholic who is suddenly cut off from his regular alcohol supplies when in hospital may get severe withdrawal symptoms (delirium tremens). They start when the blood alcohol approaches zero and include agitation, shaking, confusion, seeing things, (more often creeping insects than pink elephants) or hearing voices. This may go on to major fits within 24 hours of abstinence.

Alcoholics may be thought of as suffering from an illness or being locked into destructive patterns of behaviour which provide emotional pay offs for the individual (games). They have a need for emotional 'strokes'. These vary from physically being touched and held to symbolic ones such as praise or recognition. Those who cannot get a warm 'Hello, how are you' may settle for a 'Go to hell' rather than receive nothing. Steiner (1971) describes three types and suggests therapeutic approaches.

(1) Drunk:
'Drunk and proud of it'

He makes any rescuer feel foolish or angry. He rarely drinks at home, but under the influence of alcohol will engage in extracurricular activities such as gambling and extramarital affairs. The game is often played by executives and salesmen to punish a dominating partner. Young men may use it to get back at an overprotective/angry mother. This alcoholic rarely seeks treatment, but may be pushed into it by their partner. Family therapy, or serious threats of divorce unless the drinking stops, are often the only effective alternatives.

(2) Lush:
'Nobody loves me'

The middle-aged, suburban wife, the ageing male homosexual or the downtrodden hardworking white collar worker may lack affection/emotional 'strokes' or be sexually deprived. This alcoholic drinks at home then goes out in search of 'strokes'/emotional fulfilment. Treatment may be accepted, the 'strokes'/attention of the therapist substituting for those missing from the partner. Not surprisingly, the lush turns back to drink as therapy draws to a close. Both partners need to be treated or a new mutual 'stroking' relationship set up which may mean they divorce and marry others, or attend self-help groups, which provide a source of 'strokes' from group members.

(3) Wino:
'Ain't it awful'

The commonest picture of the alcoholic, bent on self-destruction, using body tissue damage to get attention. He plays 'ain't it awful' over the police arrest and court appearance when in fact the night in a cell has provided a roof over his head and breakfast. When sober, he can decide not to play this game. Treatment is unlikely to be successful without a place to live, an occupation and the will to be sober. To smile at the tales of drinking binges reinforces the self-destructive pattern. Avoid expressing pity or empathy and instead insist the alcoholic take responsibility for his own behaviour.

Alcoholics who respond to treatment achieve a long period of abstinence or moderate social drinking. They lose their preoccupation with alcohol and change the pattern of their activities away from pubs, clubs or drinking places to non-alcohol based enjoyment.

Some alcoholics join a self-help organisation such as Alcoholics Anonymous. Its members consider alcoholism a disease, and help each other follow 12 steps to recovery. It seems to be more effective for the type of person who accepts authority. Alanon groups are available to help the families of alcoholics deal with the problems of living with an alcoholic.

General assessment areas

Volume of fluid drunk each day
Type of fluid drunk, alcohol, calorie content
Likes and dislikes, allergies/sensitivities
Religious or cultural beliefs about drinking
Urine output, continence
Thirst
Swallowing difficulties
Discomfort when swallowing
Ability to raise hand to mouth
Ability to grip a glass or cup
Body position
Pain associated with drinking
Ability to close mouth/suck
History of head/neck or oesophageal surgery
Colour of oral mucosa
Condition of tongue and gums
Emotional response when offered fluids
Feelings of weakness or lethargy

Problems

	Page
Unable to drink sufficient fluid to balance fluid loss	127
Frightened to swallow fluids	128
Dehydration	130
Unable to swallow due to local obstruction or loss of swallowing reflex	133
Unable to drink independently	136
Drinking excessive amounts of alcohol	137
Drinking excessive amounts of non-alcoholic fluids (polydipsia)	139
Learning to restrict daily fluid intake	141
Dependence on intravenous fluids	142
Dependence on naso-gastric feeding	145

Potential problems

Cheating on therapeutic fluid intake prescription	148
Risk of sodium imbalance	149
Risk of potassium imbalance	151
Risk of renal damage from low fluid intake	152
Risk of dehydration	154
Risk of alcohol withdrawal symptoms	156

Problems

Problem	**Unable to drink sufficient fluid to balance fluid loss.**

Assessment findings Increased loss of fluid in: glycosuria
sweating
diuresis
drainage
vomiting
rapid respirations

Fluid output exceeds intake
Dry skin, decreased perspiration
Dry mouth making swallowing or speaking difficult
Rising body temperature
Body weight falls
Thirst
Headache
Specific gravity of urine over 1.030
Low urine output
Constipation
Glycosuria
Recent large alcohol intake
Fluid likes and dislikes
Certain oral fluids unsuitable

Information for the patient

The body needs water every day so that the blood can circulate oxygen and food to the tissues. The cells in the tissues need water to be able to work normally. We all lose water as sweat and water vapour when we breathe out, as well as in urine which carries away waste products. If the amount of water lost from the body is greater than that taken in, then the body takes emergency action. Thirst prompts the person to drink more. The water available in the body is moved from the skin to keep up the fluid content of the blood. If water loss is severe, the skin loses its elasticity and can be pinched into folds.

Drinking little and often will help replace the fluid and keep up with the loss from sweating and breathing. It is important that the minimum water intake matches the water lost from the body.

If the brain becomes short of water, a headache can start. A hangover is partly caused by a shortage of water in the brain.

Nursing actions

1. Discuss fluid preference and medical advice on the suitability of oral fluids with the patient, or a relative acting for the patient. Request their co-operation in planning intake.

RE. Monitor their level of co-operation and their understanding of which fluids are suitable.

2. Estimate the minimum oral fluid intake required for 24 hours. Divide the total by the number of hours the patient is expected to be awake to work out how much they will need each hour. Plan to offer small frequent drinks of at least 100 to 200 ml per hour.

RE. Record the patient's fluid intake and compare it with output and the urine specific gravity. Plan the daily pattern of drinks to maintain the fluid balance. Readjust if necessary every 6–12 hours. Record the body weight and total volume drunk each day.

127

3. Provide variety in the temperature and type of fluids. Iced water, squash or fruit juice can be more refreshing than hot, milky drinks.

RE. Observe for signs of reluctance to drink proffered fluids.

4. Provide mouthwashes until fluid replacement reverses dry mouth.

RE. Observe the mouth every 6–12 hours to see if dryness decreases. Ask the patient to report on changes in swallowing or speaking.

5. Provide a quiet, darkened area with cold compresses to the forehead to soothe any headache.

RE. Ask patient to report change in their headache.

Further action	1. Intravenous fluid prescription will depend on the degree of dehydration and its likely duration. For the short term, alternating 500 ml 5% dextrose with 500 ml 0.9% saline will be sufficient. For regimes lasting over 48 hours, the electrolyte content may need to be adjusted.

RE. Record all fluid intake and output. Blood samples may be taken to monitor electrolyte balance, particularly potassium (K^+) and sodium (Na^+).

2. Rapid rates of infusion carry a risk of circulatory overload if renal function is poor, or of water intoxication in the elderly.

RE. For patients at risk, check blood pressure and pulse rate at least hourly for any increase. If an epileptiform fit occurs slow the infusion to a sufficient rate to 'keep the vein open' and call medical aid.

3. Naso-gastric feeds may be prescribed if gastric absorption is satisfactory. A fine-bore naso-gastric tube may be passed into the stomach, or into the jejunum. If it is to the jejunum, the position should be checked by X-ray. Up to 2.5 litres of fluid may be given by continuous drip feed at room temperature. A volumetric pump may be used to control the rate of flow. Oral fluids may continue, as the fine tube rarely interferes with swallowing.

RE. Record fluid intake and output, and, if nausea or vomiting occurs, stop the feed for an hour. If symptoms subside, check the tube is in the stomach by insufflating air, restart the feed and observe for re-occurrence every ¼ hour for the next hour.

Associated medical diagnoses	Diabetes mellitus Diabetes insipidus Dysentery Oesophageal stricture Oral carcinoma Paralytic ileus Senility

---

Problem	**Frightened to swallow fluids**

Assessment findings	Low fluid intake Tense facial expression when fluids offered Limits intake to small sips Able to swallow saliva Recent swallowing difficulties

Recent episode of choking
Treatment for neuro-muscular disorders
Marked distress over urinary incontinence
Extreme fear — suspect rabies/tetanus
Severe dyspnoea

Information for the patient

Most people do not have to think about swallowing except when they have an illness which interferes with the way the throat and gullet work. The brain controls the different steps involved in swallowing. If something stops the nerves passing on the messages correctly then fluid might go down the wrong way. The doctor will not give permission for fluids to be taken until it is safe to do so. It is wise to try taking fluids slowly and carefully. Small amounts of water, not too hot or cold, are the safest way to get started. The patient should take their time, concentrate and remember that if saliva can be swallowed, so can water. A nurse will be happy to stay with the patient until they feel confident that everything is working well.

Nursing actions

1. Discuss what sensations the patient experiences when asked to drink. Suggest that cool water is the safest fluid to drink if there is a fear of choking.

RE. Observe for facial or body tension during discussion. Assess whether the patient accepts a suggestion of cool water.

2. Stay with the patient when fluids are being swallowed. Sit the patient upright to drink. Have suction equipment near bed. Suggest small amounts (15–30 ml) are taken at a time. A dessertspoonful may be more acceptable than a cup. Record the amount swallowed on a fluid chart.

RE. Observe swallowing as it takes place. Describe and report specific difficulties if they occur. Record fluid intake and output. Assess whether the daily fluid intake from all routes reaches the minimum level required.

3. Provide encouragement before and after swallowing is attempted, but do not distract the patient's concentration while swallowing.

RE. Assess whether the patient's level of confidence changes.

4. Increase the range of fluids as their confidence level increases. Slowly withdraw encouragement before swallowing attempts, and then increase the distance from the patient as drinking becomes less of an emotional matter.

RE. Assess the level of the patient's confidence in their ability to cope unaided while drinking.

5. Make a plain water ice lolly with a plastic medicine glass (water expands on freezing and could crack a glass one) and orange stick. Suggest that the frozen water will numb the back of the throat, so making swallowing more comfortable. It is also easier to control the rate and amount of fluid taken.

RE. Assess the patient's response. If positive consider adding jelly, ice cream and other semi-solids to the diet. Record the volume taken on the fluid chart.

Further action

1. Essential drugs may be prescribed as injections, suppositories, or aerosols.

RE. Review the patient's drug chart with the doctor at least weekly to keep the number of injections to a minimum.

2. Intravenous therapy or enteral feeding may be required if oral fluid intake fails to supply sufficient fluid volume and nutrients to meet the body's requirements.

RE. Weigh the patient at least twice a week. Observe for signs of developing dehydration.

Associated medical diagnoses

Bulbar palsy
Carcinoma of oesophagus
Cerebral vascular accident
Dementia
Globus hystericus
Glossopharyngeal nerve damage
Hiatus hernia
Myasthenia gravis
Oesophago-tracheal fistula
Oesophageal stricture
Paranoia
Parkinson's disease
Tracheostomy

Problem

Dehydration

Assessment findings

Thirst
Dry skin, perspiration ceases
Skin can be pinched into folds
Eyes appear sunken
Low urine output (under 300 ml in 24 hours)
Urine dark in colour, high specific gravity (1.030 or over)
Mouth feels dry — may look dry, with brown tongue
Hard, dry stools
Rising body temperature
Falling blood pressure
Pulse weakens
Increased haemoglobin and haematocrit
Increased serum potassium
Confusion
Aggression
Ability to hold and raise a glass or cup
Unable to hold and raise a glass or cup.

Information for the patient

When the body becomes short of water it affects the volume of the blood. As this could have a drastic affect on the circulation, it moves water out of the body cells and starts to decrease the normal water loss. Thirst is one way of trying to encourage fluid replacement!

To save water, sweating stops and without its cooling action the body temperature goes up and the skin feels dry. The amount of water in the urine starts to fall so it looks darker and more concentrated. The bowels reabsorb more water so the stools get hard and dry. As water moves out of the cells, they lose their normal firmness and become flabby. This can be seen by the way skin will pinch up into folds.

Nursing actions

1. Discuss the types of fluid the patient prefers. Estimate the minimum oral intake needed for the day. Plan out the amount of fluid to be offered in each

hour. Calculate the water intake from food, and include this in the estimation of total fluid intake.

RE. Assess whether the severity of the dehydration will require waking the patient to enable them to take the planned volume. Assess their level of thinking or confusion if present.

2. Select the most suitable container, according to the patient's ability to hold a cup or beaker and raise it to their lips.

RE. Observe how well the patient can pick up and drink from the chosen container. Light plastic beakers are easier to hold and lift than cups, but may be considered childish by the patient. Straws increase the amount of air swallowed, which can cause gastric distension.

3. Give the patient 50–100 ml fluid to drink at a time. Record the volume drunk on a fluid chart.

RE. Check actual intake against planned intake at least 4 hourly. Revise planned amounts if necessary.

4. If a fan is used to reduce the patient's body temperature by increasing the rate of sweat evaporation, increase the intake by at least 500 ml.

RE. Check oral or rectal temperature hourly. Stop fanning when temperature falls to 38°C, to limit water lost through sweating.

5. Calculate total fluid intake against output and insensible loss every 24 hours. (Water lost in sweat (900 ml) and as vapour from lungs (400 ml) is termed insensible loss; it is increased by fever or rapid respirations.)

RE. Intake should exceed output by 2000 ml until dehydration is corrected, and skin turgor improves. The specific gravity of the urine should be measured twice daily to see if there is a decrease. Check the pulse and blood pressure every six hours. Weigh daily to assess weight gain.

6. Clean the patient's mouth with sodium bicarbonate solution, and refresh with mouthwash. Apply vaseline or lip salve to dry lips.

RE. Inspect the mouth and tongue daily as indicators of rehydration.

7. Consider giving rectal fluids if dehydration is severe and medical aid is unavailable.

RE. This is unlikely to be successful where diarrhoea, aggression or confusion are present.

8. Avoid giving disposable enemas, high fibre foods and faecal softeners, all of which reduce the water available to the body, until signs of dehydration abate.

RE. Record the number and consistency of bowel actions. Hard, dry faeces may be passed after rehydration has been achieved.

Further action

1. Intravenous fluids will be prescribed if dehydration is severe, or if oral fluids cannot be swallowed or absorbed. If the veins of the hand or forearm are not collapsed (which they may be in old or severely dehydrated patients) they are the most likely site for the infusion. A small needle or cannula is

inserted into a vein and attached to a plastic giving set, primed with the prescribed fluid. Adhesive tape and any bandages used to keep it in place should not encircle the limb. The limb should be kept warm to promote venous dilatation.

RE. Check the site of the cannula for leakage, local swelling or discomfort at least two hourly. Make sure there is no strain on tubing, or kinking.

2. Short term rehydration (up to 48 hours) is usually achieved with a regime of 500 ml 5% dextrose alternated with 500 ml 0.9% saline. Up to 3 litres in 24 hours may be prescribed. At such rapid rates there is a risk of circulatory overload if renal or cardiac failure is present. In the elderly, water intoxication is an occasional complication.

RE. Regulate the infusion rate according to the prescription. Consider using a burette or volumetric pump if the flow rate is variable. Record fluid intake and output. Monitor the blood pressure and pulse rate for any increase at least every two hours if rapid fluid administration is under way. If an epileptiform fit occurs, slow the infusion to 'keep the vein open' and call medical aid.

3. Rehydration over 48 hours may require adjustment of the electrolyte content of the intravenous fluid.

RE. Blood samples may be taken by the doctor for sodium (Na^+) and potassium (K^+) levels or haematocrit. Normal volumes are:
Na^+ 135 to 150 mmol/1
K^+ 3.6 to 5.5 mmol/1
Packed cell-volume 47%

4. If potassium supplements are added to the intravenous fluid, mix throughly to avoid giving a high concentration at the start of the bottle, and so risking cardiac disturbance.

RE. Measure any leakage and also if the patient has diarrhoea, and record the amount on the fluid balance chart. Inform doctor so potassium intake and loss can be recalculated.

5. Subcutaneous fluids may be given occasionally if no peripheral veins are available. The administration sets are attached to small needles inserted under the skin. Hyalase may be added to increase tissue permeability by dissolving the cementing material (hyaluronic acid) between the connecting tissues.

RE. Monitor the rate of flow at frequent intervals. Check for an increase in local swelling around needle tips or leakage, indicating reduced absorption. Observe for local infection at needle sites.

Associated medical diagnoses

Addison's disease
Alcohol poisoning
Chronic renal disease
Cerebral injury
Dementia
Diabetes insipidus
Hyperglycaemia
Senile dementia
Sunstroke

Problem	**Unable to swallow due to local obstruction or loss of swallowing reflex.**

Assessment findings

Saliva pools in mouth
Coughing or choking on fluid
Saliva dribbles from the mouth
Difficulty in opening mouth
Painful muscle spasm (such as occurs in tetanus)
Speech difficulties
No swallowing reflex
Poor or no control of tongue and palate
Muscle wasting

Information for the patient

Swallowing requires that the nerves and muscles work *together* to pass fluid back off the tongue and into the gullet. From the gullet, waves of muscle action push the fluid along towards the stomach. Damage to the nerves which control swallowing anywhere along their path from the brain to the gullet can interfere with the process. The small flap which closes over the windpipe as fluid passes into the gullet may also be affected so that the fluid 'goes down the wrong way' and causes coughing. The saliva is being made all the time, but its flow increases at mealtimes. If it cannot be swallowed it must be collected to prevent choking or coughing. The doctor will decide how food and fluid will be given.

Nursing actions

1. Position so that saliva cannot pool at the back of the mouth. Sit the patient up with their head forward if they are well enough. A lateral or semi-prone position may be adopted with the head of the bed tipped down 15–30 degrees if the patient is weak or has a reduced level of consciousness.

RE. Check the patient's position uses gravity to drain saliva towards lips, so that it does not collect in the throat. Coughing or choking should then decrease.

2. Suction apparatus with a catheter or suction tip should be available near the patient for immediate use if the patient starts to cough or choke.

RE. Record the frequency of the use of suction, and patient's reaction. Check and clean the equipment at least once a day.

3. Provide adequate nutrition by the prescribed route, and note the amount given.

RE. Weigh the patient every 2 days to check that their Calorie and fluid intake is sufficient to maintain a steady body weight.

4. Check all visitors understand that they must not give the patient fluid or food. An interpreter should be used when English is not the first language as a precaution against misunderstanding.

RE. Observe the visitors fequently if there is any doubt that they may fail to comply with the request not to feed the patient.

5. Apply petroleum jelly or lip salve to the lips and the skin around the mouth to prevent excoriation from constant wetting by saliva.

RE. Check the lips and skin for redness or early excoriation.

6. Provide soft tissues and a polythene bag for disposal or make a wick of ribbon gauze to drain saliva into a small receiver. A thick towel or pad of absorbent material under the chin can be used during sleep. (Incontinence pads have a polythene backing and could cause suffocation)

RE. Check the amount of saliva lost by weighing 20 dry tissues and a polythene bag. Weigh the bag of used tissues, subtract the weight of the dry tissues to find out the weight of saliva. (5.06 g = 5 ml saliva) or measure the volume in the receiver. Record on the patient's fluid chart.

7. Discuss with the patient how they feel about being unable to swallow. Check if there are any times of the day or activities which cause them discomfort or fear.

RE. Observe for increased tension or distress.

Further action

1. Oesophagoscopy under local anaesthetic with a fibre optic instrument may be undertaken to inspect for, and biopsy, any obstruction. The flexible instrument is less likely to cause an oesophageal tear than the rigid type.

RE. Check that the patient had understood the doctor's explanation and signed consent form. Nothing should be given by mouth until the gag reflex returns after anaesthesia; this may take up to 6 hours. Test for it by touching back of throat with a spatula.

2. Intra-gastric feeding through a fine-bore naso-gastric tube passed into the the stomach allows up to 2.5 litres of fluid to be given by continuous drip. Position of the catheter tip can be checked by X-ray. See 'Dependence on intravenous fluids' on page 142. The feed should be given at room temperature. A volumetric pump may be used to control the rate of flow. Mark the catheter where it enters the nostril.

RE. Record all fluid intake and output. Fluid cannot be aspirated from the gut through a fine-bore tube, but air can be insufflated to confirm position. Ask the patient to report any discomfort due to the temperature of their feed. Check catheter mark at least 6 hourly to identify any change in the position of the tube. Check pump is delivering the fluid at the rate set and that the tubing is not kinked or clogged with feed.

3. If nausea or vomiting occur, stop the feed for 1 hour.

RE. If symptoms subside re-start the pump. Observe for recurrence every 15 minutes throughout the next hour. Report to the doctor if symptoms return.

4. Milk-based foods prepared by the local dietetic department may be cheaper than commercial products. Continuous drip feeds through a fine-bore naso-gastric tube are less likely to cause diarrhoea than bolus feeds, especially if these are given cold.

RE. Record the frequency and consistency of bowel actions. Diarrhoea may be due to concurrent antibiotic therapy, infected feeds, malabsorption, or rarely, to lactose intolerance. (Most tinned foods are lactose free).

5. Total parenteral nutrition (TPN) may be given through an intravenous catheter. To dilute potentially irritant solutions, the tip is usually sited in the superior vena cava via the sub-clavian vein. Strict aseptic technique must be used. The position is checked by X-ray. Mark the insertion point on the catheter.

RE. Check there is no strain or kinking of catheter and that it is covered by a clean dressing. Observe for leakage from the hub, as cracking can occur. Monitor the patient's vital signs for infection; a rigor may indicate septicaemia. Pain, cyanosis, or difficulty breathing indicate pneumothorax, requiring immediate medical aid.

6. The prescription of fluid volume, electrolytes, vitamins, fats and minerals, may vary daily according to the patient's condition. Feeds need to be ordered in good time from the pharmacist.

RE. Record fluid intake and output. Test the patient's urine for glucose every 6 hours as over ½% for two successive specimens may indicate faulty infusion regulation, allowing fluid overload. Weigh the patient in the same clothes at the same time each day. Observe for oedema.

7. Gastrostomy feeding is less frequently prescribed these days. A catheter is inserted through the abdominal wall into the stomach, under a general anaesthetic. 'Stomahesive' may be used around the insertion point. Feeds may be prescribed for continuous flow or for use at intervals. A large bore tube may allow diluted pureed food or milk based foods to be given.

RE. Check at least daily for leakage around insertion point, as leakage of gastric juice can burn the surrounding skin. Record frequency and consistency of bowel actions, especially if milk based feeds are given. Assess the patient's interest in their condition as they may eventually feel strong enough to learn to feed themselves via the tube. Chewing food and spitting it out can stimulate gastric secretion.

8. Intubation of the oesophagus, using a tube with a fixed lumen, may be used to maintain a passage for fluids around an obstruction. Insertion is usually under general anaesthetic.

RE. Observe for signs of pain or discomfort after insertion. Commence fluids with the agreement of the doctor. Pureed foods may be possible later. Record the fluid intake and output.

9. Drugs may be specifically prescribed to be given in the enteral or gastrostomy feeds or by intravenous or intramuscular injection. No drugs should be given via a TPN line.

RE. Check the compatibility of the drugs and the feed with the pharmacist.

Associated medical diagnoses	Aortic aneurysm
	Bulbar palsy
	Cerebral vascular accident
	Carcinoma
	Cerebral palsy
	Cervical instability
	Enlarged mediastinal lymph nodes
	Foreign body in oesophagus
	Goitre
	Motor neurone disease
	Myesthenia gravis
	Pharyngeal paralysis from glossopharyngeal damage (9th cranial nerve)
	Poliomyelitis
	Post-oesophagectomy

Quinsy (tonsillitis, resulting in an abscess near the tonsil)
Tetanus
Vagal nerve damage

Problem	Unable to drink independently

Assessment findings

Unable to grasp container
Unable to raise container to mouth
Unable to steady container so that fluid spills
Loss of control of lips or tongue
Thirst
Low fluid intake and urine output
Concentrated urine
Constipation
Confusion
Apathy
Loss of skin turgor
Able to swallow
Usual pattern of drinks
Preferred type and variety
Age
Receiving phenothiazines

Information for the patient

The body needs regular fluids to make up for those lost in sweat, urine and the water vapour in every breath. Elderly people may be short of fluid, but not feel the warning signs such as thirst. The nurses will plan out the amounts of fluid that should normally be taken and any extra drinks needed to make up fluid shortages. They can advise on the types of fluid as anyone who tends to get overweight easily has to watch the Calories contained in sweetened fruit squashes and milk. Some types of fluid may interfere with the action of drugs. Alcohol is normally allowed only with the doctor's permission. The nurses will help with drinking and keep a check on the amount taken.

Nursing action

1. Identify the minimum desirable fluid intake for each 24 hours, and plan out the frequency and variety of fluids acceptable to the patient. Include drinks during the night time only if these are part of the usual pattern.

RE. Chart the amount of fluid given to the patient, and keep a running total until the fluid intake is sufficient to meet tissue needs. Compare intake and output. Tell the patient how close they are to reaching the agreed intake.

2. Assess the range of available containers for giving the patient fluid. Consider using a syringe, beaker, cup, spoon or invalid feeder. Provide protection for clothing during feeding.

RE. Check the acceptability of these to the patient. Record any changes in the method of feeding in the care plan.

3. If right-handed, stand slightly to the left of the patient to give fluids in small amounts, allowing pauses for breaths. (other side for left-handed nurses)

RE. Observe the patient's ease of swallowing and their willingness to drink.

4. Consider whether independence would be possible if a suitable aid was available. Seek advice from an occupational therapist.

RE. Monitor for changes in ability to drink sufficient fluids for normal hydration to be maintained.

Further action

1. Tremor may be treated by withdrawing phenothiazines, or administering levodopa combined with carbidopa (Sinemet) to raise the levels of dompamine in the brain of those with Parkinsonism. The dose is increased over about 7 days until the symptoms improve. It should not be given within two weeks of stopping monoamine oxidase inhibiting drugs. Administration should be stopped at least 8 hours before any surgery.

RE. Record blood pressure at least daily if Sinemet is given. MAOI drug usage may lead to severely raised blood pressure. Drugs to control hypertension may have their action enhanced, and postural hypotension also occur as a side effect. Check rate and character of pulse daily. Observe for other side effects such as insomnia, agitation, dizziness, anorexia, nausea, vomiting, cardiac rhythm disorders, difficulty in passing urine or incontinence.

Associated medical diagnoses

Anxiety
Arteriosclerosis
Bulbar palsy
Cerebral vascular accident
Fractured radius/ulna
Fractured humerus
Frozen shoulder
Multiple sclerosis
Myasthenia gravis
Parkinson's disease
Poliomyelitis
Prolapsed intervertebral disc
Schizophrenia
Senile dementia
Spasticity

Problem

Drinking excessive amounts of alcohol

Assessment findings

Alcohol intake exceeds equivalent of 4 pints beer a day
Smell of alcohol on breath
Broad, unsteady gait on walking
Impaired fine finger movement
Nightmares
Frequent use of stimulants such as coffee and cigarettes
Blood alcohol level over 150 mg per 100 ml blood
Hallucinations
Fits
At risk groups : journalists, printers, publicans, merchant seamen, senior business executives, doctors.

Information for the patient

The body deals with alcohol by breaking it down in the liver at a steady rate, after which it moves into the water and fat within the body tissues. It also acts on the nerves, slowing the rate at which they can pass on their messages to and from the muscles. It interferes with the dreaming type of sleep (REM sleep) so that when a high level of alcohol in the blood drops, the rebound may produce vivid dreams or even nightmares. It acts as a poison in large doses or if taken regularly in large amounts. It can lead to damage to

137

the nerves, brain, liver, heart and to stomach ulcers. Nursing staff are happy to advise any patient needing help to control a drinking problem, or they will put them in touch with specialist staff.

Nursing action

1. Warn the patient that in hospital they must not drink alcohol without the permission of the doctor as it is dangerous, because it may interact with drug treatment and test results.

RE. Observe for behaviour that may indicate the patient is not complying with the ban on alcohol. Chronic alcoholics are usually adept at hiding their supplies. Frequent visits to the toilet may indicate a bottle hidden in the cistern. Sudden changes in mood may indicate alcohol has been taken. Report suspicions to the doctor so that a blood sample may be taken for alcohol estimation and any drug therapy reviewed.

2. Provide a high protein, high carbohydrate diet if there is any indication of poor dietary habits. Drinking may blunt the appetite and snack food taken in the past may have been low in vitamins.

RE. Observe how much and what types of food the patient eats. Tissue healing rates may be delayed if malnutrition has been prolonged.

3. Provide citrus fruit juice, iced water or milk to rehydrate and reduce a hangover if the patient has been drinking prior to treatment.

RE. Watch for drinking of unusually large quantities of coffee, cola drinks or other stimulants.

Further action

1. Liver function may be assessed through blood tests to identify damage. Fasting is not required before these tests.

RE. Pressure over needle sites should continue beyond the usual 2 minutes after infection as an increased tendency to bleed for longer than normal may lead to bruising. Normal blood biochemistry levels include serum bilirubin 3–17 mmol/1, serum proteins; albumin/globulin ratio 1.2:2.4, total albumin 3.4–50 g/l and total globulin 16–37 g/l. Prothrombin time 10–14 seconds.

2. Drug therapy should be reviewed, as many drugs interact with alcohol. The anticoagulant effect of warfarin is increased, phenytoin and metronidazole produce a reaction similar to that of disulfiram (Antabuse) in which a toxic level of the drug builds up in the blood.

RE. Report any increased bruising, suddenly flushed face or rapid pulse after giving these drugs.

3. Chlormethiazole orally or occasionally by infusion may be used to control symptoms of withdrawal from alcohol, such as shaking, swelling and delirium tremens. A volumetric pump should be used to control the rate of intravenous therapy. The drug is normally given at a rate sufficient to cause sleep; if too much is given, the patient becomes unconscious, with all the risks that this entails.

RE. Report if the level of drowsiness interferes with daily activities while taking oral chlormethiazole. Observe vital signs every 30 to 60 minutes during intravenous treatment.

4. Fits due to hepatic encephalopathy may be treated with lactulose to induce diarrhoea, so limiting the absorption of ammonia from bacterial break-

down of gut contents. A dose of 30 to 50 ml can be given three times a day, and adjusted to produce three soft stools a day once diarrhoea has occurred. Neomycin is usually given to destroy the bacteria in the gut.

RE. Record the time and a description of each fit. Note the time of onset of diarrhoea so the dose of lactulose can be adjusted. Record each bowel action, describe consistency and report any marked change. Severe diarrhoea may reduce potassium levels in the body.

5. Gastroscopy or barium studies may be ordered if bleeding from the stomach or oesophagus has occurred.

RE. Record any blood in vomitus (haematemesis) or dark, tarry faeces (melaena).

Associated medical diagnoses	Alcoholic cardiomyopathy
	Alcoholic cerebral degeneration
	Anaemia
	Blackouts
	Carcinoma of oesophagus
	Carcinoma of stomach
	Cirrhosis of liver
	Duodenal ulcer
	Folate and Vitamin B deficiency
	Gastritis
	Head injury
	Hepatic encephalopathy
	Hepatitis
	Hypothermia
	Infertility
	Korsakoff's psychosis
	Myopathy
	Oesophageal varices
	Pancreatitis
	Peptic ulcer
	Peripheral neuropathy
	Polyneuritis
	Portal hypertension
	Wernicke's encephalopathy

Problem	**Drinking excessive amounts of non-alcoholic fluids (polydipsia)**
Assessment findings	Oral fluid intake exceeds 4–5 litres
	Marked thirst
	Craving for fluid is so strong that inappropriate liquids are consumed if access is limited, e.g. drinking water from a flower vase.
	Urine output exceeds 5 litres
	Sleep disturbed by thirst
	Glycosuria
	Specific gravity of urine over 1028
	Specific gravity of urine below 1003.
Information for the patient	The body has a hormone which acts on the kidneys to help keep water from being lost in large volumes. This antidiuretic hormone is influenced by the pituitary area of the brain. If too little hormone is produced, or the kidneys

no longer respond to it, water is lost in the urine. This means frequent visits to the toilet to pass large amounts of dilute urine. The body reacts to this loss by thirst. A careful watch on the amount of urine passed and the amount drunk allows the doctors to assess the response to treatment.

Nursing actions

1. Provide iced water or dilute fruit squashes. Record fluid intake and urine output. Provide more fluid than is lost in the urine.

RE. Weigh the patient daily and calculate their fluid balance. Monitor their general appearance and vital signs for dehydration. Record specific gravity of urine as this may help the doctor in diagnosis.

2. Select a bed near the toilet, or provide extra urinals/commodes/bedpans.

RE. Observe the patient's ability to reach the toilet safely, in spite of urgency to micturate.

3. Provide opportunities for extra rest periods during the day to replace hours lost overnight.

RE. Record periods of sleep during the night and day.

Further action

1. Blood glucose estimation may be undertaken at random if urinary specific gravity is over 1025 and glycosuria is present.

RE. A random blood glucose over 13.9 mmol/litre indicates probable diabetes mellitus.

2. Vasopressin (anti-diuretic hormone) may be given intravenously initially to check the response of the urinary output.

RE. Record fluid intake and output after this has been given; the latter should increase. The hormone may be obtained from the pituitary glands of ox or pig. Check there is no religious objection to a particular source.

3. Desmopressin (DDAP) is a synthetic compound which is absorbed from the mucous membranes inside the nose. It should be sniffed up rather like snuff, the dose being reduced in stages until output just exceeds a normal urine output. The maintenance dose is kept above this level.

RE. Observe that any fluid restriction is followed. Record fluid intake and output.

4. Thirst may be reduced with chlorothiazide, clofibrate or carbamazepine. Chlorothiazide increases sodium excretion so the concentration of body fluids falls. The osmoreceptors in the brain are not stimulated so thirst is reduced. The mode of action of the other drugs is not understood.

RE. Observe and record fluid intake. Clofibrate may cause diarrhoea or painful muscles (myalgia). Carbamazepine may cause nausea, double vision, rashes or dizziness.

Associated medical diagnoses

Diabetes insipidus
Diabetes mellitus
Encephalitis
Hypophysectomy
Meningitis
Panhypopituitarism or Simmond's disease

Pituitary adenoma
Syphilis
Water intoxication in the elderly (low antidiuretic hormone)

Problem	Learning to restrict daily fluid intake
Assessment findings	Oedema Low urine output: less than 100 ml in 24 hours = anuria Medical advice to limit fluid intake to a set figure

Information for the patient	The body's control of water and salts depends on how well the kidneys work. They filter water and salts from the blood (plasma), then reabsorb most of the salts. If the kidneys get damaged by disease, they may not be able to filter properly. Careful control of how much is drunk gives the kidneys less to do, and helps make the most of any undamaged tissue.
	
	   In order to filter the blood the kidneys need a good blood flow. If the heart is under strain, then the amount arriving to be filtered may be too low. The fluid may then collect in the lowest parts of the body, such as the legs, under the influence of gravity.
	
	   Fluid restriction may also be necessary when there is liver damage, as the composition of the blood changes, and fluid collects in the tissues. If the tissues become waterlogged they cannot receive all the oxygen and nutrients they need and healing slows up.

Nursing actions	1. Discuss the reasons for fluid restriction, and the types of fluid allowed. Check the level of the patient's understanding, and co-operation. RE. Observe for signs of frustration or misunderstanding. 2. Ask the patient to assist in planning how their total daily fluid volume should be spaced. Small frequent drinks may limit mouth dryness. Ensure that their drinks are offered on time. RE. Chart fluid intake and output. Monitor body weight daily to detect any 'cheating' in patients with renal failure. Report variations from the set intake. Observe skin turgor, and look for signs of oedema at least once each day. 3. Provide cold mouthwashes to refresh the mouth between drinks. If there is a suspicion that the patient is swallowing some of the mouthwash, measure volume of the mouthwash before going to the patient and then measure what remains afterwards. RE. Ask the patient to report any change in dryness of mouth. Inspect their mouth daily. 4. Provide extra activities to divert the patient from thinking about drinking. RE. Listen for any comments which indicate a preoccupation with the fluid restriction.
Further action	1. The salt, potassium and protein content of the fluids may need to be carefully controlled according to the efficiency of the patient's kidney function. A regime to meet the doctor's prescription may be agreed between the nurse, patient and dietitian. RE. Observe if the patient keeps to the agreed regime. Deviations should be discussed with the dietitian so that so that adjustments may be made in the

141

planned regime. Fluid intake records should include details of the type of fluid taken.

2. The fluid intake volume for 24 hours may be prescribed as 500 ml, plus the volume of the previous day's urinary output.

RE. Measuring cylinders should be used for accuracy. Twenty-four hour urine collections may be required to monitor electrolyte content.

Associated medical diagnoses	Anuria Ascites Cerebral oedema Congestive cardiac failure Hepatic cirrhosis Nephritis Oedema Renal failure Water intoxication

---

Problem	**Dependence on intravenous fluids**
Assessment findings	Restriction of oral fluid intake Dehydration Intravenous fluid intake is prescribed Site of intravenous cannula in relation to joints Type of administration set Type of fluid prescribed Desired rate of infusion Flow rate in relation to position of limb Presence of local redness or exudate around cannula site Pain
Information for the patient	Certain fluids can be given straight into a vein if their strength is carefully controlled. The commonest types of fluid used contain sugars or salts. The needle must lie in the vein and not rest against the vein walls. If the needle moves it may go through the vein wall into the tissues. If this happens there will be swelling, irritation and increasing discomfort. Please tell a nurse if the needle site becomes uncomfortable. It is important that the drip is treated carefully. The position of the arm can affect the rate of flow. If it slows or stops dripping please inform a nurse. Infection could occur if the needle site is touched with the fingers. The nurses will be taking special care when changing the bags/bottles for the same reason. The doctor will prescribe how much fluid is to be given and at what rate. It is important that the flow rate is not interfered with once it is set.
Nursing actions	1. Check the intravenous fluid is free from particles and check the expiry date on the pack. Clear fluids should be clear. Discard an infusion pack if it appears cloudy. Record type of fluid, volume set up, time and batch number. Calculate the flow rate required to administer the volume over the prescribed period. RE. Check the flow rate, especially during the first half hour of a new infusion being started, and after moving the patient. Check their fluid intake and output at least daily. Check the pulse volume and rhythm and the blood pressure at least four times a day if there is a risk of fluid overload.

2. Adjust the patient's limb position to achieve the best flow. If the needle is sited near a joint, use a light splint to limit movement of the limb. 'Netelast' is cooler than a crepe bandage.

RE. Check the flow does not alter when the limb is moved.

3. Ensure venous blood flow is not compressed by tight sleeves, or armholes in nightclothes, tight elastic bandages, or adhesive tape encircling the limb.

RE. Check for local or general swelling in a limb.

4. Ensure that changes in the height of the drip stand do not put tension on the giving set or limit the patient's movements.

RE. Check a safety loop is made when the giving set is anchored. Ask the patient to comment on the comfort of limb position and movement.

5. Replace the giving set at least once in 48 hours and after a blood transfusion is completed if further intravenous fluids are to be given. Cover cannula/needle site with a sterile dressing.

RE. Check the patient's temperature and pulse rate for signs of infection at least twice a day.

6. Use aseptic technique when setting up a new container of fluid. Ensure the giving set is inserted to the same point each time to avoid introducing bacteria.

RE. Check the site of cannula/needle insertion for signs of local infection or swelling at least daily, and if patient complains of pain.

7. Ensure a limb used for intravenous infusion does not become cold especially at night. Blood flow decreases and changes in flow rate occur. A heated pad may be used to warm a limb if clear intravenous fluids are being given.

RE. Check the limb has light warm covering and that the skin feels warm.

8. Assess how much limitation the presence of the infusion will have on the patient's other activities; if necessary the patient can use a mobile drip stand so that they can walk around. Adjust planned care accordingly.

RE. Ask the patient to report any difficulties in reaching items or carrying out activities.

9. Wash and dry the patient's hand at least twice a day if the infusion is sited in the arm. Cover the splint with fresh absorbent material.

RE. Check that the skin on the palm and between the fingers is not becoming macerated by trapped sweat.

Further action

1. Blood may be transfused to raise the haemoglobin level or to replace blood loss. It is given in 'units', each unit contain approximately 1 g of haemoglobin (Hb) and has a volume of approximately 450 ml. A blood giving set with a filter chamber is normally used. Each unit of blood is cross-matched with the patient's blood to ensure compatibility. The hospital policy should state the exact steps to check that the correct, cross-matched blood is set up for the patient. Avoid any temptation to hurry the checking procedure, the patient is at greatest risk of receiving the wrong blood in times of crisis.

RE. Record the time the blood is set up and the unit number, as well as on the forms related to the checking procedure. Record fluid intake and output for at least 12 hours after the transfusion is completed.

2. Record the blood pressure at least once during the administration of each unit, more frequently if there is a particular risk of overloading the circulation. Record the patient's oral temperature and pulse at the start of the transfusion, and repeat after half an hour. Record the pulse half hourly if overload is a risk.

RE. A rise in temperature and pulse with a fall in blood pressure can indicate incompatibility of blood group or of antigens on the red cell surface. More rarely, pain over the lumbar region, headache, flushing or rash occur. Slow the transfusion to a minimal rate and call for medical aid immediately.

3. Anti-histamines such as chlorpheniramine and steroids such as hydro-cortisone may be prescribed for an allergic reaction if the need for blood outweighs the risk of giving it. Increase the frequency of recording temperature, pulse and blood pressure to at least half hourly and start recording respiratory rate. Stay with the patient. Save all blood containers in case laboratory testing is required later on.

RE. Monitor the rates; if they continue to rise after half an hour inform the doctor. Record urine output.

4. Diuretics may be prescribed if several units are to be given to raise haemo-globin levels, or if cardiac function is impaired. No drug should be added to the transfusion. Offer the commode, bedpan or urinal 20 minutes after a diuretic is given by injection.

RE. Observe the character of the pulse for increasing volume. Measure and record urine output. Report the response to the diuretic.

5. Iron overload may occur with repeated transfusions, leading to deposits in the liver, myocardium and endocrine glands. Desferal (desferrioxamine) may be prescribed to increase the rate of iron excretion. Slow intravenous infusion or intramuscular injection are the usual routes of administration.

RE. A sudden fall in blood pressure may occur if the infusion of desferrioxa-mine is rapid. Report if the intramuscular injection is painful. Urine collections may be required to assess urinary iron excretion.

6. An infusion of clear fluids does not require a filter in the giving set. Each container of fluid should be checked against the prescription, and inspected for cloudiness or particles which indicate contamination. Fluids containing potassium should be inverted several times to ensure even mixing of the solution, and the rate of flow of the infusion should be strictly controlled.

RE. Record the volume administered and the batch number of the container in case of adverse reaction. Check the patient's oral temperature if fever is suspected. Check the pulse rate and regularity when potassium is being administered.

7. An intravenous catheter passed via the subclavian vein into the superior vena cava may be necessary if the infusion is to be continuous or intermittent over several weeks. Its position is checked by X-ray and insertion is under-taken with strict aseptic technique. The fluid container should be raised at least 'a head' above the patient.

RE. Observe the insertion site on at least alternate days for signs of infection. Record the patient's temperature, pulse and respiration 6 hourly, as septicaemia can occur.

8. Intermittent infusions require that the line is filled with prescribed anti-coagulant (heparin) when not in use. Use atraumatic forceps to occlude the line while the giving set is removed, the anti-coagulant injected and the sterile cap inserted. Air must not enter the line.

RE. Check the line is taped out of the way on the patient's chest when not in use.

9. The flow control on blood and fluid administration sets may be by roller or by screw clamp. The rate of flow depends on the drop size, the height of the fluid container and the state of dilation of the patient's vein. Calculate the drops per minute required to deliver the prescribed volume in the time required. Adjust the pressure on the line until the desired rate is achieved.

RE. Time the drops per minute rate with a watch held beside the chamber at least every hour. Changes in the flow rate may indicate variations in vascular dilation. A heat pad may be used to dilate the blood vessels in a limb only if clear intravenous fluids are being administered. Check the flow at five minute intervals for the first 15 minutes of use of the heat pad.

10. Electronic drop counters can be set to monitor the rate of flow. An alarm sounds if the flow stops or the rate varies.

RE. Weekly or more frequent maintenance of the equipment should be carried out by a technician. If the alarm is set off without cause obtain a substitute.

11. Volumetric pumps may be used to deliver an exact volume in a set time. The fluid flow is not dependent on gravity or the dilation of the patient's veins.

RE. The equipment should be checked at least weekly by a technician. Unless a battery operated model is available, the patient may be confined to the bed area by the need for the electricity supply to the pump.

| **Associated medical diagnoses** | Any condition where dehydration, shock, bleeding or electrolyte imbalance has occurred or is likely to occur. |
| | Intravenous antibiotics or chemotherapy may involve keeping an intravenous route open with an infusion. |

Problem	Dependence on naso-gastric feeding.

Assessment findings	Unable to swallow Skin turgor decreasing Body weight falling Calorie intake insufficient for bodily requirement Rate of tissue healing
Information for the patient	When swallowing is difficult or tiring it is still possible to take enough food for the body's needs by pouring a liquid diet through a tube into the stomach or intestine. The tube is passed up through the nose, curves down over the back of throat, along the gullet to the stomach. The liquid diet or feed is usually commercially prepared or may be milk-based with added vitamins,

145

iron and extra protein. The position of the tube will be tested before it is given. The feeds may be given at intervals during the day, or at a very slow continuous drip into the intestines.

Nursing actions

1. Estimate the patient's Calorie and fluid requirement over 24 hours. Plan water as the first feed to assess the rate of gastric emptying.

RE. Observe the frequency of bowel actions, as diarrhoea may indicate intolerance or infected feeds. Most feeds are now tinned; store opened tins in a refrigerator and label with date and time of opening. Discard opened tins after 24 hours. Tinned feeds dripped continuously into the gut do not need to be warmed first. Locally produced feeds should be stored in a refrigerator.

2. Store the feeds in a refrigerator to limit bacterial activity. Use clean or sterile containers and a thermometer. Select the feed and warm it slightly so that it is tepid, to reduce irritation of the nasal mucosa.

RE. Ask the patient to report any temperature discomfort when being fed. Mucosal damage occurs with very cold or hot fluids. Check the nostril for friction sores or burns.

3. Select the smallest tube compatible with the consistency of the feed to minimise nasal irritation and tube blockage. Measure the length required to reach the stomach and note the mark, (the tubes are usually pre-marked). Ask the patient to blow their nose or clean their nostrils with small swabs, before the tube is inserted.

RE. Observe for nasal obstruction, mouth breathing and discomfort.

4. Lubricate the tip of the tube with water or a water-soluble gel before passing it, to limit irritation if it passes into the larynx. Anchor the tube with adhesive tape. Record the size of the tube and the mark indicating that the tube has been inserted far enough.

RE. Check the position of the tube and the mark for slippage. Check that the tube is anchored firmly with minimum interference to movement or vision, and with no strain on the tube itself.

5. Ensure the tube is in the stomach by injecting 5 ml air while listening over stomach with a stethoscope for the sound of air entry, or by aspirating at least 5 ml and testing for acidity with blue litmus paper. It will turn red when the fluid is acid. Repeat before every feed.

RE. Observe for abdominal distension or nausea from air or slow absorption of feeds. Monitor the amount and content of aspirate to assess the gastric emptying rate.

6. If possible, administer the feed with the patient sitting upright. Give the feed slowly using gravity to help it down. Do *not* force down with a syringe. Record the volume given. Give a small amount of water after or between feeds to clear the tube.

RE. Compare fluid intake and output. Weigh the patient at least twice a week to assess whether nutrient and fluid intake meet metabolic requirements.

7. Replace the naso-gastric tube at least once a week using alternate nostrils if possible.

RE. Inspect nostrils daily for friction/pressure sore development. Inspect pharynx daily for tissue damage from tube. Check naso-gastric tube is complete when removed for early identification of foreign body/tube tip loss.

Further action

1. A fine bore, radiopaque naso-gastric tube may be passed into the stomach and on to the jejunum; the position is then checked by X-ray. The prescribed feed may then be given continuously by drip; up to 2 litres may be given in 24 hours.

RE. Aspiration of gastric content is not possible, but air may be insufflated to confirm the tube's position before feeding commences.

2. If displacement of the tube is suspected, it should be checked by X-ray. Stop the feed until the tube is confirmed to be in the correct position.

RE. Adjust rate of the drip to make up the volume given within 24 hours. Increase the frequency of observations for absorption/nausea during this period. The type of feed prescribed will depend on the nutritional state to be remedied. Commercially prepared feeds are regularly adjusted so the manufacturer's literature should be consulted before use.

3. Clinifeed Favour is a commercial feed containing protein isolate, glucose, maize oil, medium chain triglyceride (MCT), soya oil, water, mattodextrin, caseinate, soya, vitamins and minerals. It can be given via a fine bore tube.

RE. Diarrhoea may occur if there is lactose intolerance. Egg protein makes it unsuitable for those allergic to eggs.

4. Ensure is also a commercial product. It contains water, hydrolysed corn starch solids, sucrose, corn oil, caseinate, soya protein, isolate, minerals and vitamins.

RE. Electrolyte levels may change, as the feed contains a relatively high level of protein and sodium.

5. Isocal contains water/glucose syrup solids, soya oil, caseinate, medium chain triglyceride (MCT) oil, soya protein isolate, minerals and vitamins. The presence of MCT oil makes it suitable for use where steatorrhoea is present.

RE. Blood electrolyte and urea levels should be checked at least weekly.

6. Vivonex Standard contains glucose, solids, 17 L-amino acids, safflower oil, minerals and vitamins.

RE. This has a high osmolarity so osmotic diarrhoea may occur. The low fat content and high cost means it should be used carefully. It tastes unpleasant and may be poorly tolerated if given by mouth.

Associated medical diagnoses

Anorexia
Cerebral vascular accident
Loss of consciousness (e.g. following a head injury)
Neuro-muscular disorder
Oesophageal stricture

Potential problems

Potential problem	Cheating on therapeutic fluid intake prescription

Assessment findings	Sudden weight gain or loss Raised blood pressure Extra fluids provided by visitors or other staff Increase in oedema Resentment at fluid requirement Anger Anxiety Sudden changes in peritoneal dialysis outflow patterns
Information for the patient	The body needs fluid to replace that lost in sweat, urine and the water vapour in the breath. The amount of fluid lost from the body will depend on the heart pumping enough blood to the kidneys for filtering and urine production. If either system is damaged by disease, the fluid intake has to be limited. The liver can also influence how water is held in the body and tissues. The doctor will weigh up the body's needs and its ability to cope with the fluid. The amount of fluid prescribed forms an important part of the treatment plan.
Nursing actions	1. Ask the patient to explain the amount and type of fluid intake required, as told them by the doctor. Listen to the way the patient gives the answer, watch for non-verbal signals which indicate their mood and co-operation. Ask how the patient feels about having to follow instructions. RE. Assess the level of understanding and acceptance of the doctor's prescription. 2. Discuss the effects of not adopting the required fluid intake. Avoid sounding like a parent scolding a child; instead aim for a factual conversation. RE. Assess the level of understanding through the questions asked and by asking the patient to repeat the information given, in their own words. 3. Discuss the patient's verbal and non-verbal indications of resentment. Aim to identify if there is any change the nursing staff could make to help the patient to accept and to follow the prescribed intake. Report areas where change may be possible if the doctor agrees. RE. Monitor effect of changes on patient's compliance. Remain alert for new means of cheating. Inform the doctor of changes. 4. Agree with the patient a revised plan of fluid intake for the next 24 hours. Praise any new efforts to stick to prescribed fluid intake. RE. Record fluid intake, daily weight, blood pressure or oedema as appropriate. Report thirst to doctor. 5. Explain to visitors that the patient needs their active support in keeping to the prescribed fluids. Assess their verbal and non-verbal responses to the information. RE. Observe whether visitors comply with any request not to provide extra fluids.

Further action	1. Peritoneal dialysis regimes can be adjusted to include more hypertonic bags to remove excess fluid.
	RE. Monitor accumulative fluid balance to assess effect of change in regime. Weigh daily before new regime prescribed so that adjustment can relate to current weight (0.45 kg (1 lb) body weight = about 500 ml water).
	2. Diuretic therapy may be adjusted to increase excretion of excess water.
	RE. Record each volume of urine passed after diuretic to assess response to change in therapy.
Associated medical diagnoses	Ascites Cirrhosis of liver Congestive cardiac failure Glomerulonephritis Oedema Renal failure

---

Potential problem	**Risk of sodium imbalance**

Assessment findings	Drinking large quantities of high sodium fluids (Marmite, Bovril, Oxo, clear soups, milk, milkshakes). Receiving diuretic therapy Urine output exceeds 2000 ml in 24 hours Receiving steroid therapy Receiving intravenous fluids Receiving peritoneal or haemodialysis Fever, with increased sweating Old age Paracentesis draining large volumes
Information for the patient	Table salt which is sprinkled on food contains sodium which is also found in salty foods, prepared foods where salt is added and milk. The kidneys normally get rid of sodium if it rises above the body's needs. Some drugs and medical conditions interfere with the control of sodium. If the level goes out of control then the body tries to compensate and this produces unpleasant symptoms. The doctor will check the sodium level in the blood through blood tests. It is possible to help the body keep the balance right by watching the type and amount of fluid taken in each day.
Nursing actions	1. Identify whether an increase (hypernatremia) or a decrease (hyponatremia) in the sodium level is more likely. Advise the patient which fluids to avoid or limit. Provide alternative types of fluid, especially water, if there is a risk of hypernatremia.
	RE. Check how much the patient can remember of the advice. Chart type and volume of fluid taken in 24 hours. Monitor urine output, a temporary increase followed by a fall may occur with hypernatremia.
	2. Explain the symptoms which may indicate that an imbalance is occurring. Ask the patient to alert a nurse if they do occur. Typical symptoms include:

<table>
<tr><td>*High sodium*</td><td>*Low sodium*</td></tr>
</table>

High sodium	*Low sodium*
(i) Dry, sticky mucous membranes	(i) Headache
(ii) Thirst	(ii) Vertigo
(iii) Rough dry tongue	(iii) Fatigue
(iv) Flushed dry skin	(iv) Abdominal and muscle cramps
	(v) Falling blood pressure
	(vi) Muscle weakness
	(vii) Poor skin turgor
	(viii) Lethargy
	(ix) Confusion

RE. Check how many symptoms the patient can remember. Observe the patient for signs of electrolyte imbalance. Monitor the serum electrolyte results. Check the blood pressure daily. Monitor urine output for fluid retention or diuresis. See page 96 for 'Risk of low body sodium'.

Further action

1. If the sodium level is raised, no salt should be added to food after cooking. No bacon, ham, cheese, kippers, potato crisps, salted nuts, tinned meat or vegetables should be eaten. Diets with a sodium content below 40 mmol a day require food prepared without salt. The fluid intake may be restricted to 500 ml plus the volume of the output of the previous day.

RE. Record fluid intake and output. Check the patient's meal tray to confirm that a salt pot has not been set on it.

2. Frusemide may be given to increase the elimination of water and sodium. It acts on the loop of Henle in the kidney nephrons. Diuresis begins within one hour of oral administration. If given intravenously, the peak diuresis occurs within 30 minutes. Additional potassium may be required to make up for that lost in the urine.

RE. Record fluid intake and output and time the onset of diuresis. In elderly men with prostatic enlargement, urinary retention may occur. If high doses of frusemide are given, ask the patient to report any ringing in the ears or difficulty hearing, as deafness may occasionally occur. Observe for signs of falling potassium. (See following potential problem.)

3. Peritoneal dialysate prescriptions may need to be revised to reduce the osmolarity.

RE. Report any unusual increase in dialysate drainage to the doctor.

4. Intravenous fluid regimes may need adjustment if the sodium level changes.

RE. Observe for signs of high sodium if the regime includes saline-based solutions.

5. Low blood sodium levels may be treated with slow release sodium tablets (600 mg NaCl or 10 mmol per tablet). These must be swallowed whole with a full glass of water.

RE. Weigh the patient daily and check their blood pressure for an increase due to oedema.

Associated medical diagnoses

Addison's disease
Carcinomatosis
Cerebral vascular accident

Congestive cardiac failure
Cushing's disease
Diabetes insipidus
Glomerulonephritis
Hepatic cirrhosis
Hypertension
Ileal conduit
Myocardial infarction
Nephropathy
Renal colic
Renal failure

Potential problem	**Risk of potassium imbalance**
Assessment findings	Drinking large quantities of high potassium fluids (apricot, blackcurrant, prune or tomato juice/nectar, tinned orange, grapefruit or pineapple juice, drinking chocolate, chocolate milkshakes, strong tea, instant coffee) Receiving potassium supplements — orally or intravenously Receiving diuretic therapy Fluctuating serum electrolyte levels Receiving digitalis therapy Receiving peritoneal haemodialysis Diarrhoea
Information for the patient	The body needs potassium, which is found in many fruits and vegetables. The kidneys normally get rid of it if the level rises above the body's needs. Some drugs and medical conditions can interfere with the control of potassium. If the level goes out of control, the symptoms may be unpleasant as the body tries to compensate. The doctor will check the level of potassium in the blood by carrying out blood tests. It is generally easy to keep the balance right by watching the kinds and amounts of fluid taken each day.
Nursing actions	1. Identify whether an increase (hyperkalaemia) or a decrease (hypokalaemia) in the potassium level is more likely. Advise the patient about which fluids to avoid or limit. Provide alternative types of fluid. RE. Check whether the patient can remember the advice. Keep a fluid balance chart of the type and volume of fluid taken in 24 hours and monitor urine output. 2. Explain the symptoms which may indicate that a potassium imbalance is occurring. Ask the patient to alert a nurse if any of them do.

High potassium
(i) weakness
(ii) numbness or tingling
(iii) confusion

Low potassium
(i) weakness
(ii) apathy or depression
(iii) constipation
(iv) abdominal distension
(v) soft flabby muscles
(vi) cardiac arrhythmias or bradycardia
(vii) mental confusion

RE. Check that the patient can remember the symptoms. Observe the patient for signs of electrolyte imbalance and monitor any serum electrolyte results. Describe the character of the pulse in writing at least once daily. See page 108 for risk of developing low body potassium.

Further action

1. Intravenous fluid regimes may need to be adjusted for potassium content.

RE. Record the rate and character of the pulse 6 hourly if potassium is being given in intravenous fluids. Report immediately any change in rhythm, or a rate dropping to 60 or below.

2. If serum potassium is low, potassium in slow release or effervescent form may be prescribed. They may also be used when potassium-losing diuretics are prescribed. The patient should sit upright to take the tablets, washing them down with at least one full glass of water.

RE. Ask the patient if the tablets seem to stick in the gullet as local oeso-phagitis may result. If the bowels open frequently, ask the patient to observe for the tablets passed whole in the faeces.

3. If serum potassium is high, restrict the amount of high potassium fluids. Calcium resonium may be prescribed. This ion exchange resin in powder form may be given orally or rectally. Intravenous glucose and insulin en-courages the migration of potassium from the extracellular fluid into the body cells. Intravenous calcium gluconate may reduce the toxic effect of potassium on the heart. If these methods fail then removal by dialysis may be considered.

RE. Observe for signs that calcium levels have risen (see page 112). Check the patient's pulse rate and rhythm at frequent intervals if the potassium levels are high enough to induce cardiac arrhythmia.

Associated medical diagnoses

Addison's disease
Congestive cardiac failure
Cushing's syndrome
Diarrhoea
Glomerulonephritis
Hyperparathyroidism
Ileal conduit
Polycystic kidney
Pyelonephritis
Renal failure
Ureterocolic anastomosis

Potential problem

Risk of renal damage from low fluid intake

Assessment findings

Low fluid intake
Sulphonamide drug therapy, co-trimoxazole, trimethoprim, sulphadimidine
Haemorrhage
Shock
Prolonged bed rest
Drug overdose (especially barbiturates, salicylates)
History of renal calculi
Acid urine

The kidneys require water to be able to clear the body of waste. When too little fluid is being drunk, it can lead to the tiny tubes in the kidney becoming blocked and so damaging the kidneys. Drinking a lot of fluid will keep the kidneys well flushed and help prevent problems. Lying in one position encourages the urine to stagnate in the kidney, but moving about improves drainage.

A group of drugs known as sulphonamides contain a substance which can crystallize out into the tiny tubules of the kidney. Drinking a lot of water will ensure that this does not happen.

Nursing action

1. Increase fluid intake to at least 2.5 litres in 24 hours. Include alkaline fluids if acid urine is present during sulphonamide therapy. If fever and sweating occur, increase the patient's fluid intake to 3 litres or more.

RE. Record intake and output, monitor for decreasing urine production. Weigh the patient daily to identify a sudden weight gain. Check for oedema as it is a sign of renal damage.

2. Increase the patient's physical activity if possible, turn them from side to side two-hourly if they are confined to bed, to reduce urinary stasis.

RE. Assess the suitability of an increase in activity.

3. Test the urine at least daily for acidity, protein and blood, and measure the specific gravity.

RE. Acid urine increases risk of crystalluria in sulphonamide therapy. Protein and blood in the urine may indicate renal damage. A specific gravity below 1.020 indicates adequate fluid intake.

4. Provide a drink before the patient settles at night, as urine excretion usually falls overnight. If night sedation is given, remind the patient to call a nurse if they wake to pass urine, to reduce the risk of falls.

RE. Monitor the urine output overnight. Note if the patient fails to comply with the request to call a nurse when getting out of bed.

Further action

1. Renal function may be monitored by measuring blood urea levels, and also creatinine clearance from a 24 hour urine collection. This allows the glomerular filtration rate to be calculated.

RE. The normal range for blood urea is 2.5 to 7.0 mmol per litre. The exact time that the first urine sample was passed should be noted. The first urine sample is discarded, but all subsequent amounts are added to the collection bottle, and the time the last sample was passed should also be noted on the bottle. Check the test is accurately carried out, as the time period and urine volume form essential parts of the calculation.

2. Sulphonamides, used to treat meningitis, urinary tract infections and chest infections are excreted via the kidneys. If urine output is low and the urine acid, crystals may form in the urine. A fluid intake of at least two litres in 24 hours should be maintained, alkaline fluids being preferred.

RE. Record fluid intake and output if there is a risk of reduced output. Test urine for blood and pH level. Report any marked reduction in urine output. The newer sulphonamides and the longer acting types carry little risk of crystal formation.

3. Barbiturate or salicylate self-poisoning requires intensive nursing care. Gastric lavage is used to empty the stomach of any remaining tablets or capsules. If consciousness is impaired, an endo-tracheal tube may be needed to reduce the risk of inhalation of vomit. Forced renal diuresis is used to speed up excretion of the poison. Intrevenous infusion of dextrose/saline is given with 20 mg frusemide each hour. The bladder is catheterized and the urine pH is measured at least hourly. (See 'Sleeping excessively', page 168).

RE. Monitor the rate and character of the pulse and respiration, together with the blood pressure. Severe brain depression by the drugs may require artificial ventilation. Measure urine output each hour, and report if the rate falls below 500 ml each hour. Measure the urine pH and report if it falls below pH 7, as the amount of sodium bicarbonate may need readjusting.

Associated medical diagnoses

Bacteraemia
Cerebral vascular accident
Chronic pyelonephritis
Gout
Hemiplegia
Hyperparathyroidism
Meningitis
Overdose of drugs
Peptic ulcer
Pneumonia
Renal calculi
Urinary tract infection

Potential problem   **Risk of dehydration**

Assessment findings

Recent confusion
Recent incontinence
Reluctance to drink
Diuretic therapy
Large volumes of gastric aspirate or vomit
Frequent diarrhoea
Large volumes of fluid drainage
Raised body temperature and sweating
Difficulty in swallowing
Dependence on others for fluid
Age

Information for the patient

The body needs to take in enough fluid each day to make up for that lost in sweating, getting rid of body wastes and water vapour lost on the breath. Older people seem to be less sensitive to the body's water shortage and do not feel thirsty as quickly. If the body is losing more fluids than normal this can be a risk. More fluid than the average intake of 1500 ml a day will be needed if there is sweating, breathlessness, or diarrhoea. Taking small frequent amounts is easier than trying to get down several glasses in half an hour (unless it's beer in the pub). The nurses will help to plan out how much fluid the body appears to need each day.

Nursing actions

1. Ask the patient which fluids they prefer. Plan the type and volume of fluid to be given, when the patient is awake, over the next 24 hours. Agree

on a minimum volume of intake. Consider using a vacuum flask to keep hot fluids hot or cold fluids really cold.

RE. Record the type and volume of the fluid actually drunk. Make a note of preferred flavours, temperatures and times to incorporate in the next day's fluid plan.

2. Provide variety with flavoured ice lollies or ice cubes. If food intake is adequate, consider providing extra jellies, melon or clear soup, all of which have a high water content.

RE. Record the fluid given in this form and include in the day's total.

3. Try using different containers for the reluctant patient. A table- or tea-spoon, beaker, straw, cup or syringe may be preferred. Consider if privacy while drinking is preferred because of embarrassment.

RE. Observe the patient's non-verbal reaction to the way that the drink is offered, and the volume taken.

4. Protect clothing with absorbent material such as towelling or tissue.

RE. Assess the volume of fluid lost into the protective material and deduct this from the volume 'drunk' before recording it.

5. Measure fluid loss from the body to compare with intake,

RE. If fluid loss plus insensible loss exceeds intake, report this to the doctor. Observe for early signs of dehydration.

6. Ask visitors or relatives to remind or help the patient drink.

RE. Note which, if any, member of the family achieves an unusually good intake by the patient. There may be an increased strain in relationships, as some people demonstrate affection through the giving or accepting of fluid and food.

Further action

1. An intravenous infusion of up to 2–2.5 litres in 24 hours may be pres-cribed. The regime will vary according to the serum electrolyte results.

RE. Record fluid intake and output from all sources. Record pulse rate and blood pressure at least 6 hourly if circulatory overload is a risk. A rising pulse and blood pressure combined with a relatively low urine output requires medical advice.

2. Naso-gastric fluids may be given if intestinal absorption is present. The proportion of feed to water will be prescribed. Continuous drip feeding via a fine bore tube increases the volume which may be absorbed.

RE. Observe for nausea or vomiting.

3. Diuretic therapy may need to be reviewed, especially if frusemide or bumetanide are prescribed. The risk of drug interactions should be considered.

RE. Record fluid intake and output to assess the fluid balance.

4. Diarrhoea not due to infection or following antibiotic therapy may be controlled with codeine phosphate, kaolin mixture or loperamide. Give one hour before or after other drug therapy, as it can decrease

RE. Record the frequency and consistency of bowel actions. Observe for dizziness and rashes from codeine phosphate or loperamide treatment. Nausea, vomiting or drowsiness may be side effects of codeine phosphate. Loperamide may cause a dry mouth or headache.

Associated medical diagnoses	Carcinomatosis Cerebral vascular accident Congestive cardiac failure Diabetes mellitus Diarrhoea Gastritis Ileostomy Intestinal obstruction Pneumonia Senile dementia

Potential problem	**Risk of alcohol withdrawal symptoms**
Assessment findings	Disorientation Restlessness Agitation Hallucinations — such as seeing animals Mood swings from anxiety to euphoria Tremor Sweating Raised temperature Symptoms occur 24–48 hours after admisssion Heavy use of stimulants e.g. coffee, cigarettes Lack of concentration Convulsions Alcohol container among possessions Smells of alcohol Blood alcohol raised over 100 mg to 100 ml blood
Information for the patient	When large amounts of alcohol are taken regularly, the body's tissues become used to working with alcohol within them. When the level of alcohol in the blood drops towards zero, the brain and nerves react. In some people this reaction may be no worse than bouts of trembling hands. In others it may mean 'seeing things' and a feeling of panic. Treatment at this stage is important, as in a few cases dangerous fits may occur. Once the body has adjusted to having no alcohol in the blood, recovery starts. There is a feeling of confidence which lasts for about two weeks, then one of panic sets in. This is a risky time, as some people give in and start drinking again. Ultimately, the alcoholic must take responsibility themselves for giving up alcohol. If a person can work through the panic stage, they can stay sober and improve their future health.
Nursing actions	1. Observe behaviour for signs of onset of delirium tremens or fits as blood alcohol level falls. The 'shakes' and the 'horrors' may be thought by the patient as requiring alcohol to stop them. Observe for increasing agitation, or staring at the curtains or ceiling; keep the room well lit. RE. Report the onset of symptoms to the doctor as soon as possible. If the patient stares, ask them what they are seeing; seeing such things as 'crawling insects' is a fairly common phenomenon.

2. Maintain close observation during visiting time, as alcohol may be brought in by drinking friends and hidden by them or the patient.

RE. Observe for an unexpected decrease in symptoms of withdrawal, such as shaking, which may indicate that alcohol has been taken. Frequent visits to the toilet may indicate a bottle hidden in the cistern.

3. Provide fruit juices and water for rehydration and to reduce the severity of a 'hangover'.

RE. Record fluid intake and output.

4. Provide a high protein and high carbohydrate diet with extra thiamine for the chronic alcoholic.

RE. Record how much is eaten, as anorexia may indicate gastritis.

5. Avoid giving sympathy or colluding with the patient in games of 'ain't it awful'. Do not tell the patient off for their drinking. Maintain a matter of fact attitude and avoid being provoked. Confirm that the patient has a right to choose how they live their life and that it is their responsibility.

RE. Observe which behavioural strategies the patient follows: the information may be useful to the doctor as well as to other nurses, depending on their interpretation of alcoholism as a disease or a chosen mode of behaviour.

6. Offer to contact the social worker if the 'skid row' alcoholic has no accommodation to go to following discharge. Clothing may need to be replaced in some cases.

RE. Record the patient's response to these offers of help. Treatment is unlikely to be successful without accommodation and a job.

7. Warn the patient that once they are over the physical sickness of adjusting to a zero blood alcohol level, they will feel confident for about two weeks, but then a feeling of panic may set in. This is the danger time when they are liable to take another drink.

Further action

1. Bed rest for 24–48 hours is recommended if intoxication is severe enough to produce lack of co-ordination and the risk of accident. The level of alcohol in the blood or the breath is a more reliable guide than clinical symptoms.

RE. Observe for non-compliance as the patient sobers up. The need for a drink may be so irresistible that irregular discharge from hospital is threatened.

2. Chlormethiazole given orally is usually sufficient for withdrawal symptoms, but it may be given by intravenous infusion to control major fits. A volumetric pump should be used for exact control of the flow rate, as its effect can add to that of the alcohol left in the body.

RE. Observe for respiratory depression if the drug is given intravenously. The 'twilight' sleep may require similar nursing action to that needed for the unconscious person. Inspect the insertion site of the intravenous cannula at least once daily, as local thrombophlebitis is a risk. Side effects include tingling in the nose, sneezing, conjunctival irritation, headache, and a slight fall in blood pressure.

3. Chlorpromazine orally may aid in controlling delirium tremens once the blood alcohol level has dropped. Sunbathing should be avoided as the skin can become sensitive to sunlight. Gloves should be worn when handling the drug for injection, as rashes can occur with frequent contact.

RE. Observe for drowsiness, nightmares or insomnia. Side effects include low blood pressure and a fast pulse. Large doses may produce Parkinsonian symptoms.

4. Thioridazine tablets may be used to tranquilize the patient without the same risk of side effects from chlorpromazine. The syrup form should not be used as it contains alcohol.

RE. Observe for drowsiness. Hypersensitivity may occur in patients who have received drugs of the same group in the past. Some alcoholics might have been treated repeatedly, but they may not report it.

5. Parenteral vitamins may be used if a deficiency is present. Anaphylactic shock presents a slight risk when Parentrovite has been given repeatedly, as it may have been with the chronic alcoholic.

RE. Observe for rising pulse, falling blood presssure and respiratory distress during first 15 minutes of intravenous administration. Flushing of the face may occur due to the nicotinamide in the solution.

6. Intravenous dextrose saline may be given to correct dehydration. The infusion may be at risk if the patient becomes agitated or confused. Blood electrolyte estimations may be needed daily.

RE. Record fluid intake and output, intially high alcohol levels may cause diuresis rather than rehydration.

7. Sputum may be collected for acid-fast bacilli in the 'skid row' type of alcoholic, as poor nutrition and living conditions increase the risk of tuberculosis.

RE. Observe for coughing and expectoration. Poor social habits may put others at risk of infection before the result of the sputum specimen is available.

8. Disulfiram (Antabuse) may be prescribed once the blood alcohol returns to zero to aid the patient in avoiding impulsive drinking. It is absorbed quickly and then remains in the body for 4–5 days. The patient must be able to understand that if alcohol is then taken, the reaction is very unpleasant. Flushing, palpitation, tightness in the chest, headache and nausea follow. Cardiac arrhythmia may occasionally occur after alcohol, and a cardiac monitor should be available. Warn the patient to avoid cough medicines and Listerine mouthwash, as they contain alcohol.

RE. Check with the pharmacist that all the prescribed drugs are free of alcohol, especially cough medicines. Ask the patient to list the unpleasant effects if alcohol is taken during Antabuse therapy.

Associated medical diagnoses

Alcoholic cardiomyopathy
Alcoholic cerebral degeneration
Anaemia
Blackouts
Carcinoma of oesophagus
Carcinoma of stomach

Cirrhosis of liver
Duodenal ulcer
Folate malabsorption
Gastritis
Head injury
Hepatitis
Hypertension
Hypothermia
Infertility
Korsakoff's psychosis
Myopathy
Pancreatitis
Peripheral neuropathy
Peptic ulcer
Polyneuritis
Wernicke's encephalopathy

References and further reading

Automobile Association, The. (1980). *AA Book of Driving.* Publications Division, The Automobile Association, Basingstoke, Hampshire.

Forrest, J.A.H. *et al.* (1978). The effect of long term Cimetidine on gastric acid. In: *Cimetidine: The Westminster Hospital Symposium.* Wastell, C. and Lance, P. (eds). Churchill Livingstone, Edinburgh.

Hunt, J.H. and Knox, M.T. (1972). *The slowing of gastric emptying by four strong acids and three weak acids. Journal of Physiology,* **222.** pp. 187–208.

Manson, L., Ritson, E.B. (1984). *Alcohol and Health: A Handbook for Nurses, Midwives and Health Visitors.* Medical Council on Alcoholism. London.

Moffat, D.B. (1978). *The Control of Water Balance by the Kidney.* Carolina Biology Readers/Oxford University Press.

Reed, T.E. (1983). One man's tipple is another man's poison. *New Scientist.* 8 December. pp. 746–51.

Rix, K. (1983). Taking metabolism into account. *Nursing Times.* October 19. pp. 67–9.

Rolls, B., Phillips, P. (1983). Ready for a drink. *New Scientist.* August 25. pp. 538–40.

Royal College of Psychiatrists. (1979). *Alcohol and Alcoholism.* Tavistock Publications. London.

Steiner, C. (1971). *Games Alcoholics Play.* Ballantine Books, New York.

Strong, J. (1983). Organisation to fight alcohol abuse. *Nursing Times.* September 21, 18.

5 Sleeping

Optimum environment

For most people, sleeping requires no effort or planning, unless there are major changes in the environment such as when moving house, or taking a holiday abroad. Each person develops a personal sleep pattern, together with a set of habits or a ritual of preparation when retiring to bed for sleep. Many people have a favourite body position in which they go to sleep such as the semi-foetal position. The type of bedding and pillow often play an important part in feeling settled and ready to sleep.

If necessary, new sleeping patterns can be learnt. The first period of night duty for the nurse or shift worker entails major adjustments. It becomes necessary to learn how to stay awake at night and how to sleep during the day. If there is any difficulty in sleeping, it may become the main topic of thought. Loss of trust in the ability to sleep can increase the problem of relaxing properly, and so further reduce the likelihood of sleep.

The average length of sleep for adults is 7 to 8 hours, but the range can go from 5 to 10 hours. In the elderly, the need for sleep seems to reduce gradually to between 5 and 7 hours. Ill people require more sleep than those in good health. Emotional excitement can lead to periods running into days when much less sleep than usual seems adequate.

Sleep patterns

The human sleep pattern has three phases, two of which are repeated 5 or 6 times during the night. First there is a period of sleepiness when arousal is easy. This gives way to light sleep, during which a physical response is possible without waking to consciousness. A hand brushing away the tickle of a fly landing on the skin, for example. The period of deep sleep which follows allows little body movement, and arousal is difficult. Sleeping through the thunderstorm or fire alarm which wakes all the neighbours is possible during deep sleep.

It is during light sleep that dreams occur. Rapid eye movements (REM) occur, and work in sleep laboratories has shown that this form of sleep is accompanied by changes in the breathing pattern, heart rate, blood pressure, body temperature and in electroencephlogram tracings. As the period of sleep progresses these dreaming periods last longer and occur more frequently. If woken immediately after a period of REM sleep, the dream can usually be recalled, but many people have forgotten their dreams by the morning. Sounds and sensations during REM sleep may be incorporated into the dream, for example spoken names.

If deprived of REM sleep, the body tries to make up the apparent deficit by increasing the frequency with which it occurs when sleep is allowed. Irritation, and a feeling of discontentment or depression may be reported.

It is very difficult to judge the time you fall asleep and the length of time spent asleep. Some people do not perceive their periods of light sleep, and so give exaggerated estimates of how long they have been awake. The morning feeling of being refreshed seems to be based on the awareness of sleep. Anxiety, or a high sensory input can increase wakefulness, while boredom, warmth, comfort or a low sensory input induce sleepiness. These influence the normal pattern, or circadian rhythm (circa diem = about one day). There are slight variations in the individual pattern if ordinary cues such as the daylight/night cycle are excluded. People who have experimented with isolation underground tend to adopt a pattern of sleeping and waking of between 24 and 25 hours. It is rarely as short as 23½ hours.

Jet lag

Crossing time zones changes the external influences such as the pattern of daylight and social activities. It takes several days to adjust to the new time. This period of readjustment can be uncomfortable, and regular travellers try to allow for jet lag in their schedules. Close examination of the bodily changes which occur throughout the normal day and night help to explain why this occurs.

The body temperature is lowest at about 02.00 hours, and it rises steadily through the day, being highest between about 16.00 and 20.00 hours. It then falls quite sharply. The average peak is 36.8°C and it falls to about 36.1°C (Holdencroft, 1980). The morning person, up with the lark and mentally alert at the beginning of the day, tends to reach their temperature peak earlier in the day. The evening person, the night owl who works best towards the end of the day, tends to reach their peak temperature later in the day. (See Fig. 5.1).

The level of plasma corticosteroids also varies with the time of day as does their excretion. The lowest levels occur between 22.00 and 0.200 hours, then the level begins to rise rapidly, reaching a peak at around 08.00 hours, after which it falls again. Some night workers find the hardest time to keep going occurs between 02.00 and 05.00 hours. Jet lag can lead to several days of disturbed plasma conticosteroid levels. Other hormones have variations which may be influenced by habits or by posture.

It takes longer to readjust from a flight from east to west than from one crossing the time zones in the other direction. Measures to aid readjustment to the new time of day include planning to sleep during the flight, and shifting the time of going to bed to sleep by 2—4 hours each day until bedtime matches the normal hour in the new time zone. Keeping a second watch running at the home time can be helpful for short visits. Major international airport hotels have thick curtains and soundproofing which can help a person to sleep after a long flight to a new time zone. It may be worth considering a one night stay at a hotel to start the adjustment, before going on to stay with relatives or friends.

Relaxation

Relaxation techniques can aid rest, which may then be followed by sleep. There are two basic relaxation positions. The first is to lie flat on the back, with the ankles about 10 inches apart and with the feet allowed to fall outwards, arms resting about 6 inches away from the body, palms uppermost, fingers gently curled. The second position is to lie on the side with the lower leg straight, upper leg comfortably bent, the lower shoulder and arm resting behind the back and the upper arm comfortably bent with the hand beside the head.

Concentrate hard on relaxing one foot, noticing the feel of the skin resting on the bed. After about 20 seconds move the attention to the calf and knee. Concentrate on letting the muscles relax then allow the whole limb to feel heavy. Move the attention to the second leg and repeat the focus on each part, moving from the foot upwards. Then concentrate on the abdomen and the chest followed by the arms. Start with the fingers, concentrating on how they feel and letting go of any tension, then move on to the forearm and then from the elbow to the shoulder. Repeat with the second arm. The next step is to move the attention to the shoulders and neck muscles, which are a particular area where tension is felt.

As relaxation proceeds, the limbs and body may start to feel warm and heavy. Concentrating hard on one part of the body pushes out the sensations coming from other parts. The breathing pattern tends to slow and deepen naturally.

In deep relaxation, a limb will drop heavily if lifted by someone else. It may help to test the level of relaxation achieved by asking a friend or relative to help by lifting a hand or foot a few inches from the bed and letting it fall back.

Once relaxation is achieved, the mind should concentrate on holding a single neutral image. Some people choose to imagine a single flickering candle, others imagine black velvet. Some people fall asleep long before they get to this stage!

Strange beds

The bedding and firmness of the mattress can influence relaxation and sleep. A strange bed stimulates the nerve receptors with the position of the limbs, pressure and temperature. These keep reaching the consciousness, whereas nervous stimulation from a familiar bed does not. The body becomes accustomed to repeated types of stimulation, and only new sensations then reach the consciousness. For some people the pillow is the most important item of bedding. It may be worth packing the familiar pillow when going away on holiday, or into hospital.

Happily, it usually only takes a couple of nights to become familiar with a new bed and for sleep to return to its usual pattern. Noise, however, can be more of a problem. If it annoys, then it may interfere with sleep, for example the barking of a dog or distant party sounds. Someone else snoring can become the focus for irritation. This emotional content increases wakefulness. Ear plugs may be helpful, but they make the wearer's pulse beat audible to themselves. For some this can be a welcome steady sound, for others it just adds further annoyance. Habituation to repeated noise occurs with time, especially if the sound is felt to be welcome and reassuring. It is possible for the sleeping person to select sounds to which they respond by waking, the mother waking at the first whimper of the baby being one example.

The routine of preparing for bed and sleep is established over the years. The likelihood of falling asleep can be increased by following this routine. For some the evening bath, a late night drink or reading in bed are key steps in the personal preparation for sleep. In strange surroundings, following a familiar routine may be the essential element for sleeping soundly.

Not everyone is aware of their personal sleep pattern. Some aspects, such as the length of time spent asleep, may follow a family tendency. It is worth asking older family members about childhood sleeping patterns. Some children who rarely slept for long periods, woke early and went to sleep late, go on to be adults who need only 4—5 hours of sleep a night. It is only when the myths about everyone needing 8 hours' sleep a night are heard that such a short period of sleep gives rise to concern. Other people may get concerned about their need for longer than average periods asleep.

Older people seem to need less sleep, it is often lighter and they may take more naps. The amount of REM sleep also decreases.

The use of sedatives   The use of sleeping tablets may cause a fall in blood pressure which can reduce the blood flow to the brain. This can give rise to confusion and disorientation. A cardiac stimulant such as the caffeine in coffee or tea will increase the blood flow, and help counteract the effects of sedatives.

Drugs taken to induce sleep treat the symptom rather than the cause. Their rate of excretion may be slow, leading to a hungover, drugged sensation. Their influence on reaction times may be even more important for those who drive, operate machinery or need speed and accuracy at a keyboard. Taking alcohol at the same time increases the effect, sometimes to a dangerous degree.

Regular use of sleeping tablets leads to tolerance. The liver increases the level of the enzymes used to destroy the drug. In time the dosage needs to be increased to achieve sleep. A psychological reliance can occur, so that a person may believe they cannot sleep without the drug. The anxiety produced by its withdrawal may be sufficient to prevent sleep. Until relaxation of mind and body is achieved and confidence in the ability to sleep naturally is re-established, sleep may be broken and not refreshing.

General assessment areas

Amount of sleep
Hours of day when asleep
Length of unbroken sleep
Change in sleep pattern
Use of medication
Preparations for sleep
Age
Normal sleeping position
Normal environment for sleep
Pain
Anxiety
Depression

Problems

Page

Lack of sleep (due to disturbance from environment)   167
Sleeping excessively   168
Difficulty in getting to sleep   170
Waking with bad dreams/nightmares   172
Fear of falling asleep and not waking   173
Unable to adapt to a new sleeping environment   175
Unable to lie in a comfortable sleeping position   175
Unable to follow usual sleep habits   177
Increased sleep requirement   178
Kept awake by pain   179
Night-to-day sleep reversal   180
Kept awake by nurse intervention   182
Kept awake by night cramps   184

Potential problems

Risk of disturbance to usual diurnal sleep pattern   185
Risk of exhaustion   186

Problems

Problem	Lack of sleep (due to disturbance from environment)

Assessment findings

Wakes at intervals
Woken for frequent physiological measurements
Feels tired
Change in usual sleep pattern
Unused to firm (or soft) mattress
Unused to type of bedding
Unable to adjust to noise level
Unable to adjust to room temperature
Unable to adjust to light level
Falls asleep during daytime
Irritable during the day
Sleeps for less time than reported norm
Dark circles under eyes and puffy eyelids
Yawning
Poor co-ordination

Information for the patient

When away from home it is important to follow the normal pattern of preparing for bed and sleep. A favourite pillow and a familiar bed and bed-clothes are all subtle reminders that help sleep. Few people sleep well for their first night away from home. In hospital, patients may find they share the same ward or room as several other people, and it can take two or three nights to adjust. Sleeping tablets do not give the same quality of sleep and are best avoided. The most helpful thing to do is to try to include as many of the familiar parts of the home pattern as possible. Then if you do wake or are woken for nursing care, it should be much easier to drift back to sleep.

Nursing action

1. Ask the patient to describe their usual personal ritual for preparing to sleep. Plan to include as many of the components as possible. Key points usually include time, bathing, reading and hot drinks. Group any nursing action to keep the need to wake the patient to a minimum.

RE. Note how much of their usual ritual the patient actually follows and whether sleep occurs. Review the need to wake patient for nursing care.

2. Compare hospital bedclothes with the usual type. Consider with the patient whether a favourite pillow from home would help, or providing extra blankets to match the usual weight of bedding. Consider the bed base. Fracture boards can be used to give a firmer base, sheet foam or an additional mattress can soften a firm base.

RE. Few people sleep well for their first night in a strange bed. Note whether changes in the bed or bedding improve the length of sleeping time. Ask the patient whether they slept better.

3. Review noise levels. Squeaking doors can be oiled, banging windows wedged, noisy lavatory cisterns adjusted, and metal equipment padded with fabric. Earphones can be fitted to television sets or radios, and earplugs may help block out noise.

RE. Record which sounds wake the patient. Make a written note if earplugs are in use, as there is a risk that alarms would be ignored (i.e. fire alarms).

4. Review the light level in the sleeping area. Advise against using fabric as a cover for lights because of fire risk. Consider with patient whether a dark mask over eyes would help.

RE. Record how much sleep patient appears to achieve.

5. When awake at night, offer a warm, milky drink if the patient's diet allows, and a quiet chat.

RE. Note at what time waking occurred and what triggered it. Look back over several days for a pattern of wakefulness.

Further action

1. Nitrazepam may be prescribed as a hypnotic as it causes less confusion and hangover than barbiturates, especially with the elderly. It also avoids the risk of misuse which accompanies barbiturates.

RE. Note the time the patient goes off to sleep and wakes.

Problem	Sleeping excessively

Assessment findings

Sleep lasts for 2—4 hours longer than normal
Falls asleep after meals
Low basal metabolic rate
Falls asleep when sitting or relaxed
Recent anaesthetic administration
Receiving barbiturates, tranquillizers, muscle relaxants or antihistamines
Overdosage of sedatives
Known alcohol abuse
Previous gastric surgery
Previous irregular sleeping pattern
Known epilepsy

Information for the patient

If a person seems to be sleeping for longer than usual, it may be due to a variety of different reasons such as a hangover effect from sleeping tablets or a rapid rise in blood sugar after a meal.

Nursing action

1. Discuss with patient possible reasons for sleeping so much. Confirm that their sleep at night is unbroken and that the established medical diagnosis does not indicate a possible cause.

RE. Record patient's interpretation of cause.

2. Review the known intake of sedatives, muscle relaxants or antihistamines. Record the time during which the patient is asleep in each 24 hours. Consider whether the patient is taking unprescribed medication. Check for any safety hazards if the patient is doing so.

RE. Plot the time and dosage of the known drug intake against the time asleep during each 24 hour period, to identify any apparent pattern. Discuss this pattern with the medical staff, as dosage may need to be reduced.

3. Record the type and amount of food eaten in relation to falling asleep after meals. Include alcohol in this estimation, and consider if extra alcohol is being consumed.

RE. Check for potentiation of effect between alcohol and prescribed drugs such as antihistamines and sedatives. If sleeping follows high carbohydrate meals, discuss this with the medical staff.

4. Increase fluid intake to 2.5—3 litres if the drugs are excreted in the urine. Record intake and output.

RE. Assess the urine output. Observe how long the patient sleeps for, and check if they feel less tired.

Further action

1. Assess the blood glucose for hyperglycaemia using test strips with blood from a prick of the finger or earlobe. It may be necessary to check the level every 4 hours for 24 hours. A fasting blood sugar may be taken after at least six hours without food or any drink except plain water.

RE. Normal blood glucose levels are 2.8—8.9 mmol per litre.

2. Accidental drug overdose may occur without any other symptoms being noted. A blood or urine sample may be taken to assess whether dosage adjustment is necessary.

RE. Advise the patient to avoid activities which require a quick reaction, until their sleepiness is reduced.

3. Self-poisoning with sedatives, hypnotics or tranquillizers may be limited in its effect by prompt gastric lavage using a long, soft Ryles tube of at least 12 mm diameter. (If the patient is losing consciousness, an endo-tracheal tube may need to be inserted first to reduce the risk of inhaled vomit). Give 300 ml of warm water via a funnel attached to the tube. Create a syphon back into a bucket by moving the funnel below the level of the patient's stomach before all the fluid has left the tube. Continue until the liquid is clear (this may need up to 9 litres). Save a sample of the early fluid removed for analysis.

RE. Observe for increasing drowsiness or reducing reaction to stimuli. Check the patient's pulse and blood pressure every 15 minutes until their condition becomes stable, then reduce the frequency according to improvement.

4. If systolic blood pressure falls below 90 mmHg in someone over 50 years of age, or below 80 mmHg in a younger patient, tip the head of the bed down by 45 degrees.

RE. Check the blood pressure after 5 minutes; if it remains below 90 mmHg summon medical aid as drug therapy may be needed.

5. Intravenous fluids may be required to prevent dehydration or to increase the rate of diuresis. Alkaline fluids may be used in salicylate poisoning. If the patient is unconscious, an indwelling urinary catheter may be inserted.
   Peritoneal or haemodialysis may be undertaken instead of forced diuresis.

RE. Record fluid intake and output. Record the patient's pulse and respiratory rate to monitor for cardiac strain or circulatory overload. Report a rise in the pulse rate of over 80—90 beats per minute, or a change in the character of respirations, especially slower, noisy respirations. Test the urine pH to monitor the response.

6. Secretions may need to be removed by suction or by a fine sterile catheter applied to the trachea if the patient is unconscious.

RE. Report an increase in secretion rate which may indicate circulatory overload from forced diuresis.

169

7. Observe for falling or low body temperature which may follow paracetamol or aspirin poisoning. Maintain or increase the room temperature to 21°C or use a foil blanket to reflect back body heat.

RE. Report any fall in rectal temperature below 36°C. Check the temperature every half hour until the patient's condition is stable and their body temperature above 36°C.

8. Epileptic fits may be followed by drowsiness or post-fit amnesia and automatic behaviour. An electroencephalogram (EEG) may be performed if fits are suspected.

RE. Record any unusual changes in behaviour and the time it occurred. Observe for grand or petit-mal fits. Report their occurrence to the medical staff.

Associated medical diagnoses	Alcoholism Anaemia Diabetes mellitus Drug overdose Dumping Syndrome Epilepsy Hyperglycaemia Myxoedema Petit-mal epilepsy Salicylate poisoning

---

Problem	**Difficulty in getting to sleep.**

Assessment findings	Unable to relax Unable to fall asleep Follows usual sleep rituals Restlessness Tosses and turns in bed Lies awake Feels wide awake during normal sleeping time Age
Information for the patient	Most adults have firm habits when preparing for sleep. If these are changed by illness or by being in hospital, it may be harder to fall asleep. As people get older, less sleep is needed, so some people find that they wake earlier, while others get to sleep later. Rest is more important than sleep; deep relaxation can be helpful, and the nurses can give instruction in learning to do this. Avoid reading exciting books last thing at night. Some foods, including milky drinks, are thought to increase the chance of sleep.
Nursing action	1. Discuss with the patient their usual sleep pattern and the activities which aid sleep. Plan to include as many as possible each night before the normal retiring time. Provide for a later wakening time than usual. RE. Make a note of the time the patient does fall asleep and also the periods of wakefulness. Ask the patient whether they found their sleep to be refreshing.

2. Teach a simple relaxation technique, and make sure that it is practised each night. If the patient wishes it, assist by checking the state of relaxation in the limbs.

RE. Monitor the time the patient falls asleep after relaxing. Assess their ability to achieve deep relaxation and amend the level of supervision planned as their skills increase.

3. Provide light reading such as short stories; adjust lighting and screens so that other patients are not disturbed.

RE. Check the time the patient turns their light out, and when they fall asleep. Ask them the next morning whether their sleep was refreshing.

4. Check the bladder is emptied at the usual time, particularly if the patient is old or immobile.

RE. Consider whether fear of incontinence may be preventing relaxation.

5. Review drug therapy for stimulants such as amphetamine derivatives.

RE. Discuss possible influence of drugs with the pharmacist or doctor.

6. Provide a hot drink in a vacuum flask and biscuits by the bed. If possible spend time talking quietly with the wakeful patient.

RE. Check how often the patient helps themselves to hot drinks. Consider the content of any discussion for indications of underlying worries or fears.

7. A cup of coffee just before settling may help the elderly person whose blood pressure tends to fall after taking sleeping tablets.

RE. Note when the patient falls asleep. If there is no improvement after two nights, stop the coffee.

8. A small tot of alcohol, if allowed, can increase the sense of well-being and relaxation, brandy or whisky being the traditional choice.

RE. Note when the patient falls asleep. Exercise caution if sedative drugs or antihistamines are also being taken during the day.

9. If anxiety is a problem, discuss whether the social worker could help.

RE. Note when the social worker sees the patient.

Further action

1. A hypnotic may be prescribed to decrease anxiety and restlessness. Nitrazepam and related drugs are normally excreted fast enough for there to be no 'hangover' effect in the morning.

RE. Note the time the patient falls asleep and the length of unbroken sleep. Review the need to continue giving night sedation at least every other day. In the elderly receiving nitrazepam, observe for reduced body temperature.

2. Sedatives produce deep sleep and should be used with caution, especially barbiturates. Alcohol potentiates their action. Excretion from the body may be slow, so that administration over several nights leads to a cumulative effect.

171

RE. Note the time the patient falls asleep and the length of unbroken sleep. Observe for habituation or emotional dependence if drug therapy continues over a week. Observe for 'hangover' in the morning.

Associated medical diagnoses

Anybody with emotional problems
Carcinoma
Thyrotoxicosis

Problem   **Waking with bad dreams/nightmares**

Assessment findings

Restlessness
Talking or shouting in sleep
Sweating
Wakes with a start
Fever
Recent long term use of sleeping tablets
Sleep disturbed by frequent nursing attention

Information for the patient

The body needs two kinds of sleep; one is a deep relaxed sleep, the other is more restless sleep with a lot of dreaming (REM sleep). Many people cannot remember if they have dreamed, unless they wake as soon as the dreaming stops. This type of sleep is so important to the body that if it receives less than usual, the next time you fall asleep the restless sleep starts sooner and lasts longer, as if the body is trying to make up the amount lost. Being woken up every few hours, or taking sleeping tablets, will reduce the amount of this sleep. As soon as the body has caught up on the REM sleep the dreams will lessen. This normally takes one or two nights.

If the body temperature goes up, some people are more likely than others to have nightmares. Their dreams are so vivid that the body responds with a flight or fright reaction and puts all the systems on the alert. Dreams are usually based on everyday events or on worries. If a very unpleasant thing happens, the dreams may be vivid and be repeated over and over again.

Nursing action

1. Identify how many unbroken periods of sleep of two hours or more have occurred in the last 48 hours. Review the care plan to see if any activities which wake the patient can safely be suspended overnight, or stopped altogether. If waking the patient for nursing attention, look for signs of dreaming, such as rapid eye movement beneath lids, and if possible delay until they cease.

RE. Record the time the patient falls asleep and the time of waking in relation to nursing activities. Record if the patient wakes without stimulus.

2. Plan for extra rest periods, sufficient to provide two hours more than the patient's usual amount of sleep. Teach relaxation exercises.

RE. Ask whether the patient feels refreshed after a sleep. Ask if the relaxation exercises have helped.

3. Review drug therapy for a change in the type or amount of sedative. Discuss with the patient an increase in fluid intake to at least 2 litres in 24 hours, to aid excretion of residual metabolites of such drugs. Assure the patient that a normal sleep pattern may take 5—7 days to achieve, if sedatives have been taken for a month or more and then stopped.

RE. Report possible result of change in sedative type to doctor in time for a review of therapy before next dose is due. Monitor fluid intake. Ask whether the patient feels refreshed after sleeping.

4. Reduce any fever with cool drinks, frequent sponging with tepid water (38°C), an open window or a fan in room.

RE. Check the oral or rectal temperature to see if it is lower. Record whether the patient falls asleep afterwards. Repeat if necessary.

5. Use padded cotsides and lower the bed only if restlessness is marked (in case the patient falls out of bed). If necessary check the patient frequently in case confusion or delusions lead to them climbing over cot sides.

RE. Re-assess the need for extra safety measures each night. Stop them once restlessness decreases to a manageable level.

Further action

1. Pentazocine may cause nightmares or nocturnal confusion in the elderly. Dizziness, nausea or headaches may also occur. Mild respiratory depression may follow an injection and may increase confusion in those with existing respiratory problems.

RE. Stop administration; discuss an alternative analgesic. If possible increase the amount of fluids to at least 2 litres taken until symptoms subside.

2. Paracetamol, or aspirin orally or as a suppository, may be prescribed to reduce pyrexia which can cause delerium.

RE. Check oral temperature, observe for signs of sweating.

Associated medical diagnoses

Fever
Hyperthyroidism
Myocardial infarction
Pneumonia

Problem

Fear of falling asleep and not waking

Assessment findings

Elderly
Lies awake
Refuses to follow usual sleep rituals
Refuses sedation
Anxious
Medical prognosis poor
Unable to concentrate

Information for the patient

Refreshing sleep helps the body deal with illness. Worry can keep a person awake, as can pain. Everyone has individual habits which they follow to prepare for sleep. If these can be followed they may help.

Nursing actions

1. Discuss with the patient their normal pattern of preparing for sleep and identify any changes from their usual sleep rituals. Discuss whether there are any reasons for the change. Consider whether the effect of the drugs taken may be involved; some sedatives may cause bad dreams or discomfort.

173

RE. Observe the patient's current pattern when preparing for sleep, and compare it with their description, so that changes in planned care may be carried out, such as giving a bath at bedtime if this conforms to the patient's usual pattern.

2. If the patient seems willing, explore their understanding of their condition and prognosis for evidence of any misconceptions or fears. Watch for non-verbal indications of anxiety.

RE. Consider if any other person would be found more acceptable to the patient, if they feel unable to discuss their condition. Check the next day whether the patient can repeat any explanations given to them in case they are remembering information selectively, due to anxiety or their drug therapy.

3. Suggest that the nurses will make a regular check on the patient's condition while they are asleep, in order to provide reassurance.

RE. Observe for any change in non-verbal indications of anxiety, and whether the patient falls asleep. Record how long they sleep, and make sure that a nurse keeps the promise to visit them regularly.

4. Suggest that the patient tries to keep awake but rests in a relaxed position, eyes open with a fixed stare into the dark or with eyes closed but concentrating on an image such as black velvet or a lighted candle flickering in a dark room. This may in fact help them to fall asleep.

RE. Check whether the patient is asleep. Keep them company for a while if not; some people find they can talk and discuss fears more freely during the quiet of the night.

5. Teach deep relaxation techniques, supervise these while they are practised each evening at bedtime. Consider planning a further session each afternoon.

RE. Monitor the degree of relaxation attained, plan to reduce supervision as skill increases. Record if the patient sleeps, and for how long. Ask them if they found the relaxation refreshing.

6. Suggest moving the patient closer to the night nurse's base or sharing a room with others, particularly if they are frightened of being alone.

RE. Observe whether the patient can relax more. Listen for comments suggesting a sense of reassurance.

7. Plan rest periods during the day if that is the time that the patient feels safe and can relax more easily.

RE. Observe for the additional strain on friends or relatives as their support may be needed, or visiting times adjusted.

Further action

1. Chlorpromazine may be useful in terminal care as it enhances the effect of analgesics, reducing nausea and also the patient's anxiety. Do not use a discoloured solution.

RE. Note whether the patient complains of a dry mouth. The pulse rate may rise further if tachycardia was already present.

Associated medical diagnoses	Asthma Carcinoma Chronic obstructive airway disease Myocardial infarction Paroxismal tachycardia

---

Problem Unable to adapt to a new sleeping environment

Assessment findings Normal sleeping position
Waking when position is changed by nurses
Able to sleep in some positions but not others
Woken by unusual noises of environment

Information for the patient Most people find it hard to sleep in a strange bed for the first night or two. The different sensations from an unfamiliar mattress, new noises and the presence of other people set the primitive alarm system in a state of readiness. As time goes by these systems get used to the new sleeping area and relaxation allows sleep. A few people find it harder to adapt. Following the usual habits from home will help.

Nursing action 1. Discuss normal sleeping position, bed surface, habits to prepare for sleep. Plan to include as much of normal routine as possible. Consider use of fracture boards under mattress if bed is too soft. Suggest pillow and/or duvet brought from home, if these are felt to improve sleep. Plan extra rest periods during day.

RE. Record how much sleep is achieved after 48 hours in which to adapt to new measures. Ask patient if sleep/rest was refreshing.

2. Teach relaxation exercises to carry out before sleep, supervise these and assist by checking degree of relaxation of limbs.

RE. Assess how well the exercises are performed, plan to reduce supervision as skill increases. Observe whether sleep follows the exercises.

3. Reduce outside stimuli, such as squeaky shoes, banging doors, lights left on, talking by hospital staff, dripping taps, kitchen and sluice activities, telephone noise and use of torches. Check maintenance requests are carried out within 24 hours; if not, report situation to nursing officer.

RE. Ask patient if sleep achieved was refreshing, if not consider use of ear plugs or sleeping mask to further reduce stimulus from noise and light.

4. Provide activities for wakeful periods such as reading short stories, use of earphones and transistor radio or cassette player.

RE. Check patient's activities do not disturb the sleep of others. Record how long the patient remained awake.

Problem Unable to lie in a comfortable sleeping position

Assessment findings Normal sleeping position not possible
Waking when position is changed
Able to sleep in some positions but not others
Use of night splints for limbs/joints

Breathless when lying down
Sleeping with intravenous infusion in situ

Information for the patient

Each person has their own sleeping habits and usually a favourite position in which to go off to sleep. It usually takes at least two nights to adjust to a new sleeping position, as it does to adjust to a strange bed.

Nursing action

1. Discuss with the patient the normal length of time they spend asleep. Compare the time spent in comfortable sleeping positions with the normal amount of sleep before the problem occurred. Plan that the patient is in the comfortable position when room is quiet so that the maximum sleep is possible.

RE. Record whether the patient falls asleep at these times.

2. Consider if a low air loss or net suspension bed would reduce the need for changes of position and allow unbroken sleep.

RE. Monitor how long the patient is asleep. Try a new bed for at least 48 hours before assessing whether it is helpful, as it will take time for the patient to adjust.

3. Consider whether extra support for a limb may increase the patient's comfort. Extra pillows, foam pads or gutters trimmed to suit with a sharp knife, gel pads or a sling may help. Seek medical advice if a particular position forms part of treatment, as in cerebral vascular accident or rheumatoid arthritis.
   Discuss with the patient how much is understood about the use of night splints to limit deformity developing.

RE. Review level of comfort achieved. It may take 48 hours for new sensations induced by support to be accepted and for habituation to occur.

4. Consider whether breathlessness may be eased by sleeping in a chair and resting the arms on the bed, rather than on a bedtable. Use blankets or quilted sleeping bag for warmth. Seek medical advice if cardiac or vascular problems are present.

RE. Check ankles for oedema if the patient sleeps sitting up. Check respiratory depth and rate for change.

5. Consider if the mattress is providing the most effective form of support. Too soft a surface allows the vertebral column to become misaligned increasing backache. A firm base can be achieved with boards beneath the mattress. Where the vertebrae are fixed, extra pillows may increase comfort.

RE. Record how long the patient sleeps. Check boards at least weekly for splinters, especially at the edges.

Further action

1. Night splints may be prescribed to support the limbs during sleep and reduce the development of joint deformities.

RE. Check the splint does not cause increased local redness indicating pressure with the risk of skin damage.

Associated medical diagnoses

Ankylosing spondylitis
Asthma
Bronchitis
Cervical spondylitis

176

Chronic obstructive airways disease
Congestive cardiac failure
Decubitus ulcer
Peripheral vascular disease
Prolapsed inter-vertebral disc
Rheumatoid arthritis

Problem	**Unable to follow usual sleep habits.**

Assessment findings

Caring for a restless partner
Woken by others
Usual activities disturb others
Room mate demanding attention
Sitting up with ill relative

Information for the patient

The body needs both deep relaxing sleep and dreaming sleep. How much is needed depends on the individual. Everyone has their own habits when preparing for sleep. If sleep is broken in the middle of a normal cycle, it may take an hour or more to return to sleep. Rest and relaxation are as important as sleep, so it is best to plan to relax if woken rather than worrying about not being able to get back to sleep again.

Sharing a room with someone else can make it difficult to get off to sleep. Follow as many as possible of the usual personal routines before going to bed so that the body is prepared for sleep. New habits can be learnt, given enough time.

Nursing action

1. Discuss normal sleeping habits with the patient and compare with the present pattern to identify which changes are essential. Plan for extra rest periods if possible. Consider provision of relief for those caring for a partner or relative — eg. a rota of night sitters.

RE. Ask whether sleep is refreshing and whether the amount of dreaming appears to be increasing (the patient might not remember). A deficit of REM sleep may require further measures to be taken.

2. Include as many old habits as possible in new sleep pattern. Provide patient with written plan of new pattern.

RE. Record how much sleep occurs each night. After two nights following the new pattern ask the patient whether the sleep is refreshing.

3. Consider provision of lounger in place of chair, or the use of a neighbouring room with a simple electric bell/buzzer for patient to attract attention. Sitting up inside a sleeping bag may be warmer than blankets, which can slip off.

RE. Observe for a decrease in anxiety when the new measures are tried.

4. Suggest that if sleep is broken during the night, it may be more effective to read, get up and make a hot drink or walk around for a while before trying to settle back to sleep.

RE. Check the room has no hidden safety hazards such as trailing wires. Note how often sleep is broken and how long it is before sleep re-occurs.

Further action	1. Involve social worker and general practitioner if problems of caring for sick relatives or friends at home are causing unusual sleep habits for relatives. The local branch of the British Red Cross Society may be able to provide relief with a night sitter. The Marie Curie Fund may provide night sitters when terminal illness is due to cancer.
	RE. Ask the relatives how useful the help has been. Listen and observe for non-verbal gestures which suggest guilt feelings at trying to find relief rather than struggling to cope.
Associated medical diagnoses	Carcinoma Depression Insomnia Senile dementia Urinary tract infection

Problem	**Increased sleep requirement**

Assessment findings	Fever Muscle weakness Shortness of breath Loss of weight Rapid pulse (tachycardia) Feeling of fatigue or general tiredness Over 70 years of age
Information for the patient	When the body is fighting illness it needs to conserve energy usually used in other activities. Sleep helps the muscles to relax, slows the pulse and breathing rate and reduces the tissues' need for energy and oxygen. Extra sleep helps the body to repair itself and natural sleep is more effective and refreshing than that produced by sleeping tablets. A regular nap during the day is important. As strength returns it becomes less easy to doze off during the daytime, and this can be the body's way of indicating that less sleep is required.
Nursing action	1. Group together nursing actions to provide planned periods of extra rest. Contact those therapists involved in treating the patient in order to incorporate their visits in the plan.
	RE. Monitor how long periods of rest actually are.
	2. Provide a 'do not disturb' notice to hang on the door or bed to remind visitors, medical students or therapists of the planned rest periods.
	RE. Monitor which, if any, other staff ignore the notice so that the need for co-operation can be explained to them in greater detail.
	3. Provide a warm quiet place for sleep. Sitting in a deep armchair may be more effective than resting in bed if breathlessness causes a problem.
	RE. Note at what time and for how long the patient sleeps. Ask them whether the sleep was refreshing.
	4. A mask covering the eyes or ear plugs may help patients to sleep during the day if they are normally light sleepers, or easily woken by noise.
	RE. Note what sort of things waken the patient or interfere with their sleep.

5. Suggest to visitors that they provide sleeping aids such as a small neck cushion or a herb pillow for the patient, and that they bring a book or magazine to read themselves so the patient can feel less guilty about falling asleep during their visits.

RE. Check that visitors have a quiet activity with which to occupy themselves should the patient fall asleep during a visit. Note if the presence of particular visitors aids the patient in falling asleep.

Further action

1. Serum electrolyte and haemoglobin levels, and a white cell count may be measured, as sensitivity to some drugs may result in anaemia or a reduction in white cells.

RE. Compare the results with the local laboratory's normal range of values. A reduced white cell count may predispose the patient to infections.

Associated medical diagnoses

Anaemia
Carcinoma
Cardiac infarction
Cerebral vascular accident
Chronic bronchitis
Malnutrition
Pneumonia
Thyrotoxicosis
Ulcerative colitis
Any febrile condition

Problem	**Kept awake by pain**

Assessment findings

Lies awake at night
Falls asleep but wakes suddenly
Tired
Dark circles under eyes
Puffy eyelids
Pain
Pain increased by warmth

Information for the patient

If sleep is interrupted by pain, then the most important thing to do is to find out what sets the pain off. If the pain can be brought under control, relaxation and sleep should follow. It may take up to 48 hours to get a good enough picture to be able to work out a plan of action. A pain chart would be helpful, recording at what time the pain occurs, how severe it is, and where it occurs. This needs the help of the patient, as only the person with the pain can describe these symptoms in detail.

Nursing action

1. Record with the patient the level and site of the pain while they are awake, and their response to analgesia. Record the time and duration of sleep. Consider the use of a pain chart which is kept by the patient; placing their bed near the nurses' station may also be helpful.

RE. Compare the time of the onset of pain with the time that the last analgesia was administered. Discuss the use of longer-acting drugs or the necessity of waking the patient for a top-up dose of analgesia before the time that the pain is expected to occur. Consider the use of alcohol in small amounts to increase the effect of some drugs (but only give this with medical permission).

2. Discuss the patient's usual sleep rituals. Plan to include extra rest periods at times when pain is less severe, until the analgesia allows a more typical pain-free sleep pattern.

RE. Ask the patient if they found their sleep refreshing. Dreaming may increase for a while if a deficit of REM sleep needs to be made up.

3. Teach relaxation exercises and supervise their practice each evening; consider using them before any extra sleep/rest periods. Observe for increase in pain if the muscles have been held tensely to limit pain from movement (muscle splinting).

RE. Assess the level of relaxation achieved, and reduce supervision as the patient's skill increases. Consider supporting the body position with extra pillows, shaped foam, 'bean bags' or a fluidized sand bed in order to replace muscle splinting if pain occurs.

4. If pain is increased by warmth, try folding back some of the covers from the affected area, or using a bed cradle.

RE. Ask the patient to assess relief.

Further action

1. Discuss a change in analgesia with the medical staff. Advice may be available from staff of a hospice or Macmillan service, which provides home care of the terminally ill. Long-acting, slow release drugs may be useful.

RE. Monitor the effect of analgesia using a pain chart and noting periods of rest or sleep.

2. If sleep deficit is severe, a larger dose of analgesia may be given for two nights, and then slowly reduced to achieve a balance between pain control and side effects.

RE. Record the amount of rest and sleep gained each night. Use a pain chart with the patient to assess pain. Often after several nights' rest, the analgesia needed to keep the patient pain-free may be lower than that used before the sleeping problem arose.

Associated medical diagnoses

Carcinoma
Duodenal ulcer
Ischaemia
Peripheral vascular disease
Rheumatoid arthritis

Problem	Night-to-day sleep reversal

Assessment findings

Wide awake at night
Asleep during day
Recent journey across major time zones
Elderly
Confusion
Recent change in environment
Carry-over effect of sedatives
Recent long period working night shifts
Worried about sleeping
Time of preparation for bed
Time of falling asleep
Time of waking

Sleeping and waking times are partly controlled by the internal body clock as well as by the outside world. Daylight alternates with the dark of night-time and this together with the routine of everyday living normally keeps the body clock on time. Big changes, such as those which lead to jet lag, or a number of small ones associated with being in hospital, may throw the normal body time out of step with the night time. The elderly are more at risk. It is possible to relearn a more usual sleep pattern. It has to be done slowly and steadily if the internal clock is to be reset. One of the more easily checked signs of change in the body clock is the pattern of temperature change through the day.

Nursing action

1. Identify usual sleeping pattern before reversal occurred, especially time of going to bed with rituals followed to prepare for sleep and time of waking.

RE. Compare usual pattern with current one to identify changes required. If patient is unable to describe usual pattern consider asking relatives, friends or neighbours.

2. Review the current pattern of daytime activities to identify those which could act as time cues. Observe which ones seem to be noticed by the patient including meals, baths, outings. Record oral or rectal temperature hourly when awake (Fig. 5.1).

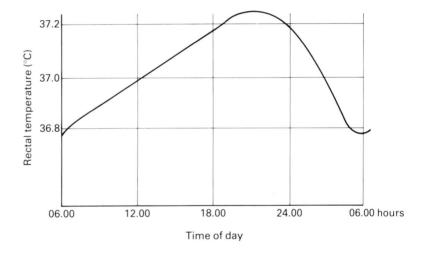

Fig. 5.1   Circadian rhythm of rectal body temperature when temperature of the environment is at 32°C, (From Holdencroft, 1980.)

RE. Compare possible time cues with those noticed by the patient. Consider if one or more evening cues could be strengthened. Compare temperature pattern with the average.

3. Plan to include at least one hour's daily exposure to natural daylight even if it is through a window.

RE. Record length of exposure to natural light.

4. Review the bed area for aspects which could be emphasized to reinforce night time cues. Consider thicker curtains to block out summer light, reducing noise levels or use of a single room.

RE. Observe whether any changes influence the patient's current sleeping pattern.

5. Plan to wake the patient two hours earlier than the current waking time and to provide stimulation to keep the patient awake throughout the day. Introduce bedtime rituals at the same time as the usual times for sleep. Repeat over at least 4 days. Record the temperature when awake.

RE. Record the time the patient falls asleep, and then wakes. If time of sleeping occurs earlier than before consider adjusting the plan by a further two hours, repeat until the usual sleeping pattern is regained. Temperature patterns may change towards normal.

6. Slowly reduce the level of daytime stimulation while noting patient's behaviour in response.

RE. Record changes in behaviour to identify whether signs of reversal re-occur. If they do then maintain the level of stimulation just above that when reversal seems to start.

7. If there is no return towards the usual pattern consider the possibility of changing the environment to allow the patient to follow their reversal pattern. Check whether the Health Authority provides a night care unit.

RE. Review the implications of night-to-day reversal for relatives and others. Discuss alternatives with the medical staff.

Further action	1. Nitrazepam given at the same time each night about half an hour before bedtime may aid re-establishment of the patient's previous pattern. Treatment may need to be continued for several weeks.

RE. Record the time it is given and when the patient fell asleep. Compare this with the previous pattern after one week, to identify whether the new pattern is acceptable. Observe for confusion.

2. A tot of brandy or whisky may help the patient relax sufficiently to aid sleep. Many people who drink alcohol tend to do so in the evening.

RE. Record the time it is given and the effect. Note when the patient falls asleep. Observe for signs of flushing of the face and trunk indicating alcohol sensitivity. Observe for a hangover next morning.

Associated medical diagnosis	Dementia

Problem	**Kept awake by nurse intervention**

Assessment findings	Woken more frequently than 2-hourly Observations of vital signs Observations of neurological state Incontinent Severe risk of skin damage Pressure lesions
Information for the patient	Nursing care often has to be carried out at times when the patient is asleep. Each person has their own pattern of alternating deep relaxing sleep and

dreaming sleep. It is easier to return to sleep if woken up when the dreaming ends and the lighter sleep is about to change to a deeper, more relaxed sleep. It takes a while for the nurses to find out someone's personal sleep pattern.

If the patient is not getting enough rest and sleep it may be possible to find alternative methods of providing the right care. These may take a while to arrange so they will only be considered if it is expected to be necessary to wake the patient for three or more nights running.

Nursing action

1. Review the need for nursing action such as turning to relieve pressure and the times it is carried out. Compare them with the patient's usual sleeping pattern. Consider modifying time of nursing action so it is carried out at the time of lightest sleep. Before waking the patient up, observe for signs of dreaming or deep sleep.

RE. Record the time that the patient falls asleep after nursing intervention. Ask them on waking whether they felt they were woken from a deep or a light sleep; mark this on a chart, together with the time.

2. Consider alternative methods of monitoring physiological change such as a thermistor for temperature recording or electronic sensors for pulse or blood pressure.

RE. Compare the likely period that monitoring will last with the cost or difficulty of obtaining the equipment and with the importance of sleep for the patient. Ask the medical staff to review the frequency of observations at least daily.

3. Consider alternative methods of changing position or relieving pressure, such as a low air loss bed, net suspension bed, fluidized sand/bead bed or gel filled pads.

RE. Monitor response of skin over pressure points after changing the method.

4. Consider alternative methods of managing incontinence such as the use of lightweight, close-fitting incontinence pads and silicone cream, or Kylie sheet, so that frequency of waking can be reduced.

RE. Monitor response of skin exposed to urine. Compare loss of habit training with the need for sleep. Consider a combination of waking the patient to use the commode with using protective pads.

5. Plan additional periods of rest and sleep.

RE. Record hours of sleep achieved in each 24 hours. Compare with usual period. Ask patient if sleep is refreshing.

Further action

1. Plan blood transfusions or intravenous drug therapy by infusion for waking hours rather than accept frequent disturbance overnight.

RE. If the transfusion/intravenous therapy runs behind schedule, discuss with the medical staff whether it is imperative to continue overnight or if a delay until the morning will be possible.

Associated medical diagnoses

Blood loss requiring transfusion
Cerebral vascular accident
Head injury
Thalassemia
Urinary incontinence

Problem	**Kept awake by night cramps**
Assessment findings	Woken by pain in foot or calf Muscle spasm distorts toes or foot Finds relief by hanging leg over bed edge Prefers to sit in a chair Sudden pain in neck muscles Limb appears pink in colour
Information for the patient	The muscles usually contract only when told to by the brain. Sometimes the counter message to relax again fails to get through, and then painful cramp or spasm occurs. If the body's salt balance is upset this can lead to cramps. Violent exercise, for example sport in hot weather, may be enough to cause this. Sometimes the pain is due not to muscle spasm but to poor blood flow in furred-up arteries. The cells need oxygen but if the flow of blood is slow they quickly remove all the oxygen available. Gravity may be helpful, and sometimes raising the limb to speed up drainage of blood in the veins helps to allow fresh oxygenated blood to enter a a faster rate.
Nursing action	1. Stretch the affected part gently but firmly. If the foot or toes are in spasm suggest that the patient pushes firmly down against the foot of the bed, or stands up or walks. Massage the affected area gently but firmly to stimulate blood flow in an otherwise normal limb. RE. Record how long it takes for the muscle spasm to subside and how frequently the spasms occur. Discuss this with the doctor. 2. Consider whether the patient should adopt a more upright or sitting position if they are not hypotensive, and where vascular changes in the lower limb are suspected. Use thick blankets or a padded sleeping bag for warmth, a wing chair for safety and check the seat edge does not press into the popliteal space (the region behind the knee). RE. Record if and for how long the patient slept. 3. If possible, teach muscle-stretching exercises that the patient can do in bed. RE. Ask the patient to report when cramp occurs. 4. Monitor salt intake to identify whether additional salt in the diet may help. RE. Estimate daily salt intake and compare with estimated loss in sweat and urine. Normal loss of salt into urine is 3–6 g/24 hours and in sweat 5–10 mmol a day.
Further action	1. Quinine sulphate may be given to reduce symptoms. It is accumulative in action and therefore normally given only once daily, in the evening. RE. Observe for hypersensitivity reactions following the first dose. Report any complaints of ringing in the ears (tinnitus) to the doctor. Monitor the pulse for arrhythmia if heart problems are known to be present. It may increase the effect of anti-coagulants. A regular blood count may be useful if treatment is to continue over several weeks.

2. Check the patient's blood serum electrolyte results for low blood sodium. Slow release sodium tablets may be useful.

RE. Ask the patient to report if whole tablets appear in stools indicating limited absorption. Serum electrolyte results should return to normal levels.

3. Antispasmodic drugs such as baclofen and mephenesin may be useful in some conditions. Give them with a glass of milk, or food.

RE. Observe for changes in the pulse rate or volume. In elderly men urinary retention may occur. Check blood pressure if dizziness occurs. Ask the patient to report any blurring of vision, especially if glaucoma is present. If high doses are given, monitor for nausea, vomiting, constipation or diarrhoea.

4. Diazepam and related drugs may be used if anxiety is present with the muscle spasm. Diazepam acts on the central nervous system and its effect is increased by alcohol.

RE. Record the frequency of spasms and any change in mood. If a variety of drugs are also being given, ask the pharmacist to check the possibility of an increased effect from diazepam. Depression, skin rash and palpitations may occur in some people. Effectiveness may diminish after two or more weeks of use.

Associated medical diagnoses	Arteriosclerosis Cerebral vascular accident Cold agglutins disease Drug abuse — drug withdrawal Hyponatraemia Hysterical hyperventilation Malaria Multiple sclerosis Peripheral vascular disease Tetany/hypocalcaemia Toxic effects of poisons Upper motor neurone disease

Potential problems

Potential problem	Risk of disturbance to usual diurnal sleep pattern
Assessment findings	Intensive nursing care Constantly lit room Constant activity in room Journey across major time zones Unusual noise in area Woken at least every two hours during the night
Information for the patient	The internal body clock which affects when people sleep and wake up relies on cues from the outside world to help keep it to time. Daylight and the darkness of night time are important, but in some circumstances it may be difficult to actually distinguish day from night. A big change to the pattern of the body clock, such as being woken frequently, or being in an intensive care unit, can upset the body clock and the sleeping pattern. This becomes

important if it lasts for more than a couple of days, so every effort will be made to keep to a normal pattern whenever possible.

Nursing action

1. Identify activities which could or do give a time cue. Plan feeding/mealtimes to move towards day times, omit naso-gastric feeding during the night unless nutrition has higher priority than sleep. If the risk of disturbance to sleep is high, record oral or rectal temperature hourly when awake.

RE. Monitor time cues, increase the emphasis on these, and ensure they are on time if the temperature pattern should start to change.

2. If possible discuss usual sleeping habits with the patient, particularly their sleeping position and times of sleeping and waking. Plan to follow these; if possible include usual rituals in preparing for sleep.

RE. Record the time that the patient falls asleep and wakes up.

3. Plan to reduce light intensity during the usual sleeping period. If light cannot be reduced, use a sleeping mask or eye pads for the night time.

RE. Observe for signs of relaxation and sleep.

4. Reduce noise and activity in area during the night time hours. If this is not possible, then use ear plugs. Ensure all staff know when these are in use so that in the event of a fire or other emergency, the patient would be warned.

RE. Observe for signs of relaxation and sleep. Ear plugs can make the pulse audible to the patient. Some people find this aids sleep, others get irritated by the sound.

Associated medical diagnoses

Head injury
Meningitis
Myocardial infarction
Tracheostomy

Potential problem **Risk of exhaustion**

Assessment findings

Lack of sleep
Weak
Intensive nursing care needed
Woken at frequent intervals
Restless
Over-active
No sleep for 36—48 hours
Severe nocturia
Fever
Hallucinations
Loss of ability to concentrate

Information for the patient

Rest is more important than sleep, but the body does need some time each night for dreams and deep relaxation. In illness the need for sleep is increased. Care and treatment can be adjusted so that rest periods are possible, however 24 to 36 hours without sleep, while unpleasant and tiring will not be harmful. It may be helpful to follow relaxation techniques and to carry out as many of the usual preparations for sleep as circumstances will allow.

Nursing action

1. Review the total care plan to identify periods when sleep is possible, and plan to provide conditions which encourage sleep. Group together nursing actions in order to increase rest periods.

RE. Record if and when the patient sleeps during their rest periods. Monitor the noise level and any unplanned disturbance of sleep, so that action can be taken to decrease it.

2. Assure the patient that rest is more important than sleep. Teach relaxation techniques if the patient is able to concentrate, otherwise teach and supervise simple relaxation exercises.

RE. Record for how long the patient rests quietly, or actually falls asleep. Assess their muscle tension level for relaxation.

3. Observe for signs of increasing tiredness, including pallor and weakness.

RE. Review the patient's condition, and the number of hours of sleep they achieved. Consider the relative importance of treatment and the need for more sleep. Discuss any adjustment of treatment with the doctor, if the sleep deficit appears to be increasing.

4. Warn the patient that dream debt may lead to a rebound, with more vivid dreams than usual occurring.

RE. Ask the patient to report whether they found their sleep refreshing, and how much they dreamed.

5. In brightly lit environments such as an intensive care unit, either dim the lights during rest periods, or provide the patient with a sleep mask to block out the light.

RE. Record whether sleep takes place. Review the amount of sleep achieved in 24 hours.

Further action

1. Plan medical examinations, treatment and physiotherapy to ensure that rest periods of at least one or two hours occur. Use a notice by the bed to remind staff that the patient is resting and should not be disturbed.

RE. Observe the patient to see whether they sleep during rest periods, and to ward off any disturbance.

2. Review the necessity for regular physiological measurements and treatments.

RE. Note whether or not the times of measurements have been altered.

3. Symptoms which increase patient's exhaustion, such as frequency of micturition, should, where possible, be relieved by medication.

RE. Record the result of treatment.

Associated medical diagnoses

Cerebral vascular accident
Cystitis
Dementia
Head injury
Myocardial infarction
Pneumonia
Thyrotoxicosis
Ulcerative colitis
Any major illness

187

Reference

Holdencroft, A. (1980). *Body Temperature Control.* Baillière Tindall Ltd, London.

Useful addresses

Nightsitting service and domiciliary nursing service for cancer patients:
   The Marie Curie Memorial Foundation, 28 Belgrave Square, London SW1X 8QG.
Support and advice for people wishing to come off medically prescribed minor tranquillizers and sleeping pills:
   Tranx (Tranquillizer Recovery and New Existence), 17 Peel Road, Wealdstone, Middlesex. Tel: 01 427 2065

Learning Outcomes for Ward Visit

AIM: To observe/assist patients with eating and drinking, and serving of meals.

OBJECTIVES: At the end of this visit the learner will be able to:

a) be aware of the patient's needs with reference to eating and drinking

b) list a minimum of five nursing activities that facilitate eating and drinking

c) identify the type of menu cards/stickers used

d) be aware of alternative methods of feeding e.g. clinifeed, intravenous infusion.

SB/SMC/May 93

6 Mobility

Optimum environment

Movement

Most people take movement for granted, having forgotten the difficulties of learning to balance, stand and walk which are so much part of childhood. The shape of the body is in part due to the pull of different groups of muscles on the underlying bones. These depend on the nervous system being able to pass on the instructions to the different muscle groups to contract or relax. Some of these instructions do not require conscious thought, particularly the protective reflexes. Touching a hot saucepan leads to a rapid withdrawal of the skin surface before severe damage can be done by the heat. It makes us 'jump'.

The skin surface has pain receptors which if stimulated, for example by the hot saucepan, send an impulse along a sensory nerve to the spinal column or the brain stem depending on which part of the body is involved. A small nerve provides a connection to the motor neurone which carries impulses back to the muscles. The impulse stimulates the muscle so it contracts. The reflex is so swift the muscle contracts before the pain reaches consciousness.

The simplest reflex pathway has just a sensory neurone and a motor neurone taking the impulse back to the muscle, eg the 'knee jerk' or patellar reflex. Reflexes have an important part to play in keeping the body upright against the pull of gravity. Stretching of a muscle is quickly opposed by muscle contraction.

The stretch receptors are called muscle spindles, they are stimulated by changes in the tension of the muscle. The spindles lie parallel to the muscle fibres. If the fibres are stretched the spindles increase the number of impulses sent to the spinal cord and the reflex which results contracts the muscle. Contracting muscle produces less stretch on the spindles so they send fewer impulses than usual. If the reflex path is interrupted the muscle becomes flaccid and has no tone. The contraction of the muscle can be monitored and controlled. Piano playing, sketching, writing, typing and many other skills can be carried out because of the precise control that is possible.

The muscles which are used in movement are under control of the thinking part of the brain. Each muscle fibre is wrapped in delicate connective tissue and bundled together with other muscle fibres in further layers of tissue. Layers of the connective tissue wrap together the bundles and connect them via the tendons to the bone. The nerves which supply the muscles divide up like a twig into many branches; at the end of each one is a specialized termination or motor end plate.

Muscles are arranged in pairs; as one contracts so the other must relax for movement to occur. Not all the muscle fibres contract at once. They contract and relax at different times so that the movement is smooth rather than jerky. Contraction requires energy and oxygen, so the blood supply to the muscle influences its performance.

Sport

Success in many sports requires muscles to contract with the minimum of effort. Training increases the blood supply to the muscles, so that oxygen and energy can be provided in greater quantities. Repeated use of a muscle leads to an increase in size of each muscle fibre. If the level of exercise decreases, the muscles get smaller again. The larger the muscle bulk, the stronger the contraction. People who go in for body building exercises use weight training to increase the bulk of specific muscle groups. Weight lifters also build up their muscle bulk. The carbohydrate for the energy supply (glycogen) stored by the muscle also increases, so that it is readily available for sudden effort. However the first part of the effort can be fuelled without using oxygen. If the oxygen supply does not keep up with the energy being used, then lactic acid collects in the muscles. This then passes into the blood stream to be picked up by the liver and converted back to glycogen. Oxygen is still needed to convert it, so the breathlessness which comes from muscular effort continues after the exercise is over, and until all the glycogen is dealt with.

The need for oxygen during exercise leads to an increased rate and depth of breathing. This provides an increased supply of oxygen within the lungs for the blood to collect and carry to the muscles. Athletic training leads to improved efficiency of the heart and lungs, so that the pulse rate does not rise as quickly when exercise starts, and it returns more quickly to normal at the end of exercise. Some schemes of training are planned according to changes in the pulse rate.

Posture

The way in which the body is held depends in part on the muscle tone. It also depends on awareness of the position of different areas of the body. The inner ear provides information on the position of the head, and hence the upper body. Three loops or semi-circular canals within the membraneous labyrinth of the inner ear contain fluid. Movement of the head swirls the fluid around, bending the tiny hairs of sensory receptors, and so sending signals to the brain. In the expanded portions of the inner ear are tiny crystals embedded among more tiny hair-like receptors. These respond to gravity, and provide more information about the position of the head. Visual information is also used, and rapid motion can lead to a feeling of nausea. Travel sickness may partly be due to conflicting information being received from the different senses.

The joints between the bones are supplied with stretch receptors in the membrane which surrounds them. Their nerve impulses join those from the skin — particularly of the feet and hands — the muscles, ligaments and tendons. Reflex adjustment of the degree of contraction of different groups of muscles keeps the body upright. If the balance is disturbed, for example by a push from behind, then other reflexes act to return the body to the upright position. New reflexes can be established for unusual positions, for example in learning to skate on ice, riding a bicycle, or for swimming.

Reflexes can also be changed, so that poor posture, especially when standing, is not corrected without conscious thought. An aching back may be the first indication of poor posture when standing for a long time, or, for example, after a spell at the typewriter. The increasingly popular 'Alexander' method develops conscious awareness of the position of the body and tension in the muscles to improve posture. The Victorian exercise of walking and sitting with a book balanced on the top of the head encourages holding the spine in more normal alignment. Yoga exercises can also be used to develop an awareness of posture and muscle tension.

Furniture

Sitting and lying in comfort depend on the type of furniture used. Choosing a bed and mattress tend not to be given the care they deserve. Few people stop to think that they will spend about eight hours in every twenty four asleep in bed. That means one third of a lifetime. The mattress can be chosen to support the normal curves of the spine, but this needs care. The type of mattress chosen so often depends on the cost, not the kind of surface it offers the body. Foam tends to break up with use, and so offers less and less support. Sprung mattresses must be chosen taking into account the weight of the person lying on them. Some firms offer mattresses for double beds with different springing — a his and hers mattress.

Those with back trouble tend to prefer a firm surface. The chainlink bedstead sags with use. A sheet of chipboard can be trimmed to fit the bed frame and provide a firm base. Care should be taken with beds advertised as 'orthopaedic' as the mattress may offer no better support than a cheaper, well-sprung mattress. It is important to test a mattress for comfort and support. The only way to do this is to lie on it. The surface should not be so soft that there is no space between the curve of the small of the back and the mattress.

It can be harmful to those with back trouble if they insist on turning the mattress. This procedure is not so necessary for a modern sprung mattress as it was for the old fashioned flock, straw or horse-hair mattresses. More important is the removal of dust from the surface. This is composed of dried skin scales and provides food for the tiny house mite. The latter can cause asthma in susceptible people.

Pillows also have a part to play in posture. One flat pillow under the head allows the curves of the neck and upper spine to remain in a normal position. Several pillows tend to push the head and neck forward. If extra pillows are needed to prop up the body during sleep to ease breathlessness, those at the base of the pile should be firm. An old fashioned bolster is useful for this.

The height and support offered by chairs can also make a big difference to posture, and to preventing backache. The height of the seat should allow the feet to rest flat on the floor without any feeling of stretching. The depth of the seat should allow the buttocks to touch the seat back, while leaving a space of about two inches between the seat edge and the back of the knee. The back of the seat should support the back in an upright position or lean slightly backwards.

If the chair cannot be changed, it is possible to improve the support in various ways. A footstool can be used to overcome too high a chair seat. Too low a seat can be improved by raising the height with a brick or wooden block under each chair leg. For safety, these should have a shallow depression into which the chairleg fits. Cushions can be used to fill the space behind the spine if the seat is too deep. Lightweight, portable backrests sold for use by car drivers make a useful alternative for those with back trouble.

Elderly people and those with stiff hips may find it easier to sit down on and get up from a chair with a higher seat than normal. An extra seat pad from another chair may be enough. A chair with arm rests is also helpful as it allows for an extra push from the arms when standing up.

The height of the table relative to the height of the body when seated also aids good posture. Those who spend several hours a day working at a table or desk should ensure that the height is sufficient for the arms to hang naturally from the shoulders without being hunched. This means that when seated, the surface of the table should be about level with the elbows. A low table can be raised by small wooden blocks, and even thick books can be used.

A typist or computer operator should ensure that the seat height is adjusted to take account of the keyboard. It is also useful to make a habit of standing and stretching, or having a brief walk around the room every half hour or so. It is very easy to get used to an abnormal posture. The muscular effort of holding the position while concentrating on the work in hand can lead to backache by the end of the day. The fashion for exercise or dance classes in the lunch break is a healthy one. Slumped postures decrease the use of the rib cage so that breathing becomes shallower and less oxygen is available. A brisk walk in the fresh air at lunch time can act as a reviver of energy and concentration.

Work surfaces and sinks should also when possible be chosen with good posture in mind. Aching feet while working at the sink may be eased by standing on a thick mat.

Feet and posture

The body's balance and therefore its posture depends on the position of the foot. The fashion for high heels tends to throw the weight forward onto the metatarsals. To maintain balance, muscles have to be brought into use in a different way from normal. It is therefore necessary to learn how to walk in high heels, or in other words to learn to ignore the normal reflexes and adopt new reflex patterns.

In walking, the toes splay out unless the shoe or boot prevents them from doing so. Fashionable shoes with pointed toes tend to push the toes into a pointed shape. The distortion gets worse with time, and pressure on the joint at the base of the big toe increases the production of fluid which would normally lubricate it. For a while this produces a cushioning effect but in time the joint becomes painful. The big toe may be pushed up over the other toes. In this way a bunion is being created. Meanwhile the small toes may be pushed back by the pressure of the toe of the shoe. The area of skin over the last joint on each toe gets thicker as a protective measure. This leads to corns that can become painful. The joints of the toes may be pushed up so that they rub on the top of the shoe. Ugly, painful feet result, and it becomes difficult to find comfortable shoes.

Foot damage from shoes can be limited by choosing footwear with a broader toe shape so that the toes can splay out to spread some of the weight of each step. The soles of the shoes should have some flexibility or 'give' with each step. Rigid wedges should not be worn for long periods. Varying the height of the heels of shoes can help limit strain on the leg muscles. A few hours wearing fashionable shoes which are not really foot shaped will do little harm if it is followed by a much longer period wearing open sandals or walking barefoot on smooth or carpeted floors. Indian style sandals with a single toe loop or shaped wooden exercise sandals encourage natural muscle action.

Tight socks can also distort the shape of the foot. Pressure from socks and shoes can press the toenails into the skin at the sides of the nail. Trimming the nails straight across rather than filing to a curved shape can help to prevent damage. Toes squeezed together do not lose sweat as easily. Combine this with footwear made of synthetic materials, and bacteria or fungal infections can occur. Absorbent cotton or wool socks are better than nylon in aiding sweat evaporation. Leather uppers on a shoe or sandals allow sweat to escape. Smelly feet usually indicate bacterial or fungal growth. Washing with a skin antiseptic can remove and prevent bacterial growth. Athlete's foot, a fungal infection between the toes, can be treated with foot powder. Comfortable feet allow comfortable walking.

Chiropody used to be thought of as a service only for the old, but unsuitable footwear can create corns and hammer toes even in the young. National

Health Chiropody services tend to concentrate on the elderly, those with diabetes, or people who are housebound. Care should be taken in selecting a private chiropodist for treatment, as it has been possible for someone to set up a service without proper training.

Exercise

Jogging is not the only form of exercise for getting and keeping fit! A brisk walk lasting 15 to 20 minutes, perhaps getting off the bus or tube one stop earlier than usual, helps improve muscle tone and breathing. Gentle stretching and bending exercises use muscles not normally given much exercise in a normal day in an office. Housework provides a wide range of stretching and bending movements, as does gardening. Walking up and down stairs also requires quite a lot of muscular effort. However all these activities tend to lack the stimulation of the company of other people. Many local authorities hold evening and afternoon keep fit classes. Dance classes have also increased in popularity. Movement in time to music in the company of others can turn dull exercises into good fun. Regular exercise should be part of everyone's body maintenance programme.

Elderly people can join in exercises, provided they start off slowly and build up the amount at a pace which does not leave them tired, or with painful muscles. Swimming or exercise classes for the older age group may be run by local authority adult education departments, or by the charity Age Concern. Dancing provides hip exercise and is less strenuous than the ice-skating which would be more suited to the young. The bones lose some of their calcium in old age, and this makes fractures more likely after a simple fall. Women are more prone to this than men. Exercise however can slow the loss of bone density, the part of the body most involved in the exercise being the one which develops stronger bones.

Activities which develop balance and muscular control of the trunk include ballet, archery, skating, and for those with a taste for the unusual, tightrope walking. Skiing, tennis and climbing develop other muscles, but are best left to the young if they have never been tried before.

Stiff muscles

Unusual, strenuous exercise can lead to painful, stiff muscles, especially the day after. A hot bath can increase blood flow by encouraging the dilation of the blood vessels on the surface. This means that waste products can be removed more rapidly, and glycogen stores in the muscles replaced. A shower after exercise removes the sweat, but does not ease the discomfort in the muscles in the same way as a ten minute soak in a hot bath.

Another way of applying heat and increasing local blood flow is to apply a rubefacient (which reddens the skin). Wintergreen oil, being rather smelly and messy to apply, has given way to creams which are absorbed into the surface layer of the skin. Salicylates, nicotinates and terpenes may be mentioned in the ingredients. Care must be taken not to touch the eyes or face with fingers which have applied the cream. A thorough wash with soap and water may not remove all traces from the skin surface.

Aerosol sprays, which can be applied over unbroken skin, cool and relieve more painful sprains and strains. Gentle massage over and around painful areas can be applied following exercise. Relaxation exercises and warmth from a well wrapped hot water bottle may also help. Discomfort after exercise should lessen within twenty-four hours, and should go within three days.

Houses safe to live in

Accidents in the home can be avoided by spotting potential hazards and making simple changes. Older people need to be especially careful about having their stairs and passages well lit. Eyesight slowly deteriorates in old age, and more light is needed to be able to see as well as in younger days. A higher wattage bulb can make a big difference. A firm stepladder should be used rather than a kitchen chair when curtains need to be hung, bulbs changed or high shelves dusted. Youth and community schemes are often willing to send someone along to carry out these tasks for the elderly or disabled.

The surface on which we walk can have a big influence on balance. A path slippery with frost or snow presents a major danger, especially to elderly women who are most prone to breaking the hip bone (head of femur) if they fall. A good neighbour may offer to do the shopping or collect the pension during such weather. Coarse cooking salt and sand can be used on a path swept clear of snow to delay refreezing of the film of water left on the surface.

Rugs on polished linoleum or wood floors may look nice but they also provide a hazard. Some carpet shops and department stores sell non-slip net which can be stitched in six inch wide strips on the short ends of rugs to anchor them. This also helps to keep the edge of the rug flat on the floor. Catching a toe on the edge of a wrinkled rug or a frayed carpet can cause a bad fall.

Special care needs to be taken with trailing electrical flex and cables. Those for televisions, record players, music centres and table lamps which do not get moved around the house can have the cable fixed to the skirting with electrician's staples. Cable should not be looped round as it will heat up when in use, instead it should be cut to size and the plug refitted by someone experienced in electrical work. The wires are colour coded and this is not a job for the colour blind.

The handyman can, with care, even up the legs of a wobbly chair so that it remains firm in use. Elderly people who hold on to furniture as they walk around a room are at particular risk, and they are also the ones whose furniture has often had years of wear and tear.

General assessment areas

Muscle strength
Limb position
Range of joint movement
Pain related to movement
Balance
Body alignment
Posture
Limb length
Daily living activities undertaken
Normal environment at home and work
Aids used to increase mobility
Awareness of body position
Age

Problems

	Page
Unable to stand without support	197
Unable to move or feel arm	200
Unable to move or feel leg	206
Unable to straighten back	210
Unable to dress unaided	212
Unable to turn over in bed	214
Unsteady gait when walking	216
Severe weakness of one side of the body	218
Loss of fine finger control	223
Loss of control of movements, with tremor	225
Increasing muscle weakness	227
Unable to use crutches correctly	229
Unable to grip with one hand	231
Unable to change position when lying in bed	232
Slow increase in activity desirable	234

Potential problems

Risk of limb contracture	235
Risk of falling	238
Risk of deep vein thrombosis developing	240
Risk of urinary infection due to stasis	242
Risk of partial pulmonary collapse (atelectasis)	244
Risk of skin damage due to loss of sensation	245

Problems

Problem	Unable to stand without support.

Assessment findings

Feels too weak to stand
Legs buckle when helped to stand
Severe pain on standing
Muscle wasting in legs
Unable to balance
Holds on to furniture
Loss of sensation in foot or leg
Foot drop (sole of foot falls downwards)
Severe deformity of the legs or hips
Loss of sensation and movement from below the waist

Information for the patient

To be able to stand, some of the muscles of the legs and back must contract and pull against the bones, other muscles relax to allow the change in position of the joints. If the muscles are weak, they cannot pull strongly enough to change and hold the body's position. The decision to stand taken in the brain must be sent to the muscles involved by the nerves. If there is a block in the nerve pathways, or the right chemicals are not in place in the nerves, then this message cannot get through. Messages about the position of the body and the stretch of the muscles also have to go back to the brain. If that return pathway is blocked then it may be very difficult for a person to keep their balance.

Nursing action

1. Discuss the pattern of the patient's daily activities to identify the number of movements from bed to chair, bath or vehicle required each day. Identify the resources available such as strong arms, adapted furniture or specific aids. Include the use of helpful aids in the care plan.

RE. Assess how the available aids are used to identify whether any modification would increase their usefulness.

2. Teach the patient and helpers how to transfer the patient from bed to chair. Place the chair at the head of the bed. Help the patient into a sitting position using a monkey pole or by crossing the leg on the far side of the bed over the nearest leg and pulling the trunk upright as the legs are swung over the bed edge.

RE. Check the bed height is low enough for the patient's feet to rest flat on the floor when sitting, with the knees bent at a right angle.

3. The helper must stand in front of the patient with the feet placed on either side of the patient's feet. The knees can then be used to prevent the patient slipping to the side. Ask the patient to rest the arms on the shoulders of the helper. Pull the patient's weight forwards from the waist, make a quarter turn and lower the patient into the chair. The helper should be taught to keep their knees slightly bent, and take the patient's weight with their legs, in order to prevent back strain.

RE. Check the chair is placed close to the bedside. If the patient pulls on the helper's shoulders, muscles may be strained. If the patient proves difficult to swivel over a quarter turn, a useful aid to try is a small flat turntable on which to stand the patient.

4. A transfer board may be used if the patient has control and sufficient strength in the shoulders to move the trunk sideways. The bed and chair should be at the same height. Place the chair or commode towards the head of the bed and remove the arm. The transfer board is then placed as a bridge between chair and bed. Help the patient sit up, help may be needed to lower the legs from the bed once the patient has shuffled from the bed over to the chair. The transfer board can then be removed and the arm of the chair replaced.

RE. Check the transfer board at least weekly for splinters so that any damage to the surface can be repaired. Several coats of varnish or polyurethane on a piece of smoothed hard wood two feet long and ten inches wide can provide a board for home use. Check that the patient develops a habit of checking that the wheels of the chair or commode are locked before transfer.

5. Lifting from bed to chair requires at least two helpers. Check the space beside the bed is cleared of furniture, place the armchair at an angle beside the bedhead. The Australian lift is the easiest if the patient has some strength in the arms. Both helpers face the patient who sits on the edge of the bed and they clasp hands beneath the patient's thighs, at the same time placing the shoulder under the patient's outstretched arms. The patient then rests the arms across their shoulders so that some of the weight is taken by the upper trunk. The helper's free hand can then be used to support the patient, or control the chair or clothing during the lift.

RE. Check the patient has control of the upper arms, so that the weight is well distributed across the helpers' backs during the lift. Check the helpers bend their knees during the lift, so the large muscles of the thighs do most of the work.

6. The basket lift may be needed if the patient has little control or strength in the arms. The two helpers stand facing each other on either side of the patient, who sits on the edge of the bed. The helpers clasp hands beneath the patient's thighs and midway up the patient's back, or reach across to the patient's waist so their arms cross. The knees must be bent during the lift so that the large muscles of the thighs are used.

RE. Observe for fatigue in the helpers as this lift requires more strength than other types of lifting. Helpers should be of similar height. If the relatives will find it difficult to use this lift at home, other means of transferring the patient should be considered. The physiotherapist can advise and the occupational therapist may be able to suggest aids and adaptations to reduce the number of times lifting will be required.

7. Moving the patient back from chair to bed is more difficult and should not be taught to relatives until they are competent at the bed-to-chair transfer. Place the patient's feet flat on the floor, about six inches apart and close to the chair. Place the patient's hands on the helper's waist, steady them by gripping just above the elbows. Lean the patient forward so the body weight is over the hips. If the helper keeps one foot in front of the other the weight can be transferred back as the patient rises. The helper's knee can also be used to support the patient's knees on standing. Turn through one quarter so that the patient's buttocks rest on the edge of the bed. From the sitting position the patient can swivel the trunk towards the head of the bed, as the helper lifts the legs on to it.

RE. Check the helper bends at the knees so that the thigh muscles are used during the lift. Check the height of the bed allows the patient to sit with the feet flat on the floor and the knees bent at right angles. Check the footwear of patient and helper provides support and does not slip easily (low-heeled shoes are necessary). Note each teaching session for the relatives, and record any comments which may indicate muscle strain.

8. A hoist lift should be considered for moving patients who are obese, uncooperative or difficult to transfer. It may be of particular help during bathing, to avoid back strain among the helpers. A canvas sling or a firm chair-type seat may be used. The former is preferable if the patient has little strength or control in the upper part of their body.

RE. Check the hoist is given a maintenance check at least every four weeks if it is in constant use. Check that each helper is able to use the hoist correctly, and develops the habit of checking the wheel brakes are on before lifting the patient with the hoist. Observe the facial expression of the patient for tension and signs of anxiety, particularly if a canvas sling is used. Check the sacral area of the back at least daily for signs of friction on the skin surface if a canvas sling is used. In obese patients, the risk of damage to the skin can be increased by the use of a hoist.

Further action

1. Investigations of the cause of muscle weakness include muscle biopsy and temporal artery biopsy.

RE. The biopsy site should be observed for bruising or bleeding during the first two hours after the biopsy. A dry dressing over the site should not be removed until the sutures are removed, unless there is an indication of infection.

2. A calico splint with rigid straps may be used to support an unstable knee, which otherwise would not allow weight bearing on one side. The physiotherapist will supply and fit the aid. It should be worn over pyjamas or other trousers.

RE. Check the straps are firm but not tight enough to interfere with the blood circulation. The calico may rub if it is secured too tightly. Inspect the skin at least daily for signs of damage. Once the knee becomes stable the splint can be discarded.

3. Moulded splints made of plastic material may be prescribed if the instability is likely to last for some time. Wash the splint with warm soapy water and dry in a warm place, away from direct heat, at least weekly. A foot splint attached to a lace up shoe may be provided for foot drop. It should be worn when standing or sitting in a chair.

RE. There is less risk of skin damage when the splint is moulded to the patient's own shape. If general weight loss occurs, the splint will need adjusting. Broken straps should be repaired quickly so the support given by the splint will remain even.

4. Physiotherapy and hydrotherapy (exercise in a shallow pool) may be prescribed to increase muscle strength, control and balance. Plan the pattern of the patient's day with the therapist and the patient so that there will be no delays in keeping appointment times in the gym or pool. Also plan rest periods to follow the more active exercise periods.

RE. Observe for signs of fatigue and for slow recovery of energy after exercise. Check the diet provides sufficient energy as activities increase.

5. A wheelchair may be prescribed if there is little likelihood of improvement. The order form requires a doctor's signature, although the physiotherapist and occupational therapist will wish to advise on the type and size of chair to be supplied. If possible, at the same time order a pressure relieving cushion to fit the chair.

RE. Check that the rooms, doorways and furniture heights of the patient's surroundings are taken into account.

Associated medical diagnoses	Acute lymphoblastic leukaemia Anaemia Ankylosing spondylitis Ataxia Cachexia Cerebral tumour Cerebral vascular tumour Dermatomyositis Guillain Barré Syndrome Huntingdon's chorea Hypotension Ménière's disease Motor neurone disease Multiple sclerosis Muscular dystrophy Myasthenia gravis Osteoarthrosis Otitis media Parkinson's disease Paraplegia Polyarteritis nodosa Prolapsed intervertebral disc Psychosis Rheumatoid arthritis Spinal cord compression Sub-acute combined degeneration of the cord Thyrotoxic myopathy Tuberculosis of the spine

Problem	**Unable to move or feel arm.**

Assessment findings	Arm in plaster cast Arm in plastic splint Arm in abnormal alignment Unable to move arm Unable to grasp with hand Loss of muscle strength Unable to lift objects Loss of coordination Unaware of position of arm on affected side Unable to tell position of index finger when moved by someone else

Flaccid (floppy rag doll) arm
Fingers curl into palm
Arm held across the body
Slumps towards affected side
Pain if arm moved by others
Pain in shoulder
Reduced muscle tone
Muscle spasm
Fails to draw affected arm when drawing a picture of a person
Drawing placed to one side of paper
Gross swelling of arm

Information for the patient

The muscles need instructions from the brain to contract or relax so that movement can take place. If there is a block in the path of the messages to the nerves from the brain, then movement cannot occur and partial blockage leads to weakness. Damage to brain cells may mean no messages can be sent. A surprisingly large area of the brain is normally devoted to sorting out all the information from the skin and muscles of the hand. If this area is damaged, all the information is left unsorted. The arm is not felt, as the messages from muscles and joints, which would provide the feeling of having an arm, are now missing. With time, new pathways may be opened up and other brain cells may take over the function of damaged cells. While this is happening the muscles on one part of the arm may be contracting, and so cause deformity. To prevent this, to increase the rate of recovery and to keep the muscles in trim, careful positioning and exercise are required. It may take up to two years to recover from the effects of a stroke which has destroyed some brain cells.

Nursing action

1. Discuss the current level of activity and agree with the patient and physiotherapist which skills will be worked on over the next two weeks. Agree a target, and if appropriate, what the reward will be for achieving it. Plan out the practice sessions, increasing the number of exercise repeats and the time to be taken. Targets may include lifting increasing weights.

RE. Assess how realistic the patient's expectations of their progress appear to be. Morale can be raised by achieving goals, so advise on those that appear likely to be achieved in the time set. Rewards may be as simple as a chocolate bar for a goal achieved, or a small sweet for every ten exercise repeats. Bigger rewards may be chosen for extra effort, such as an outing or a special meal. Progress in improving muscle tone may be slow, and not noticed by the patient. A wide variety of rewards may be needed, as too many sweets would lead to obesity.

2. Discuss with the patient and their family or close friends whether their help with the exercises would be acceptable. If so, plan out times when they will be visiting and could help. Plan teaching sessions so that both helper and patient know what to do. Repetition of exercises can get boring, so explore variations on the theme of each exercise. Enlist the help of the physiotherapist and occupational therapist.

RE. Observe for signs of loss of interest in exercising, such as avoiding exercises, not doing all the agreed repeats, not doing the exercise as slowly as recommended or giving up mid-way. Ask the helper to report back on progress and demonstrate trust and interest in their assessment by making a written note in the patient's progress notes in their presence. Loss of concentration may be a problem if there has been marked damage to the sense of position or presence of the arm.

3. Teach the patient the correct position for sitting and lying, so that any developing spasm is reduced. Encourage the patient to lie on the sound side, and use a pillow level with the shoulder, in front of the chest, so that the affected arm can be stretched forward across it. One small flat pillow under the head should be used, or no pillow at all. A small pillow or foam wedge may be placed under the affected shoulder.

RE. Check that when lying on the sound side the affected arm does not rotate inwards towards the body. Check the height of the pillow is sufficient so the shoulder does not drop forward but is supported. Check the position is comfortable for the patient.

4. The correct position when lying on the affected side has the affected shoulder pulled through with the arm stretched out on the bed, palm towards the ceiling. A pillow tucked behind the back will provide support.

RE. Check the pillow behind the back is sufficient to provide support. Check that the trunk is to one side of the bed so that there is sufficient room for the extended, affected arm to be supported on the mattress. The arm can be bent at the elbow and the hand tucked under the pillow with the palm uppermost as an alternative. Check the affected arm is not trapped under the body.

5. The correct position to be taught for the brief time that the patient should spend lying on the back, should include a pillow under the affected arm to bring the shoulder forward off the bed. The arm should be straight out with the palm facing the ceiling. The head should be turned towards the sound side. Approach the patient in this position from the affected side, to encourage head turning. One flat pillow or no pillow should be used.

RE. Check the shoulder remains lifted forward off the bed. Note the time the patient spends in this position, as it should be limited so that muscle spasm is discouraged.

6. Bed pans provide an opportunity to practise another useful exercise which will later aid sitting and walking. The patient should lie flat on the back and bend the knees so the feet lie flat on the bed. The patient's arms should lie alongside the body, palms downwards so that pushing down is possible as the trunk is raised. If muscle weakness is marked, two people need to join hands under the small of the patient's back and lift together.

RE. Check the affected arm is controlled, so that it does not suddenly slide down the bed in the middle of the lift. The position and exercise use muscles required in walking and sitting. Teach the correct way to roll which is to the affected side first.

7. Rolling during bedmaking and to reach items off the bedside locker provides further useful exercise. The more difficult roll to the sound side must be delayed until some muscle strength returns. The affected hand should be clasped and stretched out and the sound side leg bent so that the movement of the shoulder and hip produce the roll.

RE. Check the fingers are interlaced for the arm manoeuvre, and that the arms are held out straight. Check that the bed height and the position of the locker are such that items can be reached with ease and safety. Ask the patient to demonstrate their ability to reach items off the locker.

8. Use two pillows to keep the affected arm in a forward position when sitting up in bed. Place the locker on the affected side so that helpful exercise comes each time something is placed on it or taken from it. Suggest that visitors sit on the affected side to encourage head and trunk turning. Remind the patient to check the position of their arm after reaching for items.

RE. Check the shoulder is kept forward and does not droop. Observe that visitors do not limit the exercises by handing things to the patient off the locker.

9. Sitting up on the edge of the bed may be taught once muscle strength and control begin to develop. The advice of the physiotherapist should be sought. The affected arm should be used to prop up the trunk while the sound side leg is lifted across the other one. The sound hand is grasped by the helper as the patient is gently pulled into the sitting position. Two people may be needed to help at first, in order to keep the affected arm in place during the movement.

RE. Check there is adequate space around the bed, and that the affected side is nearest to the bed edge. Check that the main helper bends from the knees to use the large thigh muscles during the pulling.

10. Balance in the sitting position should be practised before moving the patient into a chair. Lower the height of the bed so that the patient's feet are flat on the floor when sitting on the bed edge. Stand in front and check their balance. Be ready to steady the patient. Ask the patient to interlace the fingers of his hands and to swing the arms up, keeping the elbows straight. If possible encourage the patient to hold them above the head before swinging them down. Once the arms can be held above the head, the patient should look up at the hands, and, with the good arm, turn the hands so the back of the affected hand points away from the body.

RE. Check the feet are not moved apart more than a few inches, as a wide base indicates poor balance. Look for signs of breath holding or rigid posture. Balance should be achieved with a relaxed posture, and movement of the trunk should be possible before movement of the hips is undertaken. This arm exercise should also be practised when sitting in a chair.

11. Choose an armchair with the seat just high enough for the patient to sit with the knees at a right angle when the feet are flat on the floor. The seat depth should allow a two inch gap behind the knees when the buttocks are touching the chair-back. A firm cushion can be used behind the patient's back if the chair is a few inches too deep. Padded arm rests should be at a height that prevents shoulder droop when the arms rest on them. A pillow can be used to correct the height if the arm rests are too low.

RE. Incorrect seating can undo hard work in practising exercises, so once the correct seat has been obtained it may be wise to place a label with the patient's name on it. Discuss suitable seating with relatives for later care at home. A so-called 'geriatric' chair rarely provides the correct type of seating and should not be used.

12. Place the armchair at the head of the bed on the patient's affected side ready for transfer. Ask the patient to interlace the fingers and put the arms

over the helper's head so that the forearms rest on the shoulders. The helper's hands are then free to direct the movement. The buttocks are 'walked' across to the edge of the bed using hip hitching movements. On standing up, the weight should be taken equally on both feet as the helper helps make a quarter turn backwards to the chair. Teach the patient to feel for the chair seat with the back of the legs before sitting down.

RE. Assess the patient's ability to transfer weight and follow instructions before a single helper transfer is attempted. Check the movement is carried out slowly, steadily and with control, to gain the confidence of the patient. Check that progress to transferring weight to the affected side is not slowed by fear of falling. Make sure the head moves to the right when the weight is transferred to the left hip, if not, gently move it, and vice versa. If progress is slow, consider planning more short rest periods on the bed so that the exercise of rolling and sitting up before transfer to the chair provides extra reasons for practice.

13. Provide an adjustable table which can be set at a height so that the patient can lean forward on their forearms with comfort. Mark the centre of the table with a straight line drawn with a chinagraph (wax) pencil or a strip of adhesive tape, so that the patient is reminded to keep the forearms parallel. The palms should be flat on the table. Meals may be eaten with the sound hand while resting on the affected arm. Reading is another activity during which weight bearing can be practiced. (Fig. 6.1).

RE. Check the patient spends time resting on the forearms with them parallel to the centre line, and transferring weight from one to the other. As much time as possible should be spent in this forearm resting position. Note how much time the patient can tolerate without becoming overtired. Check that the table does not move while in use. It may need to be anchored.

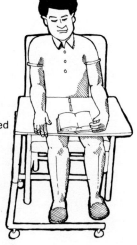

Sitting upright in a chair, weight forward through the affected shoulder to the forearm. Centre of table marked as a reminder to keep arms parallel.
Both feet flat on the floor.

Fig. 6.1 Sitting upright in a chair

14. Provide stimulation to the affected arm by passive exercises to put the shoulder, elbow, wrist and finger joints through the normal range of movements. Note in the care plan any movements which should not be attempted.

RE. Assess and report any change in muscle tone, spasm or pain.

15. Teach the patient to stretch the affected fingers gently and exercise the wrist using their other hand. Remind the patient to carry out the exercises for 5 minutes at least every two hours, when awake. Lack of awareness of the affected arm may limit the patient's ability to comply with instructions.

RE. Supervise exercises until the patient can carry them out without prompting. Brain-damaged patients may need reminding repeatedly.

16. Teach the patient and relatives/visitors that care must be taken to protect the arm from pressure. Splints should be checked for fit, and any straps should be marked to show how tightly they may be done up. Use a ball point pen or felt tip pen on velcro or leather. Check the skin for damage or redness at least once every 24 hours.

RE. Check the marks to ensure a correct fit, especially when the patient learns to adjust the splint themselves. Report any redness or bruising. Check that the padding on the splint stays in place.

17. Teach the patient and relatives/visitors that trapped perspiration can lead to maceration of the skin and fungal infection. The limb should be washed and dried at least twice a day. Clothing should not fit tightly around the armpit, elbow or wrist. Replace pillowcases on pillows supporting the arm at least once daily.

RE. Check areas where two skin folds meet for signs of maceration or increasing redness. Report these to the doctor if they occur.

Further action

1. Physiotherapy in the gymnasium will become necessary once muscle control and strength allow floor exercises and work with parallel bars to begin. Appointment times should be integrated into the care plan. Discuss whether the patient prefers to have a bath after the session in the gym. A deep warm bath may ease muscles on the unaffected side made tender by the increased exercise.

RE. Observe for increasing tiredness after sessions in the gym, which may need extra rest periods to be included in the care plan.

2. Pressure splints to reduce spasm may be used by the physiotherapist during treatments. The clear plastic splint may be inflated by blowing into the inflation tube. In some instances intermittent pressure may be used. It is applied to the arm twice a day to push fluid from the tissues back into circulation and/or into the lymphatic system. The machine is set for the prescribed pressure and for set periods of inflation and deflation. Plan for increased activity between treatments.

RE. Mechanical intermittent pressure should not be used if there is any risk of circulatory overload or deep vein thrombosis. Ask the patient to report any discomfort during use. Measure the circumference of the arm, marking the position of the tape, before and after treatment. Record the length of treatment and the result. Warn the patient that swelling may recur when treatment stops.

Associated medical diagnoses	Carcinoma of breast
	Cerebral tumour
	Cerebral vascular accident
	Cervical spondylosis
	Glioma
	Intracerebral tumour
	Lymphadenopathy
	Motor neurone disease
	Myeloma
	Neuralgic amyotrophy
	Poliomyelitis
	Polymyalgia rheumatica
	Spinal cord tumour
	Spinal nerve compression
	Sub-dural haematoma

Problem **Unable to move or feel leg.**

Assessment findings

Weakness in leg
Unable to support weight on leg
Ignores one leg
Unable to tell position of big toe when moved by someone else
Flaccid (floppy rag doll) limb
Spasm in leg
Fails to draw affected leg when drawing a picture of a person
Drawing placed to one side of paper

Information for the patient

Movement and feeling need messages to go from the skin and muscles to the brain, and for return information to go back along the nerves to the muscles. If the nerve pathway from the leg is blocked or damaged either on its way to or from the brain, then there will be problems in moving or feeling the leg. Damage in the area of the brain which controls the leg will also interfere with movement and sensation. Sometimes the area of the brain which deals with making sense of all the information coming in along the nerves gets damaged, eg due to a stroke. The leg may then be ignored unless the person's attention is directed to it. It is possible to recover movement after brain damage, but it takes months of hard work as new pathways must be opened up, and new cells in the brain taught to take over. If the spinal cord has been cut, then a permanent block on messages getting to the brain means no movement or feeling will return.

Nursing action

1. Discuss the current level of activity and agree with the patient and physiotherapist which skills will be worked on over the next two weeks. Agree a target, and if appropriate, what the reward will be for achieving it. Plan the practice sessions, increasing the number of exercise repeats and the time to be taken.

RE. Assess how realistic the patient's expectations of their progress appear to be. Morale can be raised by achieving goals, so advise against those which appear unlikely to be achieved in the time set. Rewards may be as simple as a favourite chocolate bar for a goal reached or a small sweet for every ten repeats of an exercise. Progress in improving muscle tone may be so slight it goes unnoticed by the patient.

2. Discuss with the patient and family or close friends whether their help with the exercises would be acceptable. If so plan out times when they will be visiting and could help. Plan teaching sessions so both helper and patient know what to do. Repetition of exercises can get boring so explore variations on the theme of each exercise. Enlist the help of the physiotherapist and occupational therapist.

RE. Observe for signs of loss of interest in exercising, such as missing exercises, not doing all the repeats, not doing them as slowly as recommended or giving up mid-way. Ask the helper to report back on progress and demonstrate trust and interest in their assessment by making a written note in the progress notes in their presence.

3. Teach the patient the correct position for lying and sitting so that any developing spasm is reduced. When lying in bed the affected leg should lie in front of the sound leg, both being bent slightly at the knee. A pillow may be used to support the upper leg. Turn the patient from side to side at least every two hours.

RE. Check that the patient remembers to place the affected leg in the correct position. Inspect the skin of the legs for redness due to pressure, and for increased moisture from trapped sweat.

4. Limit lying on the back to a few minutes, if possible, to discourage spasm. Use a pillow under the hip and thigh of the affected leg with the knee bent so that the leg is tipped inwards.

RE. Note the time the patient spends in this position so that the total time in twenty four hours can be limited to about 2—3 hours.

5. Bed pans provide a useful exercise for later sitting and walking. The patient should lie flat, bending the sound knee so the foot lies flat on the bed. Raise the affected leg into the same position. If there is little muscle control it may need to be held there by a third person. The trunk is then raised by the patient pushing down on the arms. A book to hold between the knees may help when loss of sensation makes it difficult for the patient to tell the position of the affected leg.

RE. Check the affected leg is controlled, so that it does not suddenly slide down the bed in the middle of the lift. The position and exercise use muscles involved in sitting and walking. A monkey pole should only be used if there is no chance of improvement, as it reduces the opportunity for correct muscle use.

6. Rolling during bedmaking and to reach items off the bedside locker provides further useful exercise. Place the locker on the affected side. The roll to the sound side is more difficult. Bending the sound leg and pushing down on the mattress helps to swing the sound hip with the movement of the arms.

RE. Check that the bed height and the locker positions allow items to be reached in safety. Check the affected leg is not hooked over by the sound foot as this interferes with the exercise of the correct muscle groups and may produce a 'bad' habit.

7. If the affected leg is ignored because of brain damage, increase the visual and verbal stimulation to draw attention to the presence and position of the leg. Approach the patient from the affected side to encourage head movement

to the affected side. Suggest visitors sit on the affected side. Give clear instructions about moving the affected leg, using the hand to point to or touch it at the same time.

RE. Warn the patient that the loss of the sense of where the affected leg is will make recovery slower, and will require extra work in practising exercises over and over again.

8. Sitting up on the edge of the bed is a good exercise to do to improve balance. The advice of the physiotherapist should be requested if balance has been poor. The arm on the affected side is used to prop up the trunk, while the sound leg is lifted by the helper across the affected one. The patient can then be helped to swing into an upright position by pulling on the sound arm. Altering the body weight from the sound side to the affected side should be practised.

RE. Check there is adequate space around the bed, and that the affected leg is nearest to the bed edge. Check the helper bends from the knees when pulling the patient upright.

9. Teach hip movement from the balanced sitting position, starting with the change of weight from one hip to the other by hitching the hips forward to 'walk' the buttocks forward across the bed. Then reverse the movement for backwards travel to the starting position. Lower the height of the bed so that the feet are flat on the floor when the knees are bent at a right angle.

RE. Check the body posture is upright and that the head moves to the right when the left hip is moved, and vice versa. These balancing exercises should be practised several times a day until the movement can be made with confidence.

10. Choose an armchair or a rocking chair with a seat just high enough for the patient to sit with the knees at a right angle when the feet are flat on the floor. The seat depth should allow a two inch gap behind the knees when the buttocks are touching the chair back. A firm cushion can be used behind the patient's back if the chair seat is a few inches too deep.

RE. An incorrect type of seat can undo the hard work involved in practising exercises, so once the correct seat has been obtained, it may be wise to place a label with the patient's name on it. Discuss suitable seating with the relatives for later care at home. A so called 'geriatric chair' rarely provides the correct type of seating, and should not be used.

11. Place the chair at the head of the patient's bed on the affected side, ready for transfer. Place a small wedge under the rocker of a rocking chair so it remains steady during the transfer. Ask the patient to use the hip hitching movement to reach the edge of the bed. On standing up the weight should be taken by the sound leg first. By placing the helper's foot on to the side of the patient's affected foot, outward movement of the affected knee can be controlled. Tell the patient to transfer their weight to the affected leg. Bare feet increase the sensory stimulation.

RE. Check the movement is carried out slowly, steadily and with control, to gain the confidence of the patient. Bare feet should not be suggested if the patient has foot disease or diabetes.

12. A quarter turn of the helper's body helps the patient to swivel towards the chair. Remind the patient to feel for the arms of the chair before bending the knees to sit down. Remove the wedges from under the rockers of the rocking chair. Suggest the patient rock forwards and backwards using the heels. This exercise helps to provide stimulation for the affected leg as well as exercise for the muscles.

RE. Observe that the heels are used when rocking. Check that the body posture remains balanced, without slumping in the chair.

13. Remind the patient to change their position at least every hour when sitting in a chair, by raising their buttocks off the seat by pushing down on the arms of the chair, and settling back in a slightly different position. Consider using a gel or shaped foam pad on the seat of the chair to increase the distribution of pressure over the buttocks.

RE. Check that the patient has remembered to change their position after each hour of sitting in the chair. Observe that their body weight is held evenly over both hips. Inspect the buttocks for red skin or other signs of prolonged pressure when helping the patient to return to bed.

14. Discuss the risk of burns from hot water bottles or sitting too close to a fire or heater. Remind the patient to use their eyes to make up for the loss of skin sensation. Provide thick covers for a hot water bottle and ensure it is placed above the top sheet. If straps are used around the affected leg, for example to hold a urinary drainage bag, mark the position on the strap so that it is not done up so tightly that it interferes with the circulation. Teach the patient to check with a finger that the strap lies flat, and is not tight against the skin.

RE. Confirm that the hot water bottle cover includes the plastic or metal stopper beneath the material. Inspect the skin surface to look for tell-tale 'corned beef' marks on the skin from sitting close to a heater. Inspect the site of any strap for redness or other signs of pressure when the appliance is removed.

15. Swelling of the ankle or whole leg may be limited by raising the leg on a foot stool with several pillows on it, while sitting. Suggest the exercises to be done while sitting are increased. Inspect the chair to confirm it is not causing pressure on the veins which drain the leg. Consider tipping the foot of the bed by 30 degrees above the horizontal when the patient is lying in bed.

RE. Measure and record the diameter of the swollen ankle before and after the patient sits in a chair, to identify whether the changes have decreased the swelling.

Further action

1. Pulsed pressure, or pressure from an inflatable splint, may be used by the physiotherapist to increase deep pressure sensory stimulation, or to reduce swelling. It may also allow exercises by limiting muscle spasm.

RE. Note the skin colour after treatment. Measuring the leg before and after treatment will indicate the effect of pressure in treating swelling. Plan activities for the periods after treatment to make the most of the time when movement is easier, because swelling is least.

2. Foot drop may make stepping forward with the affected leg rather difficult. A lightweight splint may be fitted to a well fitting lace-up shoe by the

physiotherapist. A toe spring may help to keep the toe up as the foot is brought forward during each stride.

RE. Check the skin at least daily for signs of pressure from the splint. The splint should be washed with warm soapy water, and dried away from heat, at least once each week.

3. Physiotherapy in the gym and hydrotherapy in a pool may be advised once muscle control and strength have developed. The appointments should be integrated with the other planned care. Discuss whether the patient would prefer a bath after the session in the gym.

RE. Observe for increased tiredness after treatments; extra rest periods may need to be planned.

Associated medical diagnoses	Cerebral Vascular Accident Poliomyelitis Spinal cord tumour Spinal nerve compression Sub-dural haematoma

---

Problem	**Unable to straighten back.**

Assessment findings	Kyphosis (curvature of the spine, with concavity going forwards) Scoliosis (curvature of the spine, bending to one side) Severe pain in back Pain radiating into buttocks or thighs (sciatica) Back pain worse on sneezing or coughing Unable to turn trunk Limited vision to the side Limited vision above head on standing Stiff back Rigid, poker back Pain on straight leg raising Unable to bend forward
Information for the patient	The spine is made up of a string of bones, jointed for flexibility and with pads of shock-absorbing cartilage between the bones. From the solid body of each vertebra comes an arch of bone through which runs the spinal cord. Three wings on the arch provide anchorage for the muscles which allow bending and moving of the back. If the joints between the vertebrae become stiff, then movement is limited. One or more of the pads of cartilage can be damaged, causing pain. If one of the nerves coming from the spinal cord is pinched, the pain may be felt in the buttock and down the leg. Keeping the bones and muscles in the correct position can help to reduce the pain. Then gentle physiotherapy may be used to free stiff joints and strengthen muscles in the back, so that they provide a natural corset for the bones, to keep them in the proper position.
Nursing action	1. Provide a firm bed base, with a fracture board or chipboard beneath a firm mattress. Provide a small neck pillow if the patient cannot lie flat and sleep without one. A small, thin pillow in the small of the back may be useful if the spine is not in alignment.

RE. Check the spine is held in a comfortable position. Some people may take two or more days to learn to sleep flat on their backs. Observe how much sleep is achieved. A few people find it more comfortable to sleep prone, but will need help to turn over.

2. Local heat from an electric heat pad or well-wrapped hot water bottle can be used to help relax tense muscles.

RE. Check the pad conforms to BSI (British Standard Institute) regulations and is in good working order. Ask the patient if the heat helps. Look for changes in the alignment of the spine; muscle tension may have a protective function and pain may be increased if alignment is altered.

3. Teach the patient to roll like a log, with the upper leg flexed when turning. Warn against sudden movements, or twisting the trunk. Careful, smooth movements are best.

RE. Supervise the patient when turning, until the movements are carried out correctly.

4. Place urinals within easy reach. A slipper or rubber bedpan may be used to reduce the discomfort of misalignment of the spine when passing urine, etc.

RE. Record the urine output for the first twenty four hours if there is any suggestion of pressure on the spinal cord, or any difficulty in passing urine because of the unusual position.

5. Advise the patient to take extra bran and fruit to reduce the risk of constipation from limited activity and the unusual position.

RE. Record the frequency of bowel actions. If no bowel action occurs within two days of the usual frequency, consider giving two glycerine suppositories to stimulate a bowel action.

6. Breathing exercises should be taught to the patient, with involvement of the costo-vertebral joints, to reduce the risk of decreasing aeration of the lower lobes of the lungs, and chest infection.

RE. Check that the patient can carry out the exercises correctly and at the recommended frequency.

7. If the field of vision is limited due to reduced spinal movement, or by the position in bed, consider if providing a mirror, turning the bed round, or providing special aids such as prismatic glasses, would help in maintaining involvement in activities.

RE. Check personal items and meals are placed within easy reach, and that the patient can see what is going on.

8. Discuss whether the patient's usual occupation and hobbies will need to be modified as a result of the back trouble. Loss of movement, especially turning the head easily, makes driving a vehicle or operating machinery risky.

RE. Consider whether the patient needs expert assistance in changing his employment. The Disablement Resettlement Officer at the local Job Centre has a wide range of skills and help to offer.

| **Further action** | 1. Traction may be set up to reduce pressure on a ruptured inter-vertebral disc. The patient's body weight is used to counter the weights hung over the end of the bed. |
| | RE. Check the angle of the bed is sufficient for the patient to remain balanced between the foot and head of the bed. If the weights appear to be pulling the patient towards the foot of the bed, increase the head-down tilt. If the patient appears to slide to the top of the bed reduce the tilt, or consult the doctor about increasing the weights. Inspect the pressure areas at least six hourly for signs of friction damage to the skin. |

2. Aspirin may be prescribed to reduce pain and inflammation. Check the patient is not allergic to the drug before giving the first dose.

RE. Assess the degree of pain relief by using a pain chart which is filled in by the nurse and patient. Observe for signs of gastric irritation. If high doses are given, ask the patient to report any ringing in the ears or deafness.

3. Indomethacin or other non-steroid anti-inflammatory drugs may be prescribed. They should be given after food or a glass of milk.

RE. Observe for gastric irritation, rashes, headache, ringing in the ears or dizziness. Check the patient's weight each week, if possible, as oedema may occur and first show as a sudden weight gain. It may take one to two weeks before the full effect is apparent.

4. Hydrotherapy may be used once the patient is able to take exercise without severe pain. The warm water helps to reduce muscle spasm.

RE. Note how tired the patient becomes after hydrotherapy, and whether stiffness or pain increase or decrease after the exercise.

5. A back brace may be fitted to maintain correct vertebral alignment. It may take several days of gradually increasing periods of wear, with rest periods between, before the patient can tolerate wearing it throughout the day.

RE. Check the skin for signs of pressure after the brace has been worn. Mark the fastenings once the most comfortable fitting has been achieved, so that the brace is then done up to the correct place each time.

| **Associated medical diagnoses** | Ankylosing spondylitis
Metastatic bone disease
Myeloma
Prolapsed inter-vertebral disc
Wedging of vertebrae |

| **Problem** | **Unable to dress unaided.** |

| **Assessment findings** | Poor or absent grip in one hand
Unable to use one hand and arm
Unable to stand unaided
Clothing left unbuttoned
Wears clothes inside out
Wears underclothes over top clothes |

Information for the patient

Most adults are used to getting dressed while either standing or sitting; both hands are used, and some garments need to be pulled on. Dressing can take a lot of energy and effort particularly when there is loss of limb action. There are some tricks which can be taught to make it easier for the patient, and the occupational therapist can advise on which aids may be helpful. If exercise is part of the treatment then the patient will be asked to try to put on some of their own clothes, the nurse helping them with the rest.

Nursing action

1. Assess whether the patient can understand and follow the instructions. Loss of sensation from a limb may make dressing difficult, as does brain damage, which leads to difficulty naming objects, knowing left from right or making sense of what is said. Give simple, clear instructions and allow plenty of time for them to be acted upon before repeating them.

RE. Describe the initial difficulties encountered in detail, as a baseline for progress. Consider whether a detailed assessment by the physiotherapist and occupational therapist would help in devising a suitable plan of care and treatment.

2. Assess the patient's balance when sitting and standing. Pants and trousers can be put on when lying down if sitting balance is poor and standing unaided is not possible. Assess the balance when reaching forward towards the feet. Aids for putting on stockings are available, but are difficult to use with one hand and with poor balance.

RE. If the balance is expected to be poor, a second helper may be needed for safety during the assessment.

3. Consider adapting fastenings if fine finger control is difficult. Velcro can be used to replace buttons, the button being sewn on top of the stitched-up buttonhole. Large tags on zips may provide a better grip. Check the armholes are not tight; raglan sleeves are easier to put on. When the problems are likely to be present for months or years, the specialist advice of the Disabled Living Foundation may be sought. Booklets are available giving a wide range of ideas for adapting clothing to help with different problems.

RE. Relatives may be willing to undertake the alterations to clothes with the advice of the occupational therapist. Check that the patient or relatives have the address of the DLF.

4. Plan the re-learning of dressing skills when there are likely to be few interruptions, and make sure there is no sense of urgency. Provide a choice of clothes. Concentrate on teaching the patient how to put on one garment during each session. Use the same clear, simple instructions each time. Record these in the care plan for continuity, if others should take over the sessions.

RE. Observe the facial expression for concentration or puzzlement if there appears to be difficulty in following instructions. Add learning to put on a new garment only when the first has been mastered.

5. Teach the patient to put their weaker limb into the armhole first. The fabric is gathered up in the good hand and slid over the weaker hand by grasping and raising the wrist. It can then be pulled up to the elbow and on to the shoulder. Reaching with the good hand to pull it across the back may cause a loss of balance, so be ready to give support. Buttons at the cuff of the good hand may be attached with elastic and done up before the shirt or blouse is put on.

213

RE. Check the sleeve is anchored up under the armpit before the patient tries to pull the fabric across the shoulders.

6. Teach the patient to put their weaker limb into the trouser leg first. It may be easier to put on trousers when sitting on the bed. The trousers can be spread out on the mattress and the weak leg raised by flexing the knee, the foot of the weak leg being 'lassooed' with the trousers and pulled up to the knee before the second leg is put into the other trouser leg.

RE. A semi-sitting position supported with pillows is easiest on the bed. It is easier to sit in a chair without arms than in one with arms, but requires good balance.

7. When dressing the patient follow the same pattern, allow the patient to assist as much as possible.

RE. Assess how much interest the patient shows in each step of the process.

Further action

1. Dressing practice may be provided by the occupational therapist as part of the treatment plan. Plan activities so that there is no sense of hurry and no interruptions.

RE. Observe whether the patient is tired by the effort; if so plan for additional rest periods.

Associated medical diagnoses

Cerebral tumour
Cerebral vascular accident
Dementia
Glioma
Intracerebral tumour
Motor neurone disease
Myeloma
Poliomyelitis
Spinal cord tumour
Spinal nerve compression
Sub-dural haematoma

Problem **Unable to turn over in bed.**

Assessment findings

Unable to roll
Weakness down one side of body
Skin in contact with bed is red in colour
Skin traction

Information for the patient

When a person lies in one position the tissues are pinched between the bones and the mattress, which stops the blood circulating properly. Normally the nerves pass a message back before it becomes painful, and without having to think about it the position is altered slightly. If someone does not move, then the tissues get damaged. The tissue cells die from lack of the oxygen and food normally brought by the blood. The skin starts to look red, the area is painful and a blister may appear beneath which is an ulcer. This is known as a bedsore. It can be very painful, and take a long time to heal up. To prevent this occurring the position should be changed at least every two hours, more often if possible. The nurses can help patients turn over in bed and teach them how to help themselves. The same pressures can occur when sitting in a chair, so regular changes of position will go on being important.

Nursing action

1. Provide a 'monkey pole' if the patient can raise the trunk using the arms, without pain or spasm. Teach the patient how to pull up as the hips and legs are turned over by the nurse.

RE. Not to be used after a stroke as it limits the exercise and muscle control which comes from rolling using the arms and hips. Ask the patient to report any pain or stiffness in the arms. Check the height of the handle is just within reach of the patient's outstretched hands.

2. Turn the patient every two hours or more frequently if the skin remains red for 20 minutes or more after pressure is removed. If the patient's condition permits, plan to turn the patient from side to back to other side, in sequence. If possible plan the turns so the patient is lying with the stronger arm uppermost at mealtimes.

RE. If the pattern of turning is inconvenient for mealtimes, increase the frequency of the changes of position. Two hours in one position is the maximum that tissues will tolerate without marked damage. Check the staff are aware that tissue damage may take up to 48 hours after it was caused before becoming apparent. An hour glass, watch or clock alarm may be useful as a reminder if turns are not done on time.

3. Consider providing pressure spreading devices such as a large cell ripple mattress, gel flotation pad, sheepskin or low air loss bed. If possible, the patient should lie directly on one sheet over the ripple mattress, gel pad or low air loss bed sacs, and lie directly on the sheepskin. Use of these devices except the low air loss bed, should not reduce the frequency of turning. The low air loss bed reduces the need for turning to change the site of pressure, but consideration should be given to other reasons for turning, such as lung and kidney drainage.

RE. Check the motor is in working order on the ripple mattress, and that the setting suits the body weight of the patient. Sheepskins should be combed out each day so that the surface does not get matted and reduce the pressure distributing qualities. Pressure-spreading devices should be cleaned as recommended by the manufacturer.

4. In turning the patient from the back, use the position of the patient's shoulders and hips to ease the turn. Stand on the side to which the patient is to be turned. Bring the patient's hand to the edge of the bed and the other arm across the body, turning the head towards you. Lift the far leg across the other one, bending the patient's knees slightly. Place one hand on the upper shoulder, the other on the far hip and gently roll the patient towards you. Stand on the other side of the bed to lift the patient's hips and then shoulders back to the centre of the bed.

RE. Note how much the patient is able to do, for example turning the head. If turning will still be required on the return home, discuss with the relatives and patient whether they wish to learn how to turn the patient. Plan out a teaching programme. Check that lifting is carried out so that there is no dragging of the skin across the sheet, to reduce the risk of shearing stresses on the tissues and the formation of sores from this cause.

5. A pillow may be placed behind the patient's back to maintain the position. A pillow between the knees may be used to take some of the weight of the upper leg. Keep the bottom sheet taut and free of crumbs.

RE. Inspect the skin for redness or maceration. The latter may occur if plastic pillowcases are used beneath the pillow slip, preventing the escape of perspiration. A second fabric pillowcase may be sufficient to increase the rate of evaporation of sweat. A bed cradle may also aid air circulation and the escape of moisture.

Further action

1. Physiotherapy may be useful in teaching the patient how to turn over without a helper. Muscle strength and control may need to be built up by regular exercises.

RE. Check the instructions and movements are also used by other staff so that the patient is not confused. The step-by-step instructions should be written in the care plan. Assess the ability of the patient to remember and follow the instructions.

Associated medical diagnoses

Cachexia
Cerebral tumour
Cerebral vascular accident
Glioma
Guillain-Barré syndrome
Motor neurone disease
Multiple sclerosis
Muscular dystrophy
Myasthenia gravis
Parkinson's disease
Paraplegia
Prolapsed intervertebral disc
Rheumatoid arthritis
Spinal cord compression
Sub-dural haematoma
Tuberculosis of the spine

Problem

Unsteady gait when walking.

Assessment findings

Leans to left or right when walking
Falls forward when walking
Leans backwards when walking
Feels unsteady and unsafe
Clasps furniture when walking
Uses stick or walking frame
History of falls

Information for the patient

When a person is standing or walking the brain is constantly receiving messages about the position of the limbs and whether the muscles are relaxed or tense. These messages allow small adjustments to be made to keep the body upright. If there is interference with the messages, or the brain cannot act on them, then walking becomes unsteady. If the muscles are weak, or slow to respond to the brain's message, then there may be a feeling of falling. Too much alcohol interferes with the passage of messages along the nerves to and from the brain, and so produces an unsteady walk. It is sometimes possible to

216

reopen pathways and to strengthen muscles. It means repeating movements over and over again.

Nursing action

1. Balance when sitting upright can be improved by sitting on the edge of the bed and using the hands for support, practising the transfer of weight from side to side. Stand in front of the patient's knees to supervise and encourage them. Suggest practising for a few minutes each time the patient gets up or returns to bed.

RE. Check the feet are off the floor during the exercise. Note how long the patient can continue the exercise with interest, and without tiring. Stop the exercise after five minutes, or if the balance seems to be deteriorating through tiredness.

2. Balance on standing should be achieved before walking commences. A walking frame, tripod or walking stick may be chosen as an aid to balance and safety, in consultation with the physiotherapist.

RE. Check the correct use of the aid is understood. The walking frame should be placed about 45 mm (18 inches) in front of the patient, all four legs of the frame in contact with the ground, so weight can be put on the frame during the steps towards it. A tripod should be placed just ahead and to the side of the patient, on their unaffected side, so the weight can be directed through the tripod feet to the ground. Check that the height allows this to be done in comfort, with the arm slightly flexed at the elbow. A walking stick takes less body weight through it without slipping on the ground than a frame or tripod. It provides less incentive to keep the body weight forward than the frame so it is not helpful if the patient tends to lean back.

3. Discuss and agree on the distance to be walked, check the route is cleared of trailing flex, furniture and loose rugs. Check the shoes or slippers fit closely to the feet. Firm lace-up shoes provide more support than down-at-heel slippers.

RE. Observe whether the flooring or footwear contribute to problems of balance. Consider sticking fine emery paper strips to smooth slippery soles.

4. Discuss which position for the helper will give the patient the greatest feeling of confidence, so that should they feel unsteady, falling will be prevented. Walking to one side may be preferred.

RE. Note how many times the patient loses their balance during each walk so that a comparison can be made over a period of time. Note if the patient tends to lose their concentration on walking when distracted by others, or by the helper's comments.

Associated medical diagnoses

Alcohol intoxication
Ataxia
Cerebral vascular accident
Huntington's chorea
Drug overdose
Tabes dorsalis

Problem	Severe weakness of one side of the body.

Assessment findings	Unable to move limbs Loss of muscle strength Weak grip Loss of coordination Unaware of position of limb on affected side Leg buckles on trying to stand Dropped foot on affected side Fingers curl into palm Arm held across the body Slumps towards affected side Pain Muscle spasm
Information for the patient	The muscles need instructions from the brain to contract or relax, so that movement can take place. If there is a block in the path of the messages to the nerves from the brain, then movement cannot occur, and partial blockage leads to weakness. Damage to brain cells may mean that no messages can be sent. Over a period of time, new pathways can be opened up, and other brain cells take over the function of damaged cells. While this is happening, the muscles on one part of an arm or leg may be contracting, and so cause deformity. To prevent this, to increase the rate of recovery and to keep the muscles in trim, careful positioning and exercise are required. It may take up to two years to recover from the effects of a stroke if some of the brain cells have been destroyed.
Nursing action	1. Discuss the current level of activity, and agree with the patient and physiotherapist which skills will be worked on over the next two weeks. Agree on a target, and, if appropriate, what the reward will be for achieving it. Plan out the practice sessions, increasing the number of exercise repeats and the time to be taken. Targets may include lifting weights of increasing heaviness. RE. Assess how realistic the patient's expectations of their progress appear to be. Morale can be raised by achieving goals, so advise against those that appear unlikely to be achieved in the time set. Rewards may be as simple as a favourite chocolate bar for a goal achieved, or a small sweet for every ten repeats of an exercise. Progress in improving muscle tone may not be noticed by the patient. 2. Discuss with the patient and family or close friends whether their help with the exercises would be acceptable. If so, plan out times when they will be visiting and could help. Plan teaching sessions so that both helper and patient learn what to do. Repetition of exercises can get boring, so explore variations on the theme of each exercise. Enlist the help of the physiotherapist and occupational therapist. RE. Observe for signs of loss of interest in exercising, such as missing exercises, not doing all the agreed repeats, not doing the exercise as slowly as recommended or giving up mid-way. Ask the helper to report back on progress, and demonstrate trust and interest in the helper's assessment by making a written note in the patient's progress notes, in their presence. 3. Teach the patient the correct position for sitting and lying, so that any developing spasm is reduced. Lying on the sound side, use a pillow level with

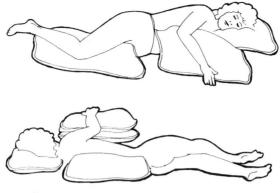

Affected arm supported by pillows
Affected shoulder forward
Affected leg slightly flexed, in front of sound leg
Small, flat pillow under head
Pillow in the back to help support position

Fig. 6.2   Lying on sound side

the shoulder and in front of the chest so that the affected arm can be stretched forward across it. The affected leg should lie in front of the sound leg, both bent slightly at the knee. One small, flat pillow under the head should be used or no pillow at all.

RE. Check that when lying on the sound side, the affected arm does not rotate inwards towards the body. Check the height of the pillow is sufficient, so the shoulder does not drop forward, but is supported. (Fig. 6.2).

4. The correct position when lying on the affected side has the affected shoulder pulled through, with the arm stretched out on the bed, palm towards the ceiling. The sound leg should lie in front, with both legs bent a little at the knee. A pillow tucked behind the back will provide support. A supporting pillow may be used under the sound leg.

RE. Check that the pillow behind the back is sufficient to provide support. Check that the trunk is to one side of the bed so that there is sufficient room for the extended, affected arm to be supported on the mattress. The arm can be bent at the elbow and the hand tucked under the pillow with the palm uppermost, as an alternative. Check the affected arm is not trapped under the body.

5. The correct position to be taught for the brief time that the patient should spend lying on the back, should include a pillow under the affected arm to bring the shoulder forward off the bed. The arm should rest lying straight out with the palm facing the ceiling. A pillow under the affected hip and thigh, with the knee bent towards the sound side, tips the leg inwards. The head should be turned towards the sound side. Approach the patient in this position from the affected side to encourage head turning. One flat pillow should be used or no pillow.

RE. Check the shoulder remains lifted forward off the bed. Note the time the patient spends in this position, as it should be limited so that muscle spasm is discouraged.

219

6. Bed pans provide an opportunity to practise another useful exercise, which will later aid sitting and walking. The patient should lie flat on the back and bend the sound knee so the foot lies flat on the bed, and should raise the affected leg alongside in the same position. If there is little muscle control it may need to be held there by a third person. The patient's arms should lie alongside the body, palm downwards, so that pushing down is possible as the trunk is raised. If muscle weakness is marked, two people need to join hands under the small of the patient's back and lift it together. As muscle strength and control return, the patient may be able to raise the buttocks off the bed by pushing down against the bed with their arms and feet.

RE. Check the affected leg is controlled, so that it does not suddenly slide down the bed in the middle of the lift. The position and exercise use muscles required in walking and sitting, so the use of a monkey pole should be avoided. Teach the correct way to roll, which is towards the affected side first.

7. Rolling during bedmaking, and for reaching items on the bedside locker, provides further useful exercise. The more difficult roll towards the sound side must be delayed until some muscle strength returns. The affected hand should be clasped and stretched out, the sound leg bent so that the movements of the shoulder and hip produce the roll.

RE. Check the fingers are interlaced for the arm manoeuvre and that the arms are held out straight. Check that the bed height and position of the locker is such that items can be reached with ease and safety. Check the affected leg is not hooked over by the sound foot, as this interferes with the exercise of the correct muscle groups and may produce a 'bad' habit.

8. Use two pillows to keep the affected arm in a forward position when sitting up in bed. A small, flat pillow, or the side of a larger one, may be used under the edge of the affected thigh to keep the leg tipped slightly inwards. Place the locker on the affected side, so that helpful exercise occurs each time something is placed on or taken from it. Suggest that visitors sit on the affected side to encourage head and trunk turning.

RE. Check the shoulder is kept forward and does not droop. Observe that visitors do not limit the exercises by handing things to the patient off the locker. (Fig. 6.3).

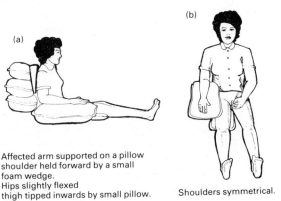

(a)

Affected arm supported on a pillow
shoulder held forward by a small
foam wedge.
Hips slightly flexed
thigh tipped inwards by small pillow.

(b)

Shoulders symmetrical.

Fig. 6.3   Sitting up in bed

9. Sitting up on the edge of the bed may be taught once the muscle strength and control begin to develop. The advice of the physiotherapist should be sought. The affected arm should be used to prop up the trunk, while the sound leg is lifted by the helper across the affected one. The sound hand is grasped by the helper as the patient is pulled into the sitting position. Two people may be needed to help at first, to keep the affected arm in place during the movement.

RE. Check there is adequate space around the bed, and that the affected side is nearest to the bed edge. Check that the main helper bends from the knees so that they use their large thigh muscles during the pulling. Observe for pallor, sweating or raised pulse, and if these occur help the patient to lie down again.

10. Balancing in the sitting position should be practised before moving the patient into a chair. Lower the height of the bed so that the patient's feet are flat on the floor when sitting on the bed edge. The knees should be bent at a right angle, with feet parallel, and the hands beside the knees. Stand in front of the patient and check their balance when moving the sound foot off the floor, or turning the trunk. Be ready to steady the patient if necessary.

RE. Check the feet are not moved apart for a distance of more than a few inches, as a wide base indicates poor balance. Look for signs of breath holding or rigid posture. Balance should be achieved with a relaxed posture, and movement of the sound foot or trunk should be possible before movement of the hips is undertaken.

11. Teach hip movement from the balanced sitting position, starting with the change of weight from one side to the other. Ask the patient to interlace their fingers and put their arms over the helper's head, so the forearms rest on the shoulders. The helper's hands are then free to direct the movement first to the affected side. One hand can support the patient's affected side just below the armpit, the other can either gently press the left side of the waist, or pat the left buttock to encourage movement. 'Walking' the bottom across the bed by alternating the weight transfer and hitching up the hip can follow later. This exercise should be practised by moving towards and back from the edge of the bed with three or four hip hitches.

RE. Check the patient's head moves to the right when the weight is transferred to the left hip; if not, gently move it. The balancing exercise should be practised several times a day until balance is established. It need not delay sitting the patient in an armchair. If progress is slow, consider planning more short rest periods on the bed, so that the exercise of rolling and sitting up before transfer to the chair provides extra reasons for practice.

12. Choose an armchair with the seat just high enough for the patient to sit with the knees at a right angle when the feet are flat on the floor. The seat depth should allow a two inch gap behind the knees when the buttocks are touching the chairback. A firm cushion can be used behind the patient's back if the chair is a few inches too deep. Padded arm rests should be at a height that prevents shoulder droop when the arms rest on them. A pillow can be used to correct the height if the arm rests are too low.

RE. Incorrect seating can undo hard work carried out when practising exercises, so once the correct seat has been obtained it may be wise to place a label with the patient's name on it. Discuss suitable seating with relatives for

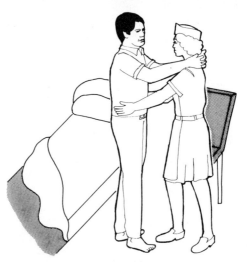

Standing up from bed, fingers interlaced, arms resting on nurse's shoulders. Weight being transferred to affected side. Chair ready at head of bed.

Fig. 6.4   Moving a person with a hemiplegia

later care at home. A so-called 'geriatric' chair rarely provides the correct type of seating, and should not be used.

13. Place the armchair at the head of the bed on the patient's affected side, ready for transfer. Use the hip-hitching movement or bring the patient's weight forward. On standing up, the weight should be taken first by the sound leg, and later, as strength returns, partly by the affected side, as the helper helps make a quarter turn backwards to the chair. By placing the feet on either side of the patient's, the knees can be used to limit any lean to the affected side. (Fig. 6.4).

RE. Check the movement is carried out slowly, steadily and with control, to gain the confidence of the patient. Bare feet increase stimulation to the affected side, but should only be encouraged if there is no foot disease or diabetes. Check that progress in transferring weight to the affected side is not slowed by fear of falling.

14. Provide an adjustable table which can be set at a height so that the patient can lean forward on their forearms with comfort. Mark the centre of the table with a straight line drawn with a chinagraph (wax) pencil, or a strip of adhesive tape, so that the patient has a reminder to keep the forearms parallel. The palms should be flat on the table. Meals may be eaten with the sound hand, while resting on the affected arm. Reading is another activity during which the weight bearing can be practised.

RE. Check the patient spends time resting on their forearms with them parallel to the centre line, and transferring weight from one to the other. As much time as possible should be spent in this forearm resting position. Note how much time the patient can tolerate without becoming overtired. Check the table does not move while in use. It may need to be anchored.

Further action   1. Foot drop makes it difficult to bring the affected leg through when walking; a lightweight splint with a toe spring may be fitted to a closely fitting, lace-up shoe. The spring helps to raise the toe as the foot is brought through with each stride.

RE. Check the skin under the splint for redness or other signs of pressure at least once a day. Wash the splint in warm soapy water and dry away from heat at least once a week.

2. Physiotherapy in the gymnasium may be commenced when muscle strength and control increase sufficiently for floor exercises and work with the parallel bars to begin.

RE. Discuss whether the patient would prefer to have a bath after treatment. Observe for increased tiredness after treatment sessions. Plan additional rest periods.

3. Pressure splints to reduce muscle spasm may be used by the physiotherapist during treatments. These are inflated either by blowing into the splint, or intermittently with a machine.

RE. Inflatable splints must be used with great caution if there is any risk of overloading the circulation, or of deep vein thrombosis.

4. Muscle spasm may be treated with diazepam 2 to 15 mg a day in divided doses.

RE. Observe for increased drowsiness; if it interferes with treatment it may be more important to reduce the dose so that activities are undertaken. Other means of reducing spasm may be considered. Note whether spasm occurs at particular times of the day, or after specific activities.

Associated medical diagnoses	Cerebral tumour
	Cerebral vascular accident
	Glioma
	Intracerebral tumour
	Motor neurone disease
	Poliomyelitis
	Space occupying lesion
	Spinal cord tumour
	Spinal nerve compression
	Sub-dural haematoma
	Transient ischaemic attack

Problem	Loss of fine finger control.

Assessment findings	Tremor at rest
	Unable to do up buttons or shoelaces
	Unable to pick up and hold small items
	Handwriting shaky or unreadable

Information for the patient	The brain has a surprisingly large area devoted to the hand, and it receives information from the skin, muscles and joints about the position of the hand. The brain also passes messages along the nerves to the muscles to contract and relax so that movement occurs. If there is a block in the pathway or damage to this area of the brain, then messages do not get through to the fingers. Picking up and holding small things requires a lot of tiny adjustments from the muscles of the fingers so the grip is neither too crushing nor so loose that the thing drops. Humans are better than chimpanzees at picking things up because they can bring the thumb and each of the fingers together with

greater control. Sometimes, although the finer finger movements are no longer easy, the fingers can still be used for most of the normal activities, and aids can be used to help.

Nursing action

1. Discuss adapting clothing by replacing buttons with large-tagged zips or velcro. The sewn-up button holes can have the button sewn on top to retain the style of dress, shirt or blouse. Pull-on shoes are easier to get on if the elastic is not tight; a small snip may be needed to loosen them. A long-handled shoe horn may help. If the grip is weak, attach a loop of wide elastic to the handle, so the hand can be slipped beneath it for extra control. Elastic shoe-laces can be bought to replace normal ones. These allow the shoe to be slipped on without them being undone.

RE. Ask the patient to demonstrate that the tag on a zip is large enough to be gripped firmly and pulled up. Note how long it takes the patient to dress unaided using the adapted clothes and shoes. Note in the care plan the time required so the patient will not be hurried.

2. Cutting finger and toe-nails may be too difficult for the patient. Consider whether the chiropodist should be asked to advise or treat the patient. Long-handled, spring-loaded clippers may be suitable as the lever effect can help a weak grip.

RE. Ask the patient to demonstrate nail care. Discuss with the patient whether a relative or friend may be able to help with nail care at home.

3. Discuss the use of an electric shaver rather than a hand razor. Arrangements may need to be made for regular cleaning, as some types require delicate handling. Advice may be sought from the occupational therapist on aids to help in applying cosmetics. Resting the elbow on a firm surface and against a heavy object may steady the forearm enough to allow makeup to be applied. A large sponge or flannel mitt may be easier to hold than a flannel.

RE. Observe for signs of difficulty, such as an uneven shave or makeup.

4. Large plastic grips can be bought to fit over the handles of cutlery. Foam rubber tubes or trimmed blocks can also be used on cutlery, pens, pencils and small handles of all sorts. A pivoted wrist support may be used if wrist control is poor.

RE. Check the handles can be held firmly.

5. Review the need to adapt splints, colostomy/ileostomy appliances or other aids which use straps or buckles.

RE. Ask the patient to demonstrate that, with the adaptations, the appliances can be used independently.

6. Practice at picking up small objects may be helpful if recovery of control is likely. Provide two bowls, one with a range of small objects. Ask the patient to pick up the objects one at a time and place them in the other bowl. Chess or draughts provide entertainment as well as practice at picking up small objects.

RE. Check the ball of the thumb is used in gripping the object. Reduce the size of the objects as finger control increases.

7. If control of finger pressure is difficult, suggest the patient practises with a disposable plastic cup, picking it up without deforming the rim.

Further action

1. Sinemet may be prescribed for tremor. Do not give it within two weeks of stopping monoamine oxidase inhibitors (drugs for depression). Several drugs interact with Sinemet (levodopa with carbidopa).

RE. Observe for gastric upsets, loss of sleep, changes in urinary output or pulse rate and rhythm.

Associated medical diagnoses

Alcoholic neuropathy
Carcinomatosis
Carpal tunnel syndrome
Cervical rib
Diabetic neuropathy
Lead poisoning
Multiple sclerosis
Parkinson's disease
Rheumatoid arthritis
Syringomyelia
Vincristine neuropathy

Problem

Loss of control of movements, with tremor.

Assessment findings

Hands shake slightly at rest
'Pill rolling' movement of the fingers
Hands stop shaking just before moving
Spasmodic jerks of the hand or arm

Information for the patient

Movement of the hands is under the control of the brain, which sends messages to the muscles and receives information back. The different groups of muscles which help to move the hand in many different ways, have to contract or relax in a set pattern for each movement. If the brain has a reduced amount of some of the essential chemicals it needs to work properly, the messages reaching the muscles get muddled. The hand may shake slightly all the time. Alcohol can act as a poison to the nerves and brain, and can also produce a tremor.

Nursing action

1. Provide melamine or other unbreakable crockery. Discuss with the patient whether a plastic-lidded drinking beaker would be preferable to a cup. Instruct the patient, staff and relatives to half fill cups or glasses. Two refills must be provided to everyone else's one, or leave two half-filled cups at a time.

RE. Check how much fluid gets spilled. If accurate measurement of fluid intake is essential and a lot of fluid is spilt on clothing, consider weighing an absorbent cloth to use as a bib and then weighing it after use, so the amount of fluid can be calculated by comparing it to the known weights and volumes.

2. A sticky plastic mat will hold plates steady and can help in safe replacement of a glass on the table. Consider using a pen clip to anchor a drinking straw to the rim of a glass, if the patient's arm movements are large or the grip is weak.

225

RE. Check the patient does not become overtired by the effort needed to suck, and that the drink is left within easy reach.

3. A plate guard or a deep rim on the plate may help to reduce spillage of food during meals. An absorbent napkin may be used to protect the clothes. Provide a wet-wipe to remove spilled food and to clean sticky hands after meals. Remind staff to remove plate heaters before offering a meal. If eating is so slow that food gets cold, suggest half the food on the plate is kept on the hot plate until the other half is eaten.

RE. Note the reaction to the offer of a napkin, as some people may feel it is childish to use one and resent the suggestion.

4. Discuss adapting clothing if there is difficulty in doing up buttons or zips and tying shoelaces. Sewing up buttonholes with the button sewn on top can hide velcro fastenings. Large pull tags or split-rings attached to zips may provide enough purchase for gross hand control. Elastic shoelaces allow shoes to be slipped on without the laces being undone.

RE. Assess the patient's ability to dress independently when these changes have been made. Occupational therapy advice may be helpful.

Further action

1. Tremor due to Parkinson's disease may be treated with levodopa with carbidopa (Sinemet) to increase the level of dopamine in the striatum pallidum and substantia nigra in the brain. The dose is increased over about 7 days until symptoms improve. It should not be given within two weeks of stopping monoamine oxidase inhibiting drugs (anti-depressants).

RE. Record the patient's blood pressure at least daily. MAOI drug usage may lead to raised blood pressure. Drugs to control hypertension may have their action increased, and postural hypotension also occurs as a side effect. Check the rate and character of the pulse daily for changes. Other side effects include insomnia, agitation, dizziness, loss of appetite, nausea, vomiting, difficulty in passing urine, or incontinence. Record the presence of tremor each day, and report when it decreases.

2. Benzhexol may be prescribed when tremor is due to drugs. It is given in increasing doses. The sustained release tablets must be swallowed whole.

RE. Ask the patient to report a dry mouth, observe them at mealtimes as swallowing becomes uncomfortable if saliva flow decreases. Ask the patient to report any decrease in urine output, or measure the urine and record the volume on a fluid chart, as urinary retention can occur. Blurred vision, nausea and vomiting may also be side effects, and glaucoma may be worsened. Record the presence of tremor each day, and report whether it decreases.

3. Orphenadrine may be prescribed in divided doses, and the dosage increased over several days.

RE. Side effects are similar to those from benzhexol, but are less likely. It may also make the patient feel more cheerful.

Associated medical diagnoses

Alcoholic
Ataxia
Drug withdrawal
Epilepsy
Huntington's chorea

Hysteria
Multiple sclerosis
Parkinson's disease
Spasmodic torticollis
Wilson's disease

Problem	Increasing muscle weakness

Assessment findings

Decreasing strength of grip
Decreasing muscle tone
Abnormal limb position
Foot drop
Drops items
Easily tired
Limbs feel heavy
Poor coordination

Information for the patient

The position of the limbs and the body is maintained by the different groups of muscles pulling in opposite directions, which lead to muscle tone. Normally there is no need consciously to tell the muscles to maintain their tone, as it is a reflex action. The inner ear feeds information about the position of the body back to the brain. In the muscles there are small stretch receptors; if the muscle is stretched, the reflex response produces contraction. If one group of muscles contracts, the opposite group must relax. Muscles become weaker if they are not used, or if the nerve pathways through which the reflex is maintained get damaged.

Nursing action

1. Discuss with the patient how much activity can be managed at one time, before tiredness sets in. Plan the day's activities so that they are followed by a rest to prevent tiredness. Agree which activities could be undertaken by the nurses on the patient's behalf.

RE. Record how much activity the patient accomplishes before becoming tired. Review the care planned, and adjust to the patient's current ability. Check the patient is allowed to make as many decisions as possible. It is easier to accept help if control is not lost. Helpers have a tendency to take over the decisions because it is quicker for them.

2. If clothes or hair look soiled or unkempt, extra help may be needed to maintain personal hygiene. Offers of such help must be tactful, as responsibility for personal hygiene is often the last responsibility individuals wish to give up.

RE. Assess whether appearance is improved. Consider whether clothes need to be reviewed for ease of dressing. Loose styles with zips or velcro fastenings are easier to put on and require less energy and strength in the hands and arms.

3. Meals should include nutritious foods which do not require a lot of chewing. Independence in feeding is usually valued, and should be an early goal in the recovery of muscle strength. Assess whether aids may reduce the effort required.

RE. Record how much the patient eats at each meal and how long it takes for the meal to be eaten. Weigh them at least weekly to check that their food intake is sufficient to maintain a steady body weight.

227

4. Fluid intake may need to be adjusted to provide frequent small amounts. Consider the use of straws if sucking is not a difficulty; a pen clip on the side of the glass can hold a straw steady, without the need for muscular effort. Advise the patient that there is a greater risk of infection or kidney stones developing if the fluid intake drops while activity is decreased.

RE. Record fluid intake; at least two litres in twenty four hours should be achieved. If the intake is lower, consider whether the use of urinals or bedpans is so tiring that the patient is trying to reduce the need for them by restricting fluids.

5. Extra bedding and clothing may be required if activity is greatly reduced by muscle weakness. Muscular activity normally helps to maintain body temperature, so when it is reduced cold temperatures and draughts should be avoided.

RE. Check the oral temperature at least daily in case hypothermia occurs. Passive exercise at frequent, regular intervals will help replace normal muscle activity without tiring the patient.

6. Discuss which activities can be continued without causing overtiredness; consider long-playing records or cassettes, radio, television or recorded books. A computer keyboard set for sensitive touch requires less muscle activity than a typewriter or handwriting. It can be combined with pivoted arm rests so that only the fingers require to be moved.

RE. Resting physically can be boring mentally; assess the patient's interest and introduce greater variety when interest wanes.

7. Discuss with relatives and friends how much the patient should be encouraged to do unaided, and which activities are too tiring. In progressive muscle wasting diseases the relatives may need a lot of emotional support, so that they can accept allowing the patient to struggle to remain independent, without feeling guilty.

RE. Assess how at ease the relatives feel, and if there is any change in the relationship with the patient. The specialist help of an appropriate self-help group or charity may be suggested.

8. Activity to improve muscle strength must be carefully planned to be increased in stages as strength improves. Agree targets with the patient; underestimating likely achievement may be better for morale.

RE. Assess how much effort the patient and nurse put into achievement of activity targets.

Further action

1. Anticholinesterase drugs such as neostigmine or pyridostigmine may be prescribed in myasthenia gravis. The dosage is adjusted according to the response of the patient, and is spread out through the day. Doses should be given on time. Pyridostigmine has a longer lasting effect, and may be used at night to prevent muscle weakness on waking.

RE. Record the time that each dose is given, and the muscle strength of the patient before the next dose, until the most effective dosage pattern has been worked out. Overdosage may occur as they are both accumulative drugs. Ask the patient to report any nausea or abdominal cramp. Vomiting or diarrhoea may also occur. Observe for increased sweating, salivation or bronchial secretions. Record the pulse and blood pressure at least four hourly, as either may fall, due to the drug. Atropine or propantheline may be used to reduce these effects.

2. High doses of steroids may be used for some patients with myasthenia gravis. A thymectomy may be considered in some cases, as enlargement or a tumour of the thymus gland is sometimes associated with myasthenia gravis.

RE. Assess muscle weakness during steroid therapy, as it may increase rather than decrease in some patients. Record the blood pressure at least daily, and test the urine for glucose every day.

3. Plasmapheresis, available in some specialist centres, may provide a good initial remission in some conditions. Discuss the use of the equipment with the patient before the first treatment.

RE. Check the venepuncture sites for bruising or bleeding after treatment. Check the blood pressure at least daily.

Associated medical diagnoses	Bulbar palsy Carcinomatosis Disseminated (multiple) sclerosis Guillain-Barré syndrome Motor neurone disease Muscular dystrophy Myasthenia gravis

---

Problem	**Unable to use crutches correctly.**

Assessment findings	Unsteady gait with crutches Weight borne under arms Leans forward when walking Uneven gait with crutches One weak or missing leg Plaster of Paris cast or a splint on one leg
Information for the patient	Crutches can be used to take part of the body weight off the leg(s) and enable it to be supported by the crutch. It is important that the right size is used to avoid pressure on the armpit, which could pinch the nerve to the arm (brachial nerve). Walking with crutches may look easy, but it takes practice to do it safely, without becoming overtired by the effort.
Nursing action	1. Measure the patient's height and deduct 40 cm (16 inches) to get the length of the crutch, or with the patient lying flat, measure from the fold of the armpit to the sole of the foot, and add two inches. RE. Check that there is a gap of four finger-widths from the armpit to the padded top of the crutch when it is in position. 2. With the patient standing, wearing lace-up shoes, measure the position of the hand grip. It should be placed so the elbow is bent by 30 degrees when the crutch is 10 cm (4 inches) to the side, and just in front of the foot. RE. Check the adjustable screws are tight once the crutch has been altered to fit.

3. The weight should be taken on the sound leg while the affected leg and the crutch on that side are moved forward; the weight can then be shifted on to that arm as the sound leg and crutch are moved up to a parallel position. This method should be used in crowded places for safety.

RE. Note how many steps can be taken before the arms tire.

4. A faster gait can be taught, where the crutches are placed ahead of the body, and the weight transferred through by pushing down as both feet are lifted off the ground to swing up to the level of the crutches. As skill, strength and balance develop, the patient may wish to swing the feet beyond the crutches to gain further speed.

RE. Check that the rubber ferrules at the ends of the crutches are replaced before they wear right through, as some adhesion with the ground aids safety. Concave ferrules increase the suction, and may be useful on smooth floors when the patient is still weak and unsteady.

5. Exercises to strengthen the leg muscles may be necessary. The physiotherapist can advise on which ones would be most useful. Lying flat on the bed, and raising the sound leg up and holding it about 30 cm (12 inches) in the air for a count of five before relaxing, will strengthen the thigh muscles (quadriceps). Repeat at least five times every two or three hours during the day.

RE. When the leg can be held without holding the breath or tiring, increase the count by five.

6. Arm strength can be increased by sitting in a firm chair without armrests, placing the hands on the edges of the seat of the chair and pushing down through the arms, lifting the buttocks off the seat and the feet off the floor.

RE. When the lift can be done without obvious effort, the position above the chair seat can be held for a count of five. The count can be increased as strength increases.

Further action

1. Elbow or gutter crutches may be prescribed when weight cannot be transmitted through the hands, as for example in joint disease. The advice of the physiotherapist is important. The whole body weight cannot be taken through the arms, so the crutches cannot be used with the rapid leg swinging methods.

RE. Ask the patient to report any increase in pain after using the crutches. Check the rate of increase in activity does not exhaust the patient.

2. Consider the use of a zimmer frame or rollator, if crutches are not needed to take the full weight of the patient, and if skill in using crutches does not develop with practice. Discuss the advantages and disadvantages with the physiotherapist.

RE. Assess the length of time during which being non-weight bearing is necessary, to identify whether a change is worthwhile.

Associated medical diagnoses

Fractured tibia
Fractured os calcis
Haemophilia
Osteomyelitis
Polio
Rheumatoid arthritis

Problem	Unable to grip with one hand.

Assessment findings	Arm flaccid Hand flaccid Hand encased in plaster of Paris cast Fingers fixed in claw-like position Weak grip Unable to bring thumb and fingers together Drops items Loss of sense of touch Unable to pick up small items Unable to judge position of limb
Information for the patient	The muscles of the hands and arms are in two groups, normally they maintain tone by balancing the contraction of one group with the relaxation of the other. The nerves pass messages back and forth as reflexes, without conscious thought. If the nerve paths are damaged, one group of muscles may contract more than the other. This can make holding anything difficult, as can the loss of the sense of touch. It may be possible to keep the muscle groups in good working order while nerve damage is healing. The position of the hand and arm are important at all times, as the contracting muscle groups can distort their shape.
Nursing action	1. Place items within reach of the patient's good hand, especially at meal times. If there is loss of awareness of the position of the poor hand, place items just on the far side of it so that the patient must lean across to reach them. Each time this is done the poor hand comes into view as a visual prompt of its position. RE. Observe if the patient can reach items with safety, and if their awareness of the poor hand increases. 2. Provide a table with the top at waist height when the patient is sitting. Advise sitting with the forearms parallel on the top, fingers curled over the far edge. Propping the weight on the poorer arm during meals can aid balance, as well as reducing spasm. RE. Check the trunk is central with the shoulders held at the same height and the forearms remaining parallel. Note the degree of spasm in the poor arm and hand. 3. Discuss the activities which are difficult for the patient to carry out with one hand, and the range of aids available to help. The occupational therapist can give advice and may have aids for loan if the difficulty is likely to last only a short while. Some activities are normally carried out with the dominant hand, and if that is the one affected it may need planned practice sessions to gain skill in using the other hand. RE. Assess the amount of help the patient needs with each activity at least weekly. Review the need for further aids as recovery increases the desire for independence.
Further action	1. Arm exercises may be devised by the physiotherapist and should be incorporated into the care plan. Flex and extend the wrist and elbow joints gently at least five times every two hours when awake. Gently extend and curl the fingers and thumb at the same time.

RE. Ask the patient to report any pain or spasm. It may be necessary to give analgesia about 20 minutes before exercise to reduce pain and make movement easier.

Associated medical diagnoses	Cerebral vascular accident Lymphadenopathy Nerve entrapment Nerve palsy Parkinson's disease Space occupying lesion Transient ischaemic attacks

Problem	**Unable to change position when lying in bed.**

Assessment findings	Feels too weak to move Red skin over pressure points Muscle weakness Loss of muscle tone Arm in splint/plaster cast Limb deformity Loss of consciousness Ability to feel pain Thin Obese

Information for the patient

The skin and tissues get pinched between the bed and the bones. The pressure squashes the blood vessels so that blood cannot flow through them. If the pressure is not limited then there is damage to the cells, causing pain at first, which would normally stimulate movement. Most people change their position every few minutes without thinking about it. If it becomes difficult to move, then it is essential either to use a special bed or mattress which limits the pressure, or for someone else to move the person. The position must then be changed at least every two hours, and the tissues given time to recover. Pressure points at greatest risk when lying in bed are the base of the spine (sacrum), the elbows, ankles, heels and hips.

Nursing action

1. Assess the aids available and discuss which ones might suit the patient's condition and life style. Ten feather pillows can be used on top of a mattress if they can be fluffed up and the patient's position changed at least every two hours.

RE. Assess whether the exertion of lifting and rolling can be tolerated by the patient and those providing care.

2. A large cell ripple mattress limits the time that pressure is applied to the tissues, but the pressures are similar to those from lying on a hard floor. Sheepskins and aids for incontinence such as draw sheets and pads reduce the effectiveness of the mattress.

RE. Check the motor of the ripple mattress works correctly, that there are no leaks and that the connecting tubing does not get squashed during bedmaking or by cot sides. The motor should be overhauled at least every three months.

3. A net suspension bed which fits on the bed-frame allows the patient to be turned by one person. A thick blanket should be used between the patient and the net. Turning from side to side should be carried out at least every two hours.

RE. Assess the patient's level of fear at being suspended in a net; an increase in height above the bed may need to be gradual so that confidence is built up. Once the patient can sit up this aid should be changed as sitting upright is difficult and uncomfortable.

4. A low airloss bed may be hired, for which a source of electricity close to the bed site is essential. The air sacs must be inflated according to the body weight so that pressure distribution is correct. Mark the correct setting with tape or chinagraph (wax) pencil. Adjustment of the pressures for sitting or use of the bedpan is easy, and this type of bed is suitable for the obese patient or when movement of any kind is painful. Teach the patient how to adjust the angle of the bed, if this will not interfere with treatment. Use cot sides for safety if the patient is obese, restless or feels unsafe.

RE. Ask the patient to demonstrate adjusting the bed, to check for correct use. If wounds are present, the air sacs should be washed over with antiseptic solution and then dried at least daily. At other times a weekly wash should be carried out. Soiled sacs should be replaced and cleaned according to the manufacturer's instructions. Monitor the amount of sleep achieved by the patient, and by any others in the vicinity as the blower motor can be noisy.

5. Provide a call bell within easy reach so that help can be summoned quickly. Remind the patient to request help to move or to adjust the aid, if lying in one position becomes painful, as this may be an early indication of tissue damage.

RE. Inspect the skin over points of pressure at least twice a day for early signs of damage including redness, bruising, breaks or roughening of the surface.

Further action

1. Aspirin may be prescribed for pain, it has the added advantage of a mild anti-coagulant effect. Paracetamol is an alternative but has less anti-inflammatory effect. Stronger analgesics may cause constipation, so a high roughage diet may be needed to counteract this effect.

RE. Confirm that the patient has no known allergy to aspirin before giving the first dose. If stronger analgesia is being used, ask the patient to report any change in bowel habit. Observe stools for signs of drying due to prolonged contact with the colon.

Associated medical diagnoses

Ankylosing spondylitis
Carcinomatosis
Cerebral vascular accident
Fractured humerus
Hemiplegia
Motor neurone disease
Multiple sclerosis
Muscular dystrophy
Obesity
Osteoarthritis

Poliomyelitis
Rheumatoid arthritis
Spinal cord compression

Problem	Slow increase in activity desirable

Assessment findings

Recent severe illness
Recent myocardial infarction
Recent bed rest for more than two days
Able to stand
Able to maintain balance on sitting
Physical support needed

Information for the patient

When the body is under stress and needs more energy and protein to repair damaged tissues or to fight infection, it may start to break down the muscles to provide them. The blood flow to the legs and their muscles decreases if they are not used. Standing up after rest in bed or an illness can give the legs a 'cotton wool' feeling, as if they are not strong enough to take the weight of the body. To help to improve the blood flow and encourage the rebuilding of muscle tissue, exercise needs to be increased slowly but steadily. The exercise plan must be designed to suit the patient so that recovery is as quick as possible without their becoming tired or feeling under stress.

Nursing action

1. Discuss with the patient and doctors the level of activity to be achieved and the timescale desired. Discharge home may depend on the ability to walk a specific distance and climb a set number of stairs.

RE. If the patient cannot remember the exact layout and distances involved at home, ask if relatives or visitors may be approached for help. The community nurse may be able to supply the information or be willing to make an assessment visit. Elderly people may need home adaptations or aids, so if the occupational therapist is to make a home visit ask her/him to check the distances and steps.

2. Assess the patient's ability to balance and support their body weight on both limbs. Discuss any muscle strengthening exercises with the physiotherapist. Draw up an initial plan with the patient and agree the activities to be achieved each day. Use measurable markers of progress such as walking to and from the ward door, or mark out measured distances with coloured adhesive tape or paint.

RE. Supervise activities and record whether they were achieved, and if there was any breathlessness, dizziness, tiredness or discomfort. Amend the plan if these occur, or when the patient achieves more than the target activity without any sign of strain. Report any chest pain to the doctor, and stop the exercise until the patient's cardiac state has been assessed by the doctor.

3. Plan rest periods between each exertion. As the muscle strength and stamina increase, reduce the length of rest periods. Record the pulse rate and blood pressure if chest pain occurs, together with the level of activity achieved before it started.

RE. Ask if the rest periods leave the patient feeling refreshed. Assess their motivation and effort to return to activity after rest. Check pulse and respiratory rate at the end of each activity; the rise from the resting level should be less as stamina increases.

4. Consider readjusting the patient's diet as activity increases. Extra carbohydrate may be needed as energy requirements increase. Review the intake of foods high in potassium and sodium if the patient feels weak.

RE. Observe how much, and what type of foods are eaten. Check serum electrolyte results for low sodium or potassium levels.

5. As strength, balance and stamina improve, increase the proportion of decisions about activity taken by the patient, in preparation for the full responsibility they will have when nursing support is no longer available.

RE. Note whether the patient's decisions are realistic, so that advice and help can be given if necessary. A copy of the agreed plan of activity for the first week at home may be welcomed, as professional approval usually leads to a feeling of security.

Further action

1. Lung function tests may be requested where treatment for chronic lung disease has been given. These are usually carried out in a specially equipped laboratory. In the ward, a Wright's peak flow meter may be used for peak flow measurements. The patient is asked to take as large a breath as possible and then to blow out into the peak flow meter as hard as possible. Three attempts should be made, each result being recorded and the dial reset between them.

RE. Check the lips fit closely to the cardboard tube of the peak flow meter so that all the exhaled air goes into the machine. The average of the three attempts should be compared with previous results. The average normal value lies between 400 and 720 litres per minute. The change from the patient's earlier readings is more important than comparison with the average figures.

Associated medical diagnoses

Chronic bronchitis
Chronic obstructive airway disease
Pneumonia
Prolapsed intervertebral disc
Myocardial infarction
Rheumatoid arthritis

Potential problems

Potential problem

Risk of limb contracture.

Assessment findings

Drooping hand
Drooping foot
Chronically bent knee
Chronically bent elbow
Turning of neck towards one side
Flexed fingers
Decreased finger movement
Scar tissue
Muscle loss
Paralysis
Spasticity
Plaster cast
Loss of consciousness
Loss of feeling in an arm or leg

235

The normal position of the arms, legs and neck is achieved by the balanced pull of two opposite sets of muscles. If one set of muscles pulls harder than usual it contracts as the other set relaxes. If the joint is not used and the pull continues, then the shape becomes deformed. The unusual pull may be due to interference with the passage of messages travelling down the nerve, so that one set of muscles is constantly being told to contract. Another reason is damage to one set of muscles so that they no longer balance the normal pull of the others. Damage may occur in an accident, or because of pressure cutting off the circulation of blood so that some of the muscle dies. A different cause comes from scar tissue across a joint shrinking and pulling both sides towards each other. To prevent any of these things happening it is important that the joints are moved several times a day, and the muscles stimulated so the normal shape is maintained. Scar tissue can be discouraged by wearing firmly fitting elasticated tubing over the joint.

Nursing action

1. Plan to put all the joints through a full range of movements every two hours during the daytime, or if the patient is unconscious throughout the full 24 hours. Position the limbs so that spasm is discouraged.

RE. Note any increase in spasm or difficulty moving the joint. The exercises are best planned to accompany changes of the patient's position in the bed or chair. Ask the patient to report any pain or increased discomfort.

2. Teach the patient to carry out the joint movements every two hours. Consider asking relatives if they wish to learn how to help the patient carry out the more difficult movements. Move those joints the patient finds difficult to exercise.

RE. Ask the patient to demonstrate the exercises and movements. Observe if the patient remembers to carry them out without being reminded. Note whether the patient can increase the number of joints they exercise unaided.

3. Provide a bedcradle to take the pressure of heavy bedclothes off the feet. Consider the use of a duvet at home as this is lighter than blankets. Check that the bedclothes are not tucked in so tightly that they restrict movement.

RE. Ask the patient if the bedclothes are comfortable. Observe that exercises are carried out when the patient is in bed.

4. Observe the colour, warmth and level of sensation present in the limb at least every hour during the first 24 hours after application of a plaster of Paris cast.

RE. Report if the limb becomes pale (arterial compression), or cold and blue (venous compression). Ask the patient to report any increase in pain, 'pins and needles' or loss of feeling. Check the staff know how to use a plaster cutting saw or shears so that the pressure can be released quickly if requested by the doctor.

5. Apply firm, elasticated tubing around a joint, extending it at least two inches beyond the edge of the scar tissue. Provide two sets of tubing so that one can be washed while the other is in use. Remind the patient that fresh tubing should be obtained when the elasticity is no longer sufficient to apply firm pressure.

RE. Ask the patient to move the joint to check that the tubing will not work loose. Check that the joint can still be put through the previous range of movements when the tubing is in place.

Further action   1. Spasm may be treated with diazepam 2 mg – 15 mg daily in divided doses, and increased up to 60 mg if muscle spasm is not reduced by lower doses. Warn the patient that their reactions may be slower, and that alcohol increases the effect. Driving or operating machinery may be difficult or dangerous.

RE. Observe for drowsiness, dizziness, impaired coordination or skin rash. Ask the patient to report if they feel depressed or have palpitations. The drug accumulates, so side effects may occur weeks after treatment commences. Elderly people tend to be more sensitive to the drug.

2. Baclofen in slowly increasing doses may be prescribed for spasticity. It should be taken with food or a glass of milk to reduce any feeling of nausea.

RE. Record the blood pressure every six hours if anti-hypertensive drugs are also being given, as a sudden fall in blood pressure may occur. Observe for sedation, confusion or fatigue. Ask the patient to report nausea or vomiting. Observe for marked changes in muscle tone, as loss may increase the risk of falls or cause difficulty when standing.

3. Dantrolene in gradually increasing doses provides an alternative drug for use in spasticity. Advise the patient not to drive or operate machinery until the dosage has been stabilized.

RE. Observe for drowsiness, dizziness or diarrhoea. Ask the patient to report an increase in fatigue or a feeling of weakness.

4. Plaster of Paris splints should be well padded, especially when the elbow or knee is involved. A tourniquet or Thomas splint also carries the risk of compression of the popliteal nerve on the outer side of the knee. (Fig. 6.5).

RE. A rubber Esmarch's tourniquet should be applied only under the strict supervision of a doctor; the time should be noted, and it should be released within one hour. Splints should only be applied by those trained in their use.

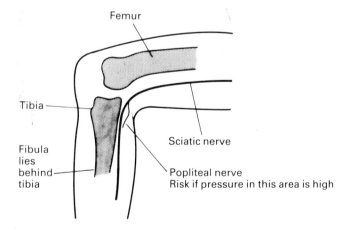

Fig. 6.5   Diagram of part of inside (medial) aspect of right knee

Associated medical diagnoses

Cerebral vascular accident
Foot-drop
Fractured neck of femur
Fractured humerus

Keloid scar tissue
Multiple sclerosis
Muscular dystrophy
Poliomyelitis
Polyneuritis
Second degree burns
Spinal cord lesion
Sub-dural haematoma
Third degree burns
Volkmann's ischaemic contracture

Potential problem	**Risk of falling.**

Assessment findings	Bruising
	Fractures
	Loss of confidence in walking
	Unsteady when standing or walking
	Dizzy
	Nausea
	Pain
	Taking tranquillizers
	Knees tend to buckle on standing
	Confused
	Wanders
	Loss of balance
	Unable to regain balance
	Poor sight

Information for the patient

Walking about safely requires good balance. This comes from the different sets of muscles relaxing and contracting together. To do this the instructions must be passed along the nerves to the muscles. Some of these instructions have to be sent by the brain, others are sent as reflexes and do not need to reach the level of the brain. If any of these nerve pathways becomes blocked, or is affected by drugs, it can make balancing more difficult. If a person feels unsteady it may not take much for them to trip up and fall. The inner ear on each side of the head includes a balancing mechanism. It provides information about the position of the head. If this gets disturbed then balance may be lost. Whirling round and round or riding on a merry-go-round at the fair disturbs the inner ear and causes loss of balance in the same way. If a person feels unsteady it is much better for them to ask a nurse to help than to risk falling over.

Nursing action

1. Check the patient's bed area for hazards such as loose cables or flex, spilt liquids, loose mats, or furniture which wobbles when leaned on. Adjust the lighting level so that the patient can see obstacles such as furniture.

RE. Remind the domestic staff to take extra care when cleaning in the patient's bed area. Ask the patient if a brighter light bulb may be helpful; elderly people need a higher level of illumination than the young.

2. Check that the patient's shoes or slippers fit closely to their feet and that the soles are not loose. Consider applying a non-slippery stick-on sole, or changing the shoes for some with composition rubber soles.

RE. Check the condition of the soles before helping the patient to put on shoes or slippers.

3. Check that the ferrules on a walking stick or on each of the legs of a walking frame have not worn through. Concave plastic ferrules can be obtained to provide slight suction and so increase contact with the floor when the frame or stick is in use.

RE. Ferrules should be checked at least once a month and replaced as soon as they begin to wear thin.

4. Teach the patient to rise slowly and carefully from a chair, and to put a hand out or feel for the chair with the back of the legs before sitting down.

RE. Ask the patient to demonstrate the correct way to rise from and sit down in a chair. Consider teaching the relatives so they can also provide reminders or supervision.

5. Walk just behind the patient if they have a tendency to fall backwards. If the helper rests a hand lightly on the patient's shoulder this may provide added confidence, reduce the need for the patient to look round to check the helper is there and provide an early warning of loss of balance.

RE. Note how often the patient asks if the helper is still there. The frequency should decrease as confidence increases.

5. Place commodes facing the bed with the brakes on and advise the patient to wait for help before trying to stand to use toilet paper.

RE. Arrange for the brakes on commodes to be overhauled at least once every six months. Take out of use any commode with faulty brakes. Check toilet paper is placed within the patient's reach, and that the patient is not left sitting on the commode once they have finished passing urine or faeces. Record if the patient fails to comply with the advice about standing. Plan to supervise them from outside the bed curtains or screens. The position of the patient's feet can indicate their activity without the nurse having to be present all the time.

6. Provide supervision and help if the patient wishes to walk to the toilet. Urgency of micturition may lead to the patient trying to reach the lavatory unaided. Provide an 'engaged' notice for the door so the patient does not need to lock it.

RE. Check that a suitable size coin or key for releasing special toilet door locks is readily available. The urge to defaecate or urinate may accompany sudden loss of blood or a drop in blood pressure, which may produce a fall or loss of consciousness. Fainting and falling may also occur after an enema.

7. Advise the patient to increase their activity in stages and without hurry after a severe illness or following ear trouble. Lower the height of the bed so the patient can sit on the edge and balance their trunk with the feet firmly on the floor. Supervise the patient during the first few days of increasing activity.

RE. Check the body position is symmetrical and that the patient appears balanced before getting up from the bed.

8. Advise the patient not to get out of bed without help after heavy sedation has been given, or when starting a course of tranquillizers.

RE. Review the dosage of tranquillizers with the doctor if the patient becomes unsteady or feels dizzy. Elderly people are sometimes particularly sensitive to these drugs. Night sedation should not be given regularly without a good reason and only after other nursing measures have been tried.

Further action

1. Postural hypotension may lead to falls during treatment with anti-hypertensive drugs, or following peritoneal dialysis. Labetalol, hydralazine, prazosin and methyldopa are particularly likely to cause hypotension. Record the blood pressure with the patient lying resting on the bed preferably for half an hour beforehand. Then ask the patient to stand. Take the blood pressure again.

RE. Report a difference of 10 mmHg between the two readings or if the patient appears or reports feeling dizzy.

2. Tranquillizers such as diazepam, chlordiazepoxide or meprobamate can accumulate in the body and lead to falls.

RE. Report any change in balance, or an increase in confusion or drowsiness, which may indicate the dose needs to be reduced.

3. Anti-emetics may be given in the treatment of inner ear disorders. Prochlorperazine may be given orally or intramuscularly. Advise the patient not to drive or operate machinery until the dosage is stabilized. Advise the patient the mouth may feel dry. Resting on the bed for half an hour after taking the drug may be helpful in reducing nausea.

RE. Drowsiness may occur at the beginning of treatment. Observe for skin reactions and ask the patient to report if mouth dryness causes discomfort.

Associated medical diagnoses

Basilar artery disease
Cerebral tumour
Cerebral vascular disease
Concussion
Drop attacks
Encephalitis
Hypertension
Labyrinthitis
Menière's disease
Myocardial infarction
Otitis media
Parkinson's disease
Sub-dural haematoma
Tinnitus
Vertigo

Potential problem   Risk of deep vein thrombosis developing.

Assessment findings   Unable to move leg
Unconscious
Poor circulation
Bed rest

Wears garters
Seat of chair presses behind knee
Prolonged sitting
Pain in legs, particularly in calves
Painful area appears red
Pillow under knee when in bed
Obese

Information for the patient

The circulation of blood in the legs is normally helped by the massaging action of the leg muscles on the thin-walled veins. If a person stays in one position for a long time, or does not use the leg muscles the flow of blood slows down. The tissues do not get enough food and oxygen from the stale blood waiting to go back to the heart and lungs. It pools in the veins which have thin walls and can be stretched to hold the extra blood. If the blood clots then it not only blocks off the vein deep in the leg, but could also cause trouble elsewhere if pieces of the clot break off and get carried to other parts of the body. To prevent clots forming, the muscles of the legs must be used to massage the blood back to the heart. Another thing that can be done to help is to take deep breaths. Inside the chest this creates a kind of suction which helps the blood flow back towards the heart. The nurses and phsyiotherapist will teach leg and breathing exercises which will be helpful if carried out frequently.

Nursing action

1. Change the position of the bed-bound patient every two hours and exercise the legs if the patient cannot do it unaided. With the leg lying flat on the bed pull the toes back towards the body, relax the pull and repeat at least five times for each leg. Provide a bedcradle to keep the weight of the bedclothes off the legs.

RE. Check the large muscles of the calf contract as the toes are pulled back.

2. Teach the patient to pull the toes up towards the body; place a hand on the top of the foot and press gently while telling the patient to try to stop you pushing the foot down. Advise the patient to repeat the exercise five times every hour when awake. Ask the patient to take deep breaths while practising the exercise.

RE. Check the patient remembers to do the exercises. Check the bedclothes are not tucked in so tightly that movement is restricted. Assess the depth of breaths by placing a hand on each side of the rib cage and observing how much the hands move with each breath the patient takes.

3. Advise the patient to press their feet down on the floor when sitting in a chair, and to relax and then repeat this at least five times every hour. Remind the patient to change their position at least every two hours.

RE. Check the patient's sitting position in the chair; if the seat is pressing against the back of the knees adjust the depth of the seat by placing a cushion behind the patient's back.

4. Advise the patient not to cross their legs when resting in bed or sitting in a chair, as this interferes with the blood circulation. Adjust pillows or other supports for the leg so that there is no pressure on the calf muscles or behind the knee. Remind staff not to lift a patient's leg by gripping the calf.

RE. Inspect the legs for redness each day. Ask the patient to report any tenderness or pain. Feel the surface of each calf to detect a rise in temperature. Check the body temperature at least once a day.

Further action

1. To reduce the risk of emboli forming, graduated compression stockings may be prescribed to provide a gradient of decreasing pressure up each leg. Measure the legs and select the recommended size and length of stocking. The stockings should be removed for bathing. Remind the patient not to turn over the edge of a stocking as this creates a tight band.

RE. Check the stockings fit as recommended by the manufacturer, ask the patient to confirm they feel comfortable. Report any swelling of the toes or above the stocking top. Provide a second pair of stockings so that one can be washed while the other is in use. Check that stockings washed by the hospital laundry are not damaged by excessive heat, producing stretching and uneven pressure.

2. Anti-coagulant therapy may be prescribed if there is a high risk of thrombosis. Heparin or warfarin may be used to decrease the likelihood of blood clotting. Aspirin also has an anti-coagulant effect as it decreases the stickyness of platelets. Explain to the patient that bruising or bleeding may occur more easily when heparin or warfarin are given. Injections should be followed by pressure over the puncture site for longer than usual.

RE. Dosages of heparin and warfarin are adjusted according to the blood clotting time. Warfarin interacts with a wide variety of drugs. Inspect the skin for bruising and report any unexpected bleeding. Test the urine for haematuria at least once a week.

Associated medical diagnoses

Arteriosclerosis
Cerebral vascular accident
Congestive cardiac failure
Fractured femur
Phlebitis
Pneumonia
Varicose veins

Potential problem | **Risk of urinary infection due to stasis**

Assessment findings

Low urine output
Loss of consciousness
Unable to move in bed
Unable to lie on one side

Information for the patient

It is important to drink a lot of fluid when resting in bed for more than a couple of days, as this helps to prevent infection. The two kidneys form urine from the waste products in the blood and water. They lie on either side of the back bone and the urine is squeezed in small amounts down a tube into the bladder. It collects in the bladder until the amount triggers off the feeling of a full bladder. Lying in one position or on one side all the time causes urine to collect where the kidney joins the ureter (or drainage tube) in the lower kidney. Salts can be deposited and can build up to form a kidney stone. In the bladder the urine begins to be broken down if there are any bacteria present. If the bladder gets overfull the large quantity of urine presses the lining of the bladder and restricts its blood supply, making it more likely to become inflamed and infected.

Nursing action

1. Plan a fluid intake of at least two and a half litres each day. Discuss with the patient which kinds of drinks they prefer. A pint of beer, lager or stout may be enjoyed whereas a pint of water may not. Ask the doctor for permission before providing alcohol as many drugs interact with it.

RE. Record fluid intake and output; allow at least one litre for loss of water in sweat and breath. Increase this amount if there is fever. Calculate the fluid balance every 24 hours. If the intake does not exceed the loss by at least 500 ml, plan to increase the intake by at least another 500 ml.

2. Turn the patient every two hours if possible, so that one kidney is not always uppermost. Discuss the use of a stryker frame or electric turning frame if the patient has to be kept flat.

RE. Record the reason why turning is not possible on a particular occasion.

3. Place urinals within easy reach of the bed bound patient. Offer bedpans to female patients at frequent intervals during the day. Provide privacy so that the patient feels less inhibited when passing urine.

RE. Test the urine for protein or blood at least once a week. Allow the urine to settle so that the amount of debris or crystals present can be assessed. Check the body temperature at least daily and report any fever. Report if the urine becomes foul-smelling or cloudy. Note any increase in the frequency of micturition not explained by an increased fluid intake.

4. Wash the genital area at least once a day, and straight away if the patient is incontinent. Advise the female patient when using lavatory paper to wipe from the front towards the back, to reduce the risk of carrying faecal bacteria towards the urinary meatus.

Further action

1. A mid-stream specimen of urine may be requested for bacteriological examination if a urinary tract infection is suspected.

RE. Check the urine sample is sent to the laboratory soon after collection, and that the time of collection is marked on it. A mid-stream urine specimen will still contain bacteria swept down from the urethra and these may multiply if the sample is delayed on its way to the laboratory, giving a false result.

Associated medical diagnoses

Cerebral vascular accident
Fibroids
Gout
Hyperparathyroidism
Prostatic enlargement
Multiple sclerosis
Myeloid leukaemia
Renal calculi
Spinal cord lesion

Potential problem	**Risk of partial pulmonary collapse (atelectasis).**
Assessment findings	Shallow breathing Bed rest Recent anaesthetic Sedated Unequal expansion of the chest Unable to move Pain on breathing deeply Fatigue Rapid pulse Poor fluid intake Ineffective cough
Information for the patient	Deep breathing is important to prevent small areas of the lung from collapsing. The windpipe divides into two (left and right bronchus) then into smaller tubes ending in tiny airsacs. If phlegm blocks one of the smaller tubes, then air cannot get into the sacs. The air gets absorbed outside the sacs and the lung tissue collapses. It then provides a site for infection. Drinking lots of fluid will help keep any phlegm thin, and therefore easy to cough up.
Nursing action	1. Teach the patient to breathe deeply by placing the hands on either side of the lower ribs and ask the patient to breathe so deeply that the hands are moved apart with each breath. Ask the patient to take at least five deep breaths each hour, when awake. An incentive spirometer may be useful if the patient finds it difficult to recognize an adequate deep breath. Raising the different coloured balls in their tubes provides a visual guide.
	RE. Note whether deep breathing causes pain or coughing. Discuss the need for analgesia and sedation with the doctor. Note whether the patient remembers to carry out the exercises as requested. Plan extra supervision if necessary. Note which coloured balls the patient can raise in their tubes.
	2. Turn the patient from side to side every two hours, and place the upper arm on a pillow so its weight does not compress the rib cage. Sit the patient up, supported with pillows, as soon as their condition allows.
	RE. Check the position of the upper arm every hour if the patient is restless.
	3. Plan out with the patient a regular drinking pattern to provide at least 2500 ml in 24 hours.
	RE. Record fluid intake and calculate the volume drunk every six hours during the day.
	4. Provide tissues and a sputum container marked with the date. Replace daily.
	RE. Measure the volume and inspect the consistency and colour of the sputum, which should be liquid. If it is thick and sticky, plan to increase the fluid intake.
Further action	1. Physiotherapy may be requested if the patient has difficulty in following instructions, or has unequal chest expansion. Plan the treatment so the patient has had time to recover energy after bathing or other activities.

RE. Discuss the need for treatment overnight. Ask the physiotherapist whether coughing has been productive.

2. Review the need for strong analgesia, as respiratory depression may occur with narcotic drugs. Pentazocine and dihydrocodeine used in moderately severe pain cause respiratory depression in high doses.

RE. Note the respiratory rate half an hour after analgesia has been given. Nalorphine may be used to counteract severe respiratory depression from morphine, pethidine or methadone.

Associated medical diagnoses	Cerebral vascular accident Cervical spinal cord injury Hepatitis Pneumonia Spinal cord tumour

---

Potential problem | **Risk of skin damage due to loss of sensation.**

Assessment findings

Injury to spine
Unable to feel leg
Unable to feel vibration from a tuning fork
Numbness
Tingling
Red areas of skin
'Pins and needles'

Information for the patient

The skin contains nerve cells to warn of too much pressure or heat which would damage the skin. If the nerves are not sending back these warning messages then the patient will have to think ahead and look for possible dangers to the skin. Too much pressure could come from sitting in one position for a long time, tight straps, ill-fitting shoes or a tight splint. Too much heat could come from such things as resting the hand against a hot plate, picking up a hot spoon, resting against a heater or from a hot water bottle.

Nursing action

1. Discuss the specific risks present in the patient's environment. Mark straps with a ball point pen, paint or nail varnish to indicate the maximum level for doing up the strap. Plan regular changes of position at least every two hours.

RE. Inspect the skin areas at risk for blisters, grazes or redness at least once every day. Check the position of straps, if they are in use.

2. Consider alternative means of providing heat, to reduce the risk of damage from heaters or hot water bottles. A thermostatically controlled electric heat pad or an electric blanket may be sufficient. Advise the patient not to sit close to an open fire or heater and to check the skin for redness which indicates damage is occurring.

RE. Arrange to have the pad or blanket checked for safety at least every six months. Observe whether the patient follows advice about sitting close to sources of heat.

3. Discuss the risks of chilling from cold weather and the use of several layers of thin warm clothing rather than thick clothes. Clothes designed for winter sports may be useful in providing insulating layers without weight. Rugs and shawls may be useful when sitting in a chair.

RE. Observe the choice of clothes in cold weather; note if they restrict movement. Check the skin temperature to see if the clothing is effective in reducing heat loss.

Associated medical diagnoses

Cerebral vascular accident
Diabetic neuropathy
Extradural neoplasm
Glioma
Head injury
Hemangioblastoma
Hydrocephalus
Medulloblastoma
Meningioma
Meningocele
Multiple sclerosis
Parkinson's disease
Peripheral vascular disease
Poliomyelitis
Polyneuritis
Prolapsed intervertebral disc
Spinal cord injury

References and further reading

Carr, J., Shepherd, R. (1979). *Early Care of the Stroke Patient.* William Heinemann Medical Books Ltd. London

Carr, J., Shepherd, R. (1982). *A Motor Relearning Programme for Stroke.* Heinemann Medical Books Ltd. London.

Johnstone, M. (1983). (2nd edn). *Restoration of Motor Function in the Stroke Patient.* Churchill Livingstone. Edinburgh.

King Edward's Hospital Fund for London (1972). *Catalogue of Garments for the Handicapped and Disabled.* 2 volumes. The King's Fund for the Shirley Institute. London.

Macartney, P. (1973). *Clothes Sense for Handicapped Adults of All Ages.* Disabled Living Foundation. London.

Ruston, R. (1977). *Dressing for Disabled People – A Manual for Nurses and Others.* Disabled Living Foundation. London.

Useful address

Disabled Living Foundation, 380 Harrow Road, London W.9.
Tel. 01-289-6111

7 Religion

Optimum environment

Throughout the world there are groups of people who share a belief in some higher, unseen controlling force or power. The historical development of such beliefs varies. However a common belief is that illness may be caused or influenced by a supernatural force. Becoming sick may be thought of as a consequence of breaking one or more religious rules.

Religious beliefs may influence the way health care services develop as well as influencing the medical sciences which underpin them. The dominant religion in a country is likely to influence the legal system, and in some instances the government. In recent years the west has become involved in the oil trade with the Middle East, and so has become more aware of the intimate relationship between Islam and the laws of countries such as Iran. In Britain the House of Lords includes both Lords temporal and Lords spiritual.

In a multi-cultural society people of different religious beliefs live and work close to each other. A detailed knowledge of each other's beliefs and religious practices can develop only through the sharing of knowledge. This can be difficult to attain if neither can speak the other's language. The temptation then is to use stereotypes to provide a general guide to a person's likely beliefs. This is a poor substitute but it may be the only available route to follow if time together is brief. Health care professionals therefore sometimes make assumptions about a person's beliefs which are far from being correct for the individual.

People from the same racial group may share a common religion, or may come from different sects which have developed widely varying practices based on similar beliefs, or they may belong to very different religious groups. If communication is poor, relationships can deteriorate because offence is caused through misunderstanding of the person's beliefs and customs. Culture shock for those moving to a strange country can be intense. It is little wonder that members of the same religious group tend to stay together to follow familiar customs and practices when living in a new country. If their experience of those from other groups is unsatisfactory there may be charges of racism.

Individual racism is due to the behaviour of one or more individuals who believe there is racial superiority of one or more groups over other groups. The caste system of the Hindus has religious sanction and is tied up with the theory of reincarnation. The belief is that each person is born into a caste according to how he or she behaved in former life. Each caste has specific roles and duties, and those duties must not be performed by someone from a different caste. People from the lowest caste perform the duties which pollute, such as cleaning lavatories. The Indian government has brought in laws against caste discrimination but beliefs change slowly, especially when they have a deeply ingrained religious origin.

Institutional racism comes about through the policies and practices of institutions. Civil rights activists suggest that the responsibility for the continuation of such conditions belongs to everyone, especially those who make no effort to understand or to change the situation. British laws have in the past discriminated against women, and women still make up the largest proportion of the lowest-paid in the workforce. Increasing awareness of the problems this can bring may help in identification with the problems suffered by racial minorities.

The culture in which a person grows up may leave them with deep-seated beliefs, which can remain long after knowledge has shown the beliefs to be untrue. In illness there is a tendency to feel vulnerable and at the mercy of others; this may result in a return to patterns of coping behaviour learnt in childhood. Deep-seated beliefs and fears may surface again, and may cause problems because they are known to be illogical and therefore the person holding them may not wish to confess them to others.

Some religions influence the person's daily activities to a very great extent. The tables which accompany this chapter try to set out in a quick reference form key points which may be useful in understanding the beliefs of some of the major religious groups likely to be found in the United Kingdom. Other aspects which may be helpful when caring for the sick are set out in the following sections. It is important to remember that individuals choose what they believe, and that the stereotypes are no more than a very rough guide.

Folk medicine

Folk remedies, especially those based on herbs, have become more popular in the west as dissatisfaction with conventional medicine has increased. The shelves of health food shops have a wide range of products. Sometimes the remedies are found to be based on plant or fungal material which has healing properties. For example, in the west of England, a bad cut might have been bound up with cobwebs from the dairy. Cheese-making used to rely on natural yeasts and moulds, and there was a good chance that penicillin type moulds might be caught in the dusty web. Many years later, around the time of the Second World War, penicillin became available in quantities large enough to save many lives at risk from infection in wounds.

In Third World countries access to conventional medicine may be very limited. Self-help is likely to be the norm. Immigrants therefore tend to bring with them tried and trusted remedies. Some remedies may contain metals. In recent years tonics containing lead were imported by the Asian community. When possible it is wise to enquire exactly what home remedies have been tried when someone is ill and seeks health care. Some people continue to take their own remedies while accepting treatment from the doctor, and this can lead to uneven absorption, or interaction between the drug and the ingredients in the home remedy.

Food and its preparation

Meat and blood products are often involved in ritual methods of slaughter and preparation, or are totally forbidden. Orthodox Jews eat only kosher meat from an animal which has been killed in such a way that it bleeds to death. Licensed slaughterhouses can be found in the major cities in Britain where this is carried out under supervision of a rabbi. Meat and milk are not eaten at the same meal. Thus care must be taken not to offer, for example, milk pudding after a main course involving meat. There are very precise rules and guidance laid down for the Jewish housewife to ensure that meal preparation is carried out in such a way that contamination does not occur.

For example great care is taken over washing and storage for crockery and cutlery so that those items used for meat are not contaminated by being used for milk products. Pork is not eaten in any form, so lard must not be used to grease baking tins. Those who hold such beliefs and realise that others may be unaware of them, go to great lengths to avoid eating in circumstances where they have no control over food preparation and its presentation.

Moslems eat only halal meat. Again this is from animals which have bled to death and where preparation of the carcass is under supervision of a religious representative. Pork products are also forbidden.

Hindus and Sikhs do not eat beef in any form, as the cow is a sacred animal. Some sects are vegetarian or vegans. In a strange country where the contents of prepared foods are not understood, the cautious may stick to a very narrow range of foodstuffs. New immigrants may therefore become low in vitamins, especially vitamin D, iron, protein and carbohydrates. They may assume that their lack of energy and lassitude is due to the change of climate. Devout Hindus may only eat food cooked by members of the same caste.

Jehovah's Witnesses and members of the Church of God do not eat blood products, so they should not be offered black puddings or spiced sausages which contain blood.

Stimulants such as alcohol are also forbidden in some religions, and for some sects. Members of the Church of God do not drink alcohol, nor do some Buddhists, some Methodists, Moslems or Mormons. Tea, coffee and cola drinks are also considered to be stimulants which would be avoided by Mormons. Rastafarians avoid wine and other products made from the fruit of the vine.

Hindus and some Sikhs believe that specific foods can influence the body, the personality and the emotions. 'Hot' foods cause over-excitement and sweating, raise the temperature and bring on giddiness and fatigue. The 'cold' foods cool the body, and bring strength and calm. The diet is therefore balanced between both types, eg perhaps in summer more foods from the cold group would be eaten. Similar kinds of belief can be found among people from Latin America and the Caribbean. The Chinese believe the cold Yin energy force must counterbalance the Yang hot energy. An illness caused by too much of one can be treated by foods of the opposite nature.

The Hindu grouping of hot and cold foods is as follows:

Hot	Cold
aubergine	apple
brown sugar	banana
carrot	cereals
chilli	chickpeas
dates	green leafy vegetables
egg	lemon
fish	milk
ginger	nuts
honey	orange
lentils	potato
meat	white sugar
onion	
tea	

Clothing

The way in which the body is to be covered during religious observances and in daily life may be laid down in detail. Some religious groups dress in such a distinctive way that it is easy to identify to which sect they belong. Clothing may be linked with beliefs about modesty and relationships between men and women. The head and its covering may have special significance, for example the turban worn by male Sikhs. Orthodox Jewish men may wish to keep the crown of the head covered with a small cap at all times while Jewish women may keep their hair covered. If it is necessary to help an ill person undress or dress, care must be taken to handle their clothing with respect, or offence may be given.

Mormons wear a sacred white one- or two-piece undergarment, which is worn at all times and should be treated with deference. Sikhs wear as one of the five symbols of Sikhism, white underpants called Kaccha. Some regard even their ordinary underpants in this way and would be reluctant to remove them fully even for a medical examination of the genital area. In such circumstances they should be left on one leg.

Moslem women keep their bodies covered at all times, and during a medical examination only small areas of the body would normally be exposed at any one time. Even during washing, one garment may be kept on. Women wear a scarf or use part of the sari as a veil when outside the home. The Moslem women may wear a yashmak, a veil which leaves only the eyes uncovered. Rastafarian women do not wear trousers, they keep the head covered and prefer to wear clothes made of natural fibres.

Asians may not have separate day and night clothes, but only clothes which are worn inside and outside the home. When ill, therefore, they may wear what look like day clothes in bed. There is also a belief that when ill it is important to rest on the bed as much as possible. This can lead to misunderstandings if health care staff wish to start active rehabilitation before the patient feels fully recovered.

Modest dress is generally expected of anyone visiting a religious house, be it church or temple. Tourists can cause great offence by entering wearing skimpy clothes, shorts, sun-dresses or very short skirts. When visiting a foreign country it is wise for women to pack a head scarf for use when sightseeing is likely to include churches etc. Long skirts or trousers should be taken when visiting countries where the women are expected to dress modestly. Many such countries also have enclosed swimming pool and sunbathing areas for tourists staying in their modern hotels. When such facilities are provided, it is good manners to follow local customs during a holiday.

Bathing

Care of the skin and hair may have religious significance, and may form part of the ritual associated with the transition between one state and the next, for example initiation ceremonies at puberty, or preparation for marriage. Body painting and use of cosmetics, perfumes or oils may also be involved. Removal of body hair may be part of a symbolic cleansing ritual, as with Moslem women, who shave at the end of a menstrual period.

The western tub bath may be considered rather a dirty habit. Showers are preferred because water which has been poured over the body does not touch it again. A Moslem faced with a tub bath is likely to stand in it and pour water over himself with a jug or small bowl. In such circumstances there is a fair chance the water will also splash on to the floor, which can cause friction with the host. It is also normal practice to wash the anal area with water after a bowel action. Lavatory paper is not considered sufficient. The left hand is used for this. Few lavatories in the west provide a wash basin in the toilet cubicle. It is therefore helpful to provide a small bowl for water. Misunderstanding can occur with others if water used for this purpose splashes on to the floor by the WC as it may be mistaken for urine.

Moslems also have a set ritual to perform in preparation for prayer, which includes washing the hands, arms, feet and face. Water is also sniffed up the nose and blown out. Hindus may also use this nasal cleansing technique in the morning. This noisy procedure may cause offence to others who do not recognise it as an acceptable activity. The left hand is used for bathing and washing by Moslems. Hindus must wash thoroughly before praying, usually at sunrise.

The facial hair of the Orthodox Jew and the Sikh men must remain uncut. Some Sikhs wear a neat hairnet to hold the beard tidy when sleeping. Rastafarian men do not cut, comb or wash their dreadlocks.

Beliefs about death and dying

Rituals to accompany the transition from life to death often include washing of the body and dressing in specific clothing, either before or after death. Specific members of the family or community may be given the task of carrying this out. The beliefs about what happens after death colour the rituals, and the anxiety, about dying. In recent years what has become known as 'spare part' surgery has also raised issues about the donation of organs, particularly for those who live in the west.

The Christian church does not have the rigid rules of some of the other religious groups. However the opportunity to discuss dying and to receive spiritual comfort may be denied some people because of the belief that the doctor decides whether a person should be told that they are dying. It can be hard to discuss the future in a meaningful way with relatives who have been told to deny that the person is dying. Conversation can become stilted and all kinds of verbal and non-verbal tactics may be used to avoid the sensitive area. What is surprising is the amount of influence given to doctors to make the decision, and for it to be followed in the face of obvious difficulties.

Roman Catholics make a confession and receive the sacrament of the sick. This has replaced the more familiar 'last rites'. Moslems say special prayers for the dying. The dying person says a declaration of faith while facing Mecca (south east direction in Britain). Sikhs recite hymns, or these may be read by a member of the family.

The body of the Christian is prepared by washing and dressing in a shroud. In Britain embalming and other preparations are usually performed by undertakers. The body of the Orthodox Jew may be touched by gentiles (non-Jews) only in so far as the eyes are closed, limbs straightened, any tubes or medical equipment removed, the jaw bandaged and the body wrapped in a plain sheet. The body will later be washed by officials of the Jewish Burial Society.

The Moslem's body is normally washed by members of the family. Men are washed either by other men, by the widow or by a woman who would have been ineligible to marry the deceased when alive. No man may see or touch the female body. Women are wrapped in five pieces of cloth, men in three. There are special burial rites.

The Sikh would be washed and dressed with the five symbols of Sikhism before being wrapped in a white cotton shroud, prior to cremation. The Hindu hopes for the eldest son to be present before, during and after death so that he can perform the death rites. After death, a man is washed by relatives, water may be poured into the mouth and the body is dressed in new clothes. A woman is washed only by other women. The marriage thread around the neck is cut by the widower. Cremation follows.

Mourning and expressions of grief are more open than would be expected by, for example, members of the Church of England. Loud wailing and moaning and the performance of death rites are now being recognised as being helpful to the family. The traditional British stiff upper lip and tight control on the expression of grief may interfere with the normal process of grief, which must be worked through.

Illness

Faith healing may be tried by some people who believe sickness comes as a punishment or because they have failed to live up to a specific standard required by their god. Others dislike western medicine or wish to try every means to achieve recovery. Roman Catholics sometimes make pilgrimages to Lourdes. The link of mind and body in some diseases has given rise to the belief that symptoms may be controlled by the mind. Psychosomatic diseases have become fashionable topics for discussion. Christian Scientists believe sickness can be cured by proper mental processes. Treatment involves prayer and counsel, with diet and manipulation of the body being acceptable. Drugs are not.

Illness may carry a stigma for the family, which may go as far as affecting the marriage chances of the children. Diseases such as tuberculosis, Hansen's disease, eczema, asthma, epilepsy and mental illness would cast a stigma on the Asian family. To be mentally ill is to the Asian an admission of insanity and reduces the marriage prospects of other members of the family. Few would therefore seek voluntary treatment in a mental hospital even if the cultural divide allowed treatment appropriate in the eyes of the patient and family. Western treatment for mental illness is often based on discussion which may be difficult if the patient and staff do not speak the same language.

Those who believe illness is caused by evil spirits may be reluctant to do anything which they think would weaken the body. Bathing may be felt to cause chills or pneumonia. Those who follow the hot-cold food balance may refuse to take cold drinks when ill; instead they may wrap up well and take hot drinks, even when their body temperature is very high.

Beliefs about blood

The Jehovah's Witness does not accept blood from another person: the conviction is so strong that life may be lost rather than saved through accepting blood. This can create conflicts for those caring for the children of Jehovah's Witnesses, and from time to time a child is made a ward of court so that the decision about the blood may legally be taken away from the parents. If the child receives blood, the parents may reject it afterwards, the strength in the religious belief being so strong that it overcomes the emotional ties of parenthood. Some people find it very hard to accept that others hold beliefs with such strength, and try to change the believer's ideas through argument. Deeply held beliefs are held at an emotional level, and therefore do not respond to argument.

A belief held with similar strength concerns termination of pregnancy. Conflict can arise for the staff who work in gynaecology wards and clinics. Some may believe it is wrong and yet are called upon as part of their job to care for those who have undergone a termination of pregnancy. Arrangements may be made so that those holding such beliefs work only with patients undergoing other types of surgery.

Specific religious beliefs

Conflict can arise when people move from one culture to another. Hospitals tend to follow beliefs founded on science. People who work, or are treated in, such hospitals may find both major and minor discomforts in maintaining long-held beliefs, or in being in the company of those who do not share the same ideas. It is helpful for a person to think through the ideas that they do or do not believe and why. Many people hold on to ideas which they received from their parents without ever being aware of the origin.

Table 7:1   Characteristics and practices of major religions of the world

Religion	Religious observances and festivals	Treatment	Diet	Terminal care and last offices	Clothing	Bathing	Miscellaneous
Baha'i		No objection to spare part or transplant surgery or blood transfusion. Termination of pregnancy only if mother's life at risk	Alcohol forbidden	Bahai's prayers are read. After death — body is washed, wrapped in silk or cotton shroud. Bahai's ring on finger. Burial		General modesty	
Buddhism Schools: Therevada Mahayana Zen	**Therevada** Buddha day — in Spring. Meditation.	No objection to spare part or transplant surgery or blood transfusion. Objection to termination of pregnancy and contraception	Some are vegetarian and do not drink alcohol.	Cremation			Wrong desire and selfishness may cause suffering.
Chinese Buddhism **Taoism** **Confucianism** } may believe in elements of all three.	Unlikely to celebrate publicly in a hospital ward but family may wish to gather round bed to burn incense. Chinese New Year Ching Ming	Helpful to give date of planned surgery to allow the Chinese Almanac to be consulted. May be fearful if day is inauspicious	Ask if meat is eaten. If in doubt serve vegetarian meals. Western food considered 'ghost' food especially by older Chinese. Not properly reincarnated souls are 'ghost'. There may be fear of control by ghosts. May wish food to be brought from home. May not eat meat on first day of Chinese New Year.	May wish to dress the body and burn joss sticks before body leaves.	May tie a written charm around neck.		Most do not give themselves a religious title. May use written charms under pillow, burnt and mixed with water to drink or made as a set of signs over water which is then drunk. Birthdays rarely celebrated, every Chinese is automatically one year older on Chinese New Year. Most speak Cantonese which is a tonal language where each sound has a set meaning so it may sound harsh. Rarely demonstra-

Denomination	Festivals / Sacraments	Medical attitudes	Alcohol / Food	Death / Rites	Other
Christianity: Orthodox		No objection to spare part or transplant surgery or blood transfusion. Termination of pregnancy only on medical grounds.	May drink alcohol.	Hear confession, anointing with oil, communion Body lies in open coffin.	tive in public even with own family. Consider their home is not worthy of a visit so prefer to meet at a restaurant or in the street; callers are unlikely to be invited in.
Protestant: Church of England Anglican	*Christmas.* 25th December *Lent:* Ash Wednesday to Good Friday, March – April. Easter Sunday: next after Good Friday *Whitsun* Sacraments: Baptism Communion Confirmation Confession Laying on of hands Anointing		May give up specific foods, alcohol or smoking for Lent.		
Church of Scotland	} Adult baptism by immersion	Individual decision on spare part or transplant surgery, blood transfusion, contraception and termination of pregnancy			
Free Church: Baptist Churches of Christ Congregation Independent Methodist Moravian Presbyterian of Wales Salvation Army Welsh Independents United Reform Wesleyan Reform	} May not practise baptism or holy communion	} Termination of pregnancy to be avoided.	May not drink alcohol		

Table 7:1 (Cont'd)

Religion	Religious observances and festivals	Treatment	Diet	Terminal care and last offices	Clothing	Bathing	Miscellaneous
Plymouth, Exclusive or other **Brethren**		Unlikely to accept spare part or transplant surgery or termination of pregnancy.	May not wish to eat with non-Brethren			May wish to wear an article of clothing	
Quaker	No form of service, liturgy or sacraments		May abstain from alcohol.				May be pacifist
Roman Catholic	Confession Communion Sacrament of the Sick (also known as Last Rites or Extreme Unction)	Totally opposed to termination of pregnancy and artificial contraception	May not wish to eat meat on Fridays	Confession then Sacrament of the Sick. May have hands placed as in prayer holding rosary, crucifix or flower.			
Mormons (Church of Jesus Christ of latter Day Saints)	Morning and evening prayers	Termination of pregnancy only on strong medical grounds.	No tea, coffee, alcohol, cola, smoking. Fast for 24 hours once a month		Sacred, religious white one or two piece undergarment to be treated with great deference and worn at all times if possible		Resurrection and life after death
Christian Scientist (Church of Christ Scientist)	Church services — Sundays and Wednesdays	May refuse analgesics, drugs and surgery. Object to spare part and transplant surgery. Termination of pregnancy only if severe risk to mother's life.					Disease can be healed by prayer alone
Church of God	Baptism by total immersion	Prefer herbal medicines. Opposed to termination of	No blood products, black pudding. No alcohol.		Modest dress		

	Schools / Festivals	Medical	Diet	Death	Dress	Washing	Beliefs
Jehovah's Witness		pregnancy. No blood transfusion or human plasma. May accept non-blood volume expanders (eg dextrose polymer). Opposed to termination of pregnancy	No smoking. No blood products — black puddings				Resurrection of the dead will occur.
Spiritualist			May be vegetarian	Burial preferred.			The spirit will survive death and communicate with loved ones. Suffering is a necessity.
Hindu	Main schools — Samkhya, Yoga, Nyava, Vaishesika, Purva-Mumamsa, Vedanta. No standard form — meditation, prayer or physical exercise. **Festivals — Shivati** (March); **Holi** (end March); **Ram Naumi** (April); **New Year** (mid-April); **Rath Yatra** (July); **Janam Ashtami** (August); **Ganesh Chaturthi** (end August); **Dwga Purja** (October); **Diwali** (mid-October)	Women prefer to be examined by female doctors and nurses. May wish to consult with father or husband before signing consent forms. Object to bovine grafts and bovine insulin.	No beef, veal, sausages, bovril, oxo or other meat extracts, jelly, consomme. May not eat meat or fish. Some are vegans and may not eat eggs or milk products. Foods include dhal (lentils), chapattis (unleaven wheat cakes), ghee (clarified butter), roti (flat round bread), pilau (rice), curries, yoghurt, white fish. Different castes may not wish to eat together. May fast regularly.	May wish for eldest son to be present before, during and after death to perform death rites. Clothes and coins touched by patient then given to poor. **Men** Relatives wash body. Water may be poured into mouth. Body dressed in new clothes. **Women** Women only wash body. Marriage thread round neck cut by husband. If a post-mortem is carried out all organs **must** be replaced. Cremation	**Women** Blouse, sari, long petticoat, glass wedding bangle only removed on husband's death. White may be worn during mourning by widows. Coloured forehead spot worn by married woman to indicate she has performed her morning prayers. Men of Swami Narayan Sect may wear bead necklace. May also have red spot on forehead.	Prefer showers. Must wash thoroughly and change clothes before praying, usually at sunrise.	Reincarnation. Non violence. Cows are sacred. 'Hot' foods — pungent, acidic, salty, produce giddiness thirst, fatigue, sweating, inflammation. 'Cold' foods — sweet, astringent, bitter, produce cheerfulness, pleasure strength, steadiness. Women responsible for religious education of children. Caste system. Bhagrad gita = holy book.

Table 7:1   (Cont'd)

Religion	Religious observances and festivals	Treatment	Diet	Terminal care and last offices	Clothing	Bathing	Miscellaneous
Jain	Not Hindus but may join in Hindu observances.		Strain all fluids. Strict vegetarians. May fast for 1 or 2 days a week				Strict austere form of Hinduism. No harm to be done to *any* living creature.
Jew: Liberal	**Rosh Hashanah** (Jewish New Year); **Yom Kippur** (Day of Atonement) 10 days later; **Succoth** (Feast of the Tabernacle). 5 days later; **Simchath Torah** (Rejoicing in the law); **Chanukah** (Festival of lights) December; **Purim** (Feast of Esther) March; **Pesoch** (Passover) March or April; **Tishah B'Av.** Sabbath starts at sunset on Friday and ends at sunset on Saturday	No porcine insulin or skin grafts. No objection to spare part surgery and blood transfusion. Termination of pregnancy left to mother — usually only if risk to life.	Fast for 24 hours for Yom kippur Passover – no unleavened bread for 8 days, omit cake. Kosher meat.* No pork, ham, bacon, sausages. No shellfish. No meat and milk at the same meal. May not eat cheese. May not use hospital cutlery or crockery	Prefer cremation			*In London hospitals kosher meals service available Rabbi may give dispensation to allow non-kosher food.
Orthodox	No work done on Sabbath	Object to porcine insulin, skin grafts. Termination of pregnancy on strict medical grounds only.		Prayers recited by rabbi or family Gentiles allowed to straighten limbs, remove tubes, etc., bandage jaws, wrap in plain sheet. The body is washed by officials from Jewish Burial Society. Burial.	Skull cap and prayer shawl when praying. Men may wear a phylactery (small box of prayers). Some Jews keep head covered at all times.	Facial hair remains unshaved.	

Muslim/ Moslem						
Al-Whudhu (ablution) before prayer at least 5 times a day, may use prayer mat and face Mecca (south east). Fajr — sunrise Zuhr — mid-afternoon Mahgrib — sunset Isha — night Dates of festivals based on lunar calendar (12 × 28 days) *Birthday of Prophet Mohammed* *Lailat ul-Mi'raj* *Lailat Ul-Bara'at* *Ramazan (Ramadhan)* *Eed-ul-Fit* (end of Ramadhan) *Eed-ul-Azha* Muharram	No porcine insulin or skin grafts. No non-medical drugs Opposed to spare part or transplant surgery and termination of pregnancy. May refuse to take drugs between dawn and sunset during Ramadhan.	No pork, bacon, ham, sausages, or any food made with pig fat. Hallal meat. Large breakfast then fast from dawn* to sunset at Ramadhan (30 days). No alcohol. Wash before eating. Right hand used for eating. Rinse mouth with plain water after food.	Special prayers said for dying. Patient says declaration of faith facing Mecca. **Men** Washed by men, wife or woman who would be ineligible to marry man if he was alive. Alternative — washing face and hands with dust or sand. Wrapped in 3 pieces of cloth Kaffan. **Women** No man can see or touch a female body. Washed by women, wrapped in 5 pieces of cloth. Special burial rites. Display of strong emotion an expected part of mourning. Post-mortem to be avoided — a moslem is not the owner of his body, it should not be harmed.	Women must keep bodies completely covered. **Pakistani** Tapered trousers, long shirt tunic, scarf. **Middle East** Long black dress or skirt and blouse, black veil, yashmak. **Indian** Sari, blouse. Some moslems may wear verses of the Koran in a lock or pouch. Talismans may be worn to give strength during illness or hospital stay. Nose jewel may be worn, only removed on husband's death. **Men** High-collared coat, brimless hat.	Women prefer to undress in private, may keep on a garment for modesty, may shave off body hair at end of menstrual period. Ritual washing is extremely important before prayer. Left hand used to wash body after using toilet even after cleansing with toilet paper. Water poured over the body should not touch it again. Showers preferred, otherwise a bath and jug to pour over water while standing up. May rub in scented oils afterwards, (which can mark bed linen).	Pain is god's will. One god — Allah *Dispensation may be given by Imams. May wish to keep separate from Hindus and Buddhists. Holy book — Koran. May use prayer beads. Mosque also acts as a community centre. Right hand used to shake hands. Nurses have low prestige. Moslem boys circumcised before puberty.

Table 7:1 (Cont'd)

Religion	Religious observances and festivals	Treatment	Diet	Terminal care and last offices	Clothing	Bathing	Miscellaneous
Sikh	Rise early, pray at sunrise, sunset, before bed. Baptised Singh. **Birthday of Guru Gobind Singh** (18 January); **Holi** (March); **Bai Saki (Amrit Parchar)** (13 April); **Martyrdom of Guru Arjan Dev** (June); **Rakhi** (July/Aug); **Dassera** (Oct); **Diwali** (Oct/Nov); **Birthday of Guru Nanak** (Nov/Dec)	**Women** prefer to be examined by female doctor and nurse. No bovine insulin	No beef, veal, sausages, bovril, oxo or other meat extracts, consommé, jelly. No smoking, no meat. No food of which another person has already eaten a part. May fast.	Hymns recited by patient or family. Washed and dressed with the five symbols of Sikhism. Body wrapped in white cotton shroud. No religious prohibition on postmortem. Cremated.	**Amritdari Sikhs** **Men** Kangha small comb worn under turban. Kara – steel bangle on right wrist. Kirpau – small dagger. Kacha – white shorts/underwear **Women** Sari or long dress, scarf to cover head.	Hair must not be cut. Women may wear glass wedding bangle which is only removed on husband's death. May wear coloured forehead spot to show she has performed morning prayers.	Dispensation may be given by local Sikh temple. One god. Guru Grant Sahab = holy book.
Rastafarian		Use cannabis – 'ganja' No spare part or transplant surgery or termination of pregnancy. May refuse blood transfusion. Contraception limited to sheath or rhythm method.	Mostly vegetarian, some eat all meats except pork. No currants, grapes, sultanas, wine		Natural fibres. **Women** Woollen socks, not nylons. No trousers. Head covered.	Hair must not be cut, combed or washed; 'dreadlocks'	

General assessment areas

Religious denomination
Ethnic group
Special dispensations required
Dietary taboos
Religious rites to be followed when ill
Festivals occurring
Contact with other believers
Personal beliefs about illness

Problems

Page

Unable to follow usual diet   263
Unable to follow usual clothing beliefs   264
Unable to follow usual religious rites   266
Conflict in beliefs   267

Problems

Problem	Unable to follow usual diet
Assessment findings	Eats little of what is offered Drop in body weight Refuses food Diabetic diet prescribed Reducing diet prescribed Low protein diet prescribed High protein diet prescribed Low fat diet prescribed Different ethnic group from hosts Different religious group from hosts
Information for the patient	In illness the body needs three main types of food; protein to build new cells, with carbohydrate and fats for energy. Some kinds of disease are treated by changes in the amounts of these three types of food. In British hospitals the diet tends to follow the usual British pattern. If a patient wishes to follow a different pattern to suit their religious or other belief, the dietitian will be able to help. Relatives may bring in food if it is in keeping with the patient's treatment.
Nursing action	1. Consider whether there is a language barrier between the patient and staff which will make detailed discussion and understanding of the diet difficult. Consider arranging for an interpreter to be present during the discussion with the dietitian. RE. Record the name of the interpreter. Plan at least one hour of quiet, uninterrupted time for the discussion. Ask if the main cook in the family would also like to be present. 2. Ask the patient or relative to describe in detail the food eaten at home each day. RE. Record the diet in detail. Compare the likely proportions of protein, fat and carbohydrate with those desired during the period of illness. Identify which items need to be changed. 3. Plan with the patient, relative and dietitian which foods the hospital can supply that the patient is willing and able to eat. Plan which foods the family will supply and when they can bring them. Ask the interpreter to confirm in writing the full plan for the family and patient. Plan the foods that the hospital can supply and when they can be provided. Arrange for the special diet description sheets to be translated into the language of the patient and family if they are able to read. RE. Record the discussion and the agreed action. Adjust the diet ordered from the hospital to prevent food being wasted. Inform the medical staff of the plan. 4. Inform domestic and other staff if relatives have been given permission to bring in food at meal times. Request facilities for heating and serving food if necessary. Consider advising the family to use wide-necked vacuum flasks to carry hot food.

RE. Note if the family arrive with the food at the times planned. Check that the composition of the food follows the doctor's prescribed diet. Weigh the patient at least weekly to confirm that the diet is sufficient to keep the weight steady, or that weight loss is occurring if this has been recommended. Note if the patient eats all the food supplied by the hospital.

5. Special ethnic diets may be available, either in pre-packed portions, or made by the hospital kitchen according to ethnic recipes.

RE. Ask the patient if the food is to their taste. Note how much of the food is left at the end of a meal.

6. Discuss with the patient whether there are any customs associated with eating that they wish to follow. Include these in the care plan.

RE. Check that the staff are aware of the customs and follow the agreed plan. Note if the patient's appetite improves.

Further action

1. Information about the diet actually eaten by the patient may be needed for the interpretation of blood tests, especially glucose, albumin, globulin and folate levels.

RE. Monitor the amount and types of food eaten if the family provide part of the diet.

Associated medical diagnoses

Anaemia
Cholecystitis
Colitis
Diabetes mellitus
Diverticulitis
Hepatitis
Malabsorption
Obesity
Renal failure
Steatorrhoea
Tuberculosis

Problem

Unable to follow usual clothing beliefs.

Assessment findings

Preparation for operation
Weak
Unable to dress self
Incontinent
Religious constraints, eg:
   Plymouth Brethren
   Mormon
   Hindu
   Orthodox Jew
   Moslem
   Amritdari sikh

Information for the patient

In British hospitals the patients are asked to wear night clothes during the day, if they are very ill or too weak to dress in ordinary clothes. Part of the preparation for an operation is the removal of fabrics which could cause a spark of static electricity, and thus the risk of explosion from some of the anaesthetic gases. Jewellery and watches also have to be removed or covered with adhesive tape, as there is a small risk of burns from the electrical equipment used in the surgery (diathermy). If a patient has strong religious beliefs about the clothing they wear they should tell the nursing staff so that necessary changes can be kept to a minimum.

Nursing action

1. Consider whether there is a language barrier which might hinder a full discussion. If there is, arrange for an interpreter to be present.

RE. Record the name of the interpreter.

2. Ask the patient to explain which, if any, custom they wish to follow. Explain the reason for any variation needed because of treatment. Review the care plan to describe any changes from British practice which other staff may need to know about. Examples may include wearing clothing during a bath or blanket bath, keeping the head covered at all times, or changing clothes before prayers.

RE. Check that staff are aware of the changes requested. Ask the patient if the changes are being carried out to their satisfaction.

3. Provide a long operation gown which reaches to the ankles for Moslem women. Inform the theatre sister and the recovery room staff, so that extra care is taken not to expose the patient unnecessarily.

RE. Record the use of a long gown, check whether there is an adequate supply of long nightdresses for the immediate post-operative period, if the patient's own night clothes will not be suitable.

5. Provide a long gown for X-rays where the clothing must be removed. Inform the radiographer of jewellery of religious significance which should not be removed if at all possible.

RE. Check the X-ray request form mentions the reason for requesting that jewellery remains in place.

6. Consider using incontinence pads held directly against the body by close fitting pants for urinary or faecal incontinence to protect the clothing so that the number of changes is kept to a minimum. Ask the patient if extra changes of clothes can be brought in from home and if they can keep up with the washing.

RE. Check the supply of clean clothing is adequate for the likely number of changes required.

Further action

1. Discuss whether pre-operative skin preparation which requires exposure of the body and is usually carried out in the ward can be undertaken in the theatre when the patient is under the anaesthetic.

RE. Record the decision and adjust the care plan.

Associated medical diagnoses

Anaemia
Chronic renal failure
Malnutrition
Tuberculosis

Problem	Unable to follow usual religious rites.

Assessment findings	Weak
	Low blood sugar
	Confined to bed
	Unable to use hands
	Skin preparation for surgery requires removal of body hair
	    Moslem
	    Orthodox Jew
	    Hindu
	    Sikh

Information for the patient	While a person is ill it may not be possible for them to follow their usual religious practices. They should inform the hospital staff of how they can help them when they are well enough. Most religious teachers or priests will provide a dispensation on health grounds.
Nursing action	1. Discuss with the patient or their family which religious rites would give most comfort to the patient if they could be modified for use while the patient is ill. Make detailed notes in the care plan on the usual nursing activities which could be adapted. RE. Note the changes. 2. Consider if blanket bathing or other bathing activities can be adapted. Time bathing before usual prayer time for Moslems, use the left hand for cleansing the genital area, and pour water over their hands and feet if possible during washing or showers, if the patient is fit enough. Hindu patients may prefer a thorough wash early in the morning, before sunrise, so they are ready for prayer. Note if the patient wishes to keep some clothes on during washing. RE. Ask the patient if the nursing care given is acceptable and if not what changes they would like to be made if possible. 3. Check if any religious festivals important to the patient will occur during the time that the patient is in hospital. Note those which would normally require a period without food. Consider if starving will affect the patient's physical condition. Arrange for food to be available after sunset for Seventh Day Adventists, and Moslems during Ramadhan. RE. Note if following the usual religious rites affects the morale of the patient. Observe the patient while they are going without food.
Further action	1. Intravenous therapy may be used to maintain blood sugar for diabetic patients who wish to fast. Plan teaching sessions in how to adapt the pattern of insulin and food intake for diabetics who wish to follow fasting rites. RE. Suggest the patient tries a fast while in hospital or under the supervision of the community nurse, so that both health care staff and patient are confident that a safe balance can be maintained.
Associated medical diagnoses	Anaemia Severe burns Cerebral vascular accident

266

Chronic bronchitis
Diabetes mellitus
Pneumonia

Problem	Conflict in beliefs.

Assessment findings	Uneasy with some staff Unable to make a decision Refuses treatment Refuses drugs Offered blood transfusion Offered transplant surgery Offered contraception

Information for the patient

Illness which means seeking help from a doctor or a hospital can lead to uncomfortable decisions having to be made. The patient may well feel torn between what they have always believed was the right and proper way of doing things, and the advice the doctor offers them to improve their health. Many people find it helps just to try to put the feelings into words and to talk through the situation with their religious representative. It may be possible for a person to be granted a dispensation because of their illness. The staff can try to make the arrangements for them, if they wish. They should be willing to discuss the problem with them. In the end the decision is the patient's.

Nursing action

1. Check the general list of beliefs for the patient's religious group. Ask the patient which things are particularly important to them. Try to use this to start a discussion with the patient on how they see the problem. Provide factual information rather than giving an opinion.

RE. Note whether there are signs of non-verbal discomfort, and try to judge the willingness of the patient to discuss the problem. Note any misunderstanding of the situation.

2. Ask if there is any other person with whom the patient would find it helpful to talk. Provide time and privacy for any such discussion.

RE. Record any request made on the patient's behalf.

3. Observe if there is a common factor among those who appear to make the patient uneasy. Women may prefer to be treated by female staff. Men from some cultures consider nurses to be of low status and prefer to deal with doctors.

RE. Note if there is a common factor, adjust the care plan as much as possible to limit or avoid contact with those who induce discomfort.

Further action

1. Insulin and other hormones from unacceptable animal sources may be substituted with those from alternative sources. Human type insulin is now available.

RE. Check the patient's prescriptions stipulate the type of product and that a warning not to give a product from the unacceptable animal is clearly attached to the prescription chart.

2. Check the ingredients list of prescribed drugs with the pharmacist if alcohol is unacceptable. Syrups, linctus and tinctures may contain alcohol.

RE. Note if drugs are refused, and the reason given by the patient. Consider if there are nursing measures which may ease pain or discomfort for the patient in these circumstances.

3. Provide an interpreter other than a member of the family for a woman if contraception or termination of preganancy are to be discussed.

RE. Observe for signs of undue pressure on the patient to make a decision without full information and the opportunity to discuss the doctor's advice with others.

Associated medical diagnoses

Anaemia
Carcinoma
Cardiac failure
Diabetes mellitus
Duodenal ulcer
Pancreatitis
Rubella
Severe burns
Varicose ulcer

References and further reading

Henley, A. (1979). *Asian Patients in Hospital and at Home.* King Edward's Hospital Fund for London. Distributed by Pitman Medical Publishing Co. Ltd. Tunbridge Wells. Kent.

Sampson, C. (1982). *The Neglected Ethic – Religious and Cultural Factors in the Care of Patients.* McGraw-Hill Book Co. (UK) Ltd. Maidenhead.

Wolf, L., Weitzel, M., Fuerst, E.V. (1983). 7th edition. *Fundamentals of Nursing.* Chapter 9 – Belief systems: religion, culture and ethnicity. J.B. Lippincott, Philadelphia.

8 Social role

Optimum environment

The way we think about ourselves depends to a large extent on the way we interact with others. This self-image may depend on the job that we do, the neighbourhood in which we live or were brought up, the clubs to which we belong, the hobbies which fill our spare time, and our place within the family. In each of these spheres we play a slightly different role. Each role demands changes in behaviour towards other people. Busy executives tend to leave their high-powered ways behind when visiting their mother for the day, when they may act more like a child than like a boss.

We tend to copy people we look up to and admire, and to take on their opinions and attitudes, or at least to keep quiet about our different views. This starts early on in childhood, and parents tend to be the people on whom we model ourselves. Try listening to the clichés and sayings that seem to slip off the tongue with ease; very often these are the same sayings as those used by our parents. Attitudes towards other people can also be adopted from others, and we may feel uneasy about someone without any logical reason. We have accepted or absorbed the views of our parents (Berne, 1964).

Some psychologists suggest that parental views form part of the mental makeup of us all, along with the natural child-like, fun-loving side of our personalities and the more factual adult part. They talk of parent, adult and child — three different levels within the one person. In some people, the parent is uppermost for a large part of the time. Law, politics, medicine and teaching attract people who feel they know better than others and therefore have a right to tell them what to do, just as parents do with their children. Parental personalities tend to control themselves, their outward emotions and other people.

People with the adult part of their personality uppermost tend to deal in facts, figures and logic. Researchers, economists, statisticians, bankers and accountants use the evidence to decide how to behave, rather than feeling that they already know the answers. Perhaps those with the childlike personalities may be found in the arts — the painter, actor, dancer, writer, craftsman — having fun, enjoying the feel of their work materials.

Many people do not get set into one of these three levels. Instead, they fluctuate between them, depending on the circumstance at the time. Parental at home, adult at work, and child when having an evening out on the town. Illness can upset this pattern, and then we tend to say that someone acts 'out of character'.

The personality we show to the outside world can be likened to the character in a play, with the true feelings hidden from others. Some people have a very clear idea of how they will go through life, and have a lifescript already drawn up in their minds. Job, career, family, house, are all mapped out. The lifescript may have come from the parents' ideas. Why else should sons follow fathers into the same type of job, or daughters copy the way that their mothers work or run the household? It can feel very risky indeed to break away and to write your own, different, script.

Adolescence and young adulthood tend to be the time when we break away from the habits of our parents, at least for a while. The college student is seen to have a different role from that of school friends who went straight into jobs. Students are thought of as experimenting and trying out new life styles, of getting involved in protests and social causes, as well as studying. However, parental ideas often seem to reappear in the late twenties, when setting up a home, and choosing a marriage partner and a career.

Social class and imagined roles

Social class tends to be made much of in Britain. One popular political image tends to depict workers as sweating, muscular people, working in factories, living in towns and exploited by the well-paid boss. This ignores the evidence of the steadily growing proportion of the working population who are employed in office-based jobs. The so-called white collar workers are out-numbering the blue collar workers. At the other extreme are the upper class, portrayed as having lots of money without needing to work; hunting, fishing and shooting or jetting off to the sun. This image ignores the fact that even the owners of stately homes usually have to earn money to run their houses by opening them to the public and providing entertainment and car parking in order to earn enough money to pay the bills. The shooting now tends to be done by syndicates of businessmen. More fishing is done in the canals and rivers by 'ordinary folk' than by the upper classes, and summer holidays in the sun are regularly taken by office workers; yet these images persist.

Social surveys tend to place their subjects in social classes according to the type of occupation followed by the man of the house — another out-of-date idea, when many households are of single-parent families, or where the working woman is the main money earner. Advertisers aim their products at people they feel fit particular images, trying to make them feel that to buy product 'X' will enhance status or image. Why else should 'designer' or makers' labels sewn on to the outside of clothes not only be tolerated but even sought-after? The glamour of another social class, from wearing Gloria Van . . . . jeans!

Body image

How we feel about ourselves depends on how we see ourselves in comparison to others. At present it is fashionable to be slim. We buy expensive slimming products instead of eating less, choose clothes which given an optical illusion of leanness, and apply cosmetics like stage make-up to accentuate cheek bones or to slim a chubby face. The way the body is presented may become so important to some individuals that cosmetic surgery is used to lift the face, flatten wrinkles and create an illusion of youth. A change in the image we hold of our bodies can feel devastating. To lose a leg or a breast from accident or illness produces a visible change, and the grief of such a loss may be as bad as that of losing a spouse.

Growing old

In industrialised societies a major change in social role comes with retirement from work. It also brings loss of status and different expectations of life. Pensioners tend to be portrayed as poor, and bus passes, parcels at Christmas, cut-price rates at hairdressers, at the cinema and theatre, all tend to underline this assumption. In fact, many who have been retired for only a few years can manage comfortably on their income, and their main problem may be one of limited social contacts, unless they join in clubs and societies to fill the gap from loss of workmates. Using work skills on behalf of local groups or charities, such as acting as a treasurer, secretary, event organiser, scene painter or dressmaker, provide new ways of meeting other people. Evening classes, hobbies, sports, coach trips and package tours can provide new interests.

More large organisations now sponsor their employees on pre-retirement courses to help them plan for, and mentally adjust to, the change ahead. Moving to a retirement home at the seaside soon after leaving work is rarely a good idea. It increases the gap in social contacts, and may not seem so attractive an idea after the first few months. Forward planning can lead to a weekend cottage in the chosen area, so that a social network is built up in the new area well before the move.

Health in old age depends in part on the foundations laid in youth. The eating habits of youth tend to influence not only the state of the body's tissues, but the way money is spent when the budget gets tighter. Some grocery stores provide small tins and packets for the single person, but these cost more weight for weight than the larger sizes. Retired people who have not learnt to cook should consider cookery classes as an investment. The death rate increases with advancing age, and having to learn new skills immediately after the death of a spouse is likely to be very difficult. There is also an advantage from having more time; raw ingredients can be used instead of packaged, convenience foods which cost more. Fruit and vegetables which are plentiful at certain times of year, can be bought cheaply and turned into jams or chutneys, deep-frozen, or made into prepared meals for the future. New skills can be turned into cash by selling bottled goods through local markets or health food stores.

Disability and social roles

The social role of the disabled person can be uncomfortable. Not only is there the change in self-image, but other people behave differently towards the disabled person (Bond and Bond, 1980). It is no accident that a radio programme for the disabled is called 'Does he take sugar?'. Physical imperfection tends to produce the assumption that the disabled person is damaged mentally as well as physically. Other people seem embarrassed to talk directly to disabled people and tend to talk to them through another person.

A congenital handicap, or one that develops in early childhood may colour a person's attitude to other people throughout life. If the parents felt guilty about the handicap they may be over-protective and always treat the handicapped person as a child. If they felt inadequate in their ability to cope with the demands of a handicapped child they may either be over-protective or set unrealistic goals. Parents who become irritated by the child's slowness or poor performance because of the handicap will create a lifelong sense of rejection.

There seem to be a large number of deep-seated myths which influence the way we behave towards those who have physical imperfections. The blind tend to have things explained to them in a very loud voice as if their hearing had gone as well. The deaf are isolated because no one talks to them, although many are skilled lipreaders when other people take the trouble to face them in a good light and speak slowly. Those who have stomas may not be allowed to work in kitchens or food preparation areas, as if their stoma made them dirty all over. The neat plastic stoma bags provide a waterproof seal but are somehow seen as 'leaking germs all over the place'.

Those with the misfortune to suffer from skin diseases may get treated as if they are infectious. The handicapped people can be regarded as if they had no emotions, are incapable of feeling love and certainly should not be allowed to experience sex. The personality seems to get hidden by the disability. Other people feel uncomfortable about how to treat someone who is no longer in full physical working order. One way the handicapped can tackle these problems is to join together and act as a pressure group to achieve change. A list of the pressure groups, associations for the handicapped and those charities which focus on the needs of special groups can be found in the local library.

Stress and role change

Major changes in lifestyle or events may sometimes be followed by illness. It is as if the mental stress of the change causes strain which shows as physical illness. Such major change may also come with a change in social role. Marriage or divorce require a variety of different alterations — to life style and even to the name one is known by.

Some people increase the stress on themselves almost to breaking strain by trying to achieve targets way beyond their reach. They take work home every day, work most of the weekend, skip holidays, miss meals and take little time to relax. Diseases linked with high stress include raised blood pressure, heart disease and duodenal ulcers.

Stress control includes planning regular holidays or weekends away, spaced out through the year. There are two helpful ways of making the most effective use of each working day. One is by drawing up a list of the most important things to be done, and including at least two relaxing activities. Working through the list, task by task, brings satisfaction from the things achieved and guilt-free time to relax. The second way is to set aside specific times for each activity and to stop at the end of the set time whether the job is finished or not. Such time structuring makes the most of the hours of the working day and should include planned meal breaks. Sport or a walk in the fresh air can also help, providing they are enjoyed and not strongly competitive.

Job loss changes roles

How a person feels determines how they think and act. Getting to know how someone else feels can help us see them in a different light, and understand why they behave as they do. Someone who is used to being in control of their life may feel a sense of guilt if they are made redundant through no fault of their own. The feeling of being unwanted may be so strong that the obvious economic facts are ignored. Depression and lethargy set in. The need to get a job may be felt so strongly that job applications are sent off for posts which are obviously unsuitable, but this is ignored and disappointment increased by the inevitable rejection. The feeling of guilt and self-blame is fed by such experiences.

Some unemployed men revert to childish behaviour. They look to their wives for mothering, competing with the children for attention and so increasing family tensions. The loss of confidence may lead to refusal to retrain or learn new skills although these are well within the individual's capability. The loss of money may also be of great emotional significance. It may have been used as a token of love by parents, in the form of presents and pocket money. Its loss may also be tied up with feelings of being grown up, strong, or adequate as an adult.

Joining a group for retraining may be helpful. It provides a chance to talk through how it feels to be unemployed. The opinions of others can be useful in spotting the no-hope job applications and so reduce disappointments.

Treating getting a new job as a job in itself may help. Working regular hours at scanning the advertisements, up-dating knowledge, doing the background reading about a firm, getting experience at interviews, going to evening classes to learn new skills, all help improve the chance of getting a job and increase morale.

Family role changes

The family relationships can help explain how its members react to big changes such as sudden unemployment or chronic illness. Responsibility for family finances, companionship, discipline of children, recreation and religious practices may be shared. In some families the father plays the leading role, in others it is mother who makes all the decisions. In a few families neither parent takes responsibility. If there is a big change affecting one partner, it is helpful to consider how the other partner reacts. Do they take over with uncertainty, shown by hesitation or irritation when confronted with the new state of affairs? Is it with a marked protest and hostility towards the other person who is seen as having let them down? The dependent wife suddenly faced with a very sick husband may feel he has broken his marriage vows by not looking after her.

Sometimes the other partner will take over the responsibilities readily and be pleased to do so. There may have been a growing frustration at not being allowed to take the decisions and once the chance comes it is taken with great enthusiasm. The unlucky partner may be quite upset about the new state of affairs. Family rivalry, especially among the sons, may occur, each trying to take over what they see as the male role once held by the father. For other couples, taking on more of the family responsibilities may be uncomfortable, but both partners adapt to the new situation.

For people who find adapting to the new situation difficult, the most important thing can be that both partners feel able to talk to each other, and explain how they feel. This can be very hard to do if family friction has already reached the surface. It may then be helpful to involve someone from outside the family. Professional helpers skilled in helping others to express how they feel include nurses, social workers, health visitors, counsellors, marriage guidance counsellors and some general practitioners. Real friends who are good listeners may also be helpful, and give support during difficult times.

The helper's role

Helping others to sort out their problems rarely means directly telling them what to do. The person with a problem needs to work out what the right course of action will be for themselves. It must feel right to them if it is to work well. Having someone else with whom to bounce ideas around often helps, as does having an interested listener who asks probing questions that open up new lines of thought. To be a helpful listener certain social skills are useful. Looking at the other person, nodding, smiling, saying 'uh huh', or 'mmm' help keep the conversation flowing. Phrases which also help to do this include 'I see', 'yes, go on', 'well', 'so', 'and then' and when appropriate 'no!'. It is also important for the helper to look as if they are listening, as well as occasionally repeating what has just been said, asking questions and summarizing the comments. All these show interest and that the person really was listening.

Sometimes just talking about a problem makes it seem less difficult. Many people write to the problem page of a magazine, especially if they feel their problems are so embarrassing that they could not tell anyone face to face. It can be difficult to ask the all-important but 'silly' question when feeling unsure about the reaction of the other person.

Helpers also need support, especially if they undertake a lot of difficult counselling work. An experienced supervisor helps the counsellor sort out their own feelings and may provide suggestions for a different approach if problems crop up. Counselling courses not only provide theory but help course members build up their own support network.

Patient roles

Illness brings with it a change in role. The sick person is expected to seek help. Those who fail to do so may produce irritation in others, including health care staff, especially if the illness is serious. For example the woman who delays consulting her doctor about a breast lump through fear that surgery would be advised. The sick person is allowed — even expected — by others, to give up normal activities while ill. Staying in bed resting may be encouraged. Small gifts may be given to the ill person, such as grapes, other fruit, chocolates or flowers. Anyone who does not follow the expected role makes other people feel uncomfortable.

Sick people are expected to take the advice of health care staff and to try to get better. Those who are not co-operative in trying to return to health may be disapproved of; the unpopular patients. Many health care staff gain emotional reward from helping sick people, those who do not wish to get well therefore deny others their expected reward. Staff may stop trying to help and almost ignore the patient, giving only the minimum of attention. The 'moaners' and 'grumblers' are also seen as unpopular patients. Fellow patients may also be openly critical if they feel another patient is asking for extra attention from the staff. There seems to be an understood level of behaviour which makes up the sick person's role. Those who overdo it, or do not follow the role may become unpopular with other patients and staff.

The role of the hospital patient means behaving differently from usual. It may well mean spending all day in night clothes and having to ask permission to leave the ward area. Communal living in 'nightingale style' wards can be very difficult to accept. The presence of other patients who 'know the ropes' provides the new patient with ideas of how to play the patient role. The behaviour of the staff towards the patient also influences the patient.

The setting itself may increase the pressure to behave in the hospital patient role. It may also help the staff feel comfortable in carrying out intimate procedures for others. The internal examination of a woman could be seen as an assault if it were not carried out in a serious way, the emphasis being on the need to find medical signs and symptoms of disease. The drapes, instruments, disinfectant smells and uniform of the staff all provide a setting in which such an examination is acceptable, at least for those who understand the setting. People from other cultures or religions may not share the same understanding and therefore fail to behave in the patient role. Foreign people can therefore become unpopular patients through not behaving in the expected way. They make the staff and others feel uneasy. If there are language difficulties it may also be difficult for the staff to find out how the patient feels, so they cannot understand their behaviour.

General assessment areas

Size of personal space 'bubble'
Willingness to make eye contact
Occupation
Family members and relationships
Housing conditions
Dependants
Pets
Friends and personal contacts
Contact with social agencies
Perceived level of self-esteem
Non-verbal gestures

Problems

Unable to adapt to sick role   277
Changed sexual behaviour   278
Inappropriate behaviour   279
Difficulty adjusting to chronic illness   280
Difficulty in accepting temporary dependence on others   282
Unable to express anger   283
Unable to express fear   284
Unable to control anger   286
Loss of contact with family or friends   287
Unable to share information about diagnosis/prognosis   288
Poor housing   289
Change in home environment desired   291
Socially unacceptable habits   293
No fixed address   294

Potential problem

Risk of aggression towards staff or other patients   295

Problems

Problem	Unable to adapt to sick role

Assessment findings

Does not follow medical advice or prescriptions
Denies presence of symptoms
Hides signs such as haematuria
Refuses to plan for the period of illness
Makes unrealistic plans for the future
Accuses staff of sexual interference during medical examinations
Refuses treatment

Information for the patient

Some people find it hard to get used to thinking of themselves as ill, even if it is only for a short time. The staff will try to explain exactly what is involved in each step of the treatment, but it is up to the patient to decide if they wish to accept it and follow instructions. If they do not wish to do so they should say so as it can be upsetting for the staff if the patient backs out of what was thought to be their agreed role in the treatment.

Nursing action

1. Explain clearly and without using jargon each step of the treatment. Use an adult manner and indicate that the patient is expected to act as an adult in the discussion.

RE. Record the topics discussed and the patient's reaction. Observe if questions are asked and the way in which the information seems to be received by the patient.

2. Provide a chaperone if any physical examination is to take place. Confine the discussion during the examination to matter-of-fact instructions, and behave as if the activity is a serious occasion.

RE. Record who was present and the patient's reaction. Report any complaint to the senior staff so that more detailed records can be made and advice given.

3. Record any signs or symptoms observed so the medical staff will have a more complete picture of the patient's condition than that which is given verbally by the patient.

RE. Compare the observations made by the staff with those reported by the patient.

4. Involve the patient and the family in the planning of nursing care and treatment. Provide pyjamas, washing things and towels if the patient failed to bring them in. Ask the family to collect the personal articles and bring them in to the patient.

RE. Observe whether the patient gains confidence from being asked to make decisions about care and treatment.

5. Introduce the patient to another patient who has been in the ward longer, so that the new patient can be 'shown the ropes'.

RE. Observe if there is any change in behaviour.

6. Discuss with the family whether there is any urgent need for decisions to be made about affairs at home. If so ask the medical social worker for advice or help.

RE. Ask the family whether matters have been sorted out.

Further action

1. Plan out the investigations and treatments so that the patient has a clear idea of the probable length of the stay in hospital. Whenever possible discuss treatment in such a way that the patient feels there is a choice to be made. Explain any drug treatment and the proposed pattern of doses.

RE. Review the plan with the patient every day. Observe for signs of increasing cooperation or positive comments about the hospital stay.

Associated medical diagnoses

Any illness requiring a stay in hospital.

Problem

Changed sexual behaviour

Assessment findings

Reports loss of potency
Talks constantly of sex
Makes sexual remarks
Reports increased libido
Exposes genitals to others
Masturbates in view of others
Tries to fondle staff

Information for the patient

Some people find it hard to accept intimate care from hospital staff; they tend to think that the image created by pornographic films and books is true. That is unfair to staff, who are professional people who are carrying out responsible jobs. An adult person is expected to use self-control and not to embarrass others.

Nursing action

Ignore physical advances the first time; if it happens again look the patient straight in the eye and tell the patient to stop their behaviour. Behave in a calm, quiet, matter-of-fact manner.

RE. Discuss the patient's behaviour with the other staff so all are aware of the problem and do not feel embarrassed if it happens to them. Record the incident.

2. If the advances are repeated, record the problem in the care plan.

RE. Note if there are any further incidents. Review the care given to the patient to see if there are activities which could be misinterpreted by a confused mind, for example catheter care. Discuss the treatment plan with the doctor.

3. If the patient is seen to be masturbating tell the patient firmly that he should have asked for the curtains to be drawn. Draw the bed curtains and leave the patient for ten minutes. Plan times for privacy in the bathroom or behind drawn bed curtains. Tell the patient for how long they will be left alone and do not return until after the stated time.

RE. Record the incident in the progress notes. Check with the other patients whether they find such behaviour so disturbing that they wish to be moved to another bed area.

Further action	1. Neurological or psychiatric advice may be sought by the doctor. If the behaviour is severe a course of female hormones may be offered to male patients to reduce testosterone activity. In severe cases, with the written consent of the patient 'cyproterone acetate' may be prescribed. It will not work if alcohol is taken. Advise the use of a male sheath during intercourse as malformed sperm may cause abnormal embryos.
	RE. Blood is taken every four to six weeks for haemoglobin estimation and liver function tests. Record body weight weekly as weight gain may occur. Ask the patient to report any breast enlargement, tiredness or feeling of depression. Other side effects include headache, skin reactions and changes in blood pressure.
Associated medical diagnoses	Frontal lobe disease Senile dementia Subarachnoid haemorrhage

---

Problem	**Inappropriate behaviour**

Assessment findings	Throws food about at mealtimes Refuses to use cutlery when eating Spits on the floor Walks around naked when others are present Constantly uses swear words Avoids washing and bathing Clothing left unbuttoned, exposing body
Information for the patient	It is always difficult to get used to living in close contact with other people, especially when feeling unwell. There are a number of types of behaviour which annoy others, such as swearing, spitting and throwing things about. It is helpful if the patient considers the feelings of the other people on the ward, and remembers that they are in the same situation.
Nursing action	1. When inappropriate behaviour occurs, take the person aside, if possible, and ask why they are behaving in this way. Explain what it is that annoys others, and ask the patient to think about how other patients might feel, and to stop the behaviour.
	RE. Observe the patient's facial expression for an indication that the disapproval is understood. Record that the inappropriate behaviour occurred, and the response to the discussion and the request. Swear words may be an everyday form of language in some environments.
	2. Observe whether there are triggers for the behaviour, consider if it is a means of gaining attention. Talk with the patient at various times during the day to reduce any need to obtain company through inappropriate behaviour.
	RE. Record any possible causes; note if, with added attention, there is a decrease in the inappropriate behaviour. If there appears to be a pattern, make a note of the times of the patient's difficult behaviour.
	3. Suggest that the patient eats alone if their table manners annoy others. Consider providing small amounts of food at a time.
	RE. Assess how much food is being eaten each day and calculate whether this will meet daily requirements for energy and protein. Consider weighing

the patient twice a week if intake is below that required to maintain a normal body weight.

Further action

1. Review drug therapy for those drugs which may increase confusion or, like alcohol, reduce the usual social inhibitions. Barbiturates, diazepam, phenothiazines, antidepressants and anticholinergic drugs may be involved.

RE. Compare any pattern of clusters of inappropriate behaviour in relation to the times drug therapy is given. Consider if alcohol or other drugs are being taken in secret.

Associated medical diagnoses

Alcoholism
Psychosis
Space occupying lesion

Problem | **Difficulty adjusting to chronic illness**

Assessment findings

Refuses to use aids provided
Cheats on fluid restriction
Cheats on special diet
Refuses to plan ahead
Sits silently and appears apathetic
Refuses to allow family to deal with urgent business
Avoids discussing situation
Blames self for situation

Information for the patient

Illness influences how someone will plan their future, so staff and patient need to spend time talking about the patient's feelings. Later they must plan how the patient and the family are going to deal with the situation. The nurses can give advice but the patient must decide what is right for them.

Nursing action

1. Ask the patient to explain what they know about the illness and how they think it might affect them in the next few months. Discuss how they feel about the news that the illness is not going to go away. Listen carefully to what is said and the way in which it is said.

RE. Record the patient's feelings. If relief is expressed at having talked about their condition, consider moving on to the next step.

2. Ask the patient if they have ever experienced similar news or been in a similar situation; ask how it felt and what happened. Listen for clues to a possible approach to this situation.

RE. Note the patient's feelings, consider if any previous reaction indicates a repeat of the present difficulties. Suggest useful coping behaviour used before which could be tried in solving current problems.

3. Correct any misunderstanding about the situation, provide relevant facts and discuss how the patient feels. Go on to provide new ideas and to discuss the pros and cons of each one. Leave the patient to decide which ones seem most suitable. Provide suitable aids but leave it to the patient to decide when to try them.

4. Discuss with the family why the patient may be behaving in a negative way. Ask how they feel about the situation. Suggest that they discuss how they feel with the patient.

RE. Observe how the patient and family react to the exchange of feelings. Consider if they are now making realistic plans.

5. Draw up a plan of how the patient is going to make adjustments to their life, how the family is involved, and what help, information or advice is required. Suggest which services are available for help. If the patient is unable to make contact directly, offer to contact them on behalf of the patient, or suggest that a family member does so.

RE. Record the plan. Discuss the patient's readiness to make firm plans with other professionals involved.

6. Discuss which methods of learning the patient has found most effective in the past. Ask what level of schooling was achieved. Plan teaching programmes for new skills in small steps, checking what has been learnt before adding the next new items of information. Praise each achievement.

RE. Record the level of skills achieved. Re-plan if the steps appear too big for the patient to achieve with ease.

7. Discuss with the family which nursing and other skills they need to learn. Plan out teaching programmes and time for practice. If the community nurse will be involved in helping to support the patient and family arrange a meeting, and if possible a joint planning session.

RE. Assess the level of performance achieved. Suggest a weekend at home if the patient and relatives appear ready to manage without close supervision.

8. Make arrangements with the community nurse and other services for a trial run at home. Assure the patient that they may return at any time during it if things go wrong.

RE. If the patient returns, record the date and time. Ask the patient to describe how things went, how they felt and praise how well the patient and family coped. Ask the family members for their reaction. Plan further teaching if skills need improving. Consider planning further longer periods at home.

Further action

1. The community physician may be informed of the patient's disability and any long term implications. Support may be needed in rehousing or in obtaining planning permission for a temporary building to house home dialysis equipment.

RE. Note whether the contact has been made. Check the patient is aware of what is being done on their behalf. Ask for the patient's permission to release personal information if it is requested.

2. The medical social worker can offer special counselling skills and practical help in contacting the Local Authority and Social Services. Discuss the patient's reactions to what has happened so far and make sure they are happy with the decisions agreed upon. Provide a quiet, private place for discussions if counselling is required.

RE. Note the patient's reactions after their discussion with the medical social worker and any decisions made.

Associated medical diagnoses	Alzheimer's Disease Amputation of a limb Cerebral vascular accident Crohn's disease Chronic obstructive airways disease Coeliac disease Colostomy Diabetes mellitus Emphysema Hemiparesis Ileostomy Incontinence Multiple Sclerosis Muscular Dystrophy Paraplegia Pneumoconiosis Peripheral Vascular Disease Quadriplegia Renal failure Senile dementia Silicosis Steatorrhoea Urostomy

---

Problem	**Difficulty in accepting temporary dependence on others**

Assessment findings	Refuses help Reluctant to request bedpan or commode Does not comply with staff requests Does not rest in bed as advised Loses temper Rude to staff Quiet and withdrawn Constantly complains Repeatedly calls for attention 'Clock-watches' for drugs or treatments
Information for the patient	Many people find it very difficult to have to depend on others for help when they are ill. To some it reminds them of being a child and of the unhappy events in their lives. Nurses generally appreciate that it can be difficult for patients to accept advice from people younger than themselves, However, it is sometimes necessary for people to accept the help of others, until such time as they are able to look after themselves.
Nursing action	1. Describe any pre-test preparation and after-care which will mean the patient will have to rest in bed. Explain how long the time in bed is likely to last and the reason why it is necessary. RE. Record any comments from the patient that indicate the period of bedrest will be a difficult time for them. 2. Explain the reason for each nursing or medical request, and why failing to meet it may hinder recovery. Treat the patient in an adult manner, and give the patient a choice of accepting or refusing to comply.

RE. Record the patient's response, both verbal and as indicated by the degree to which they comply with the request.

3. Ask the patient to describe how they feel about having to rely on others. Remind them that the dependence is only temporary. Speak in a way that indicates you expect them to take full responsibility for their behaviour both now and in the future. Review the care plan with the patient. Identify if any of the care can be adjusted to make it more acceptable to them. Amend the plan as agreed.

RE. Record any change in the patient's behaviour. Ask them how they feel they will cope with the rest of the time during which they will have to rely on others.

Further action

1. If the use of a bedpan or commode for bowel actions will cause distress to the patient discuss whether for short periods it may be beneficial to induce constipation. Codeine phosphate or propantheline may be used to reduce gut motility.

RE. Note whether the drug induces constipation. Note how much the patient eats. Stop the drug 24 hours before the bedrest is due to end so gut motility returns towards normal. When the bedrest is over check if the bowels have moved within the next 24 hours. If not consider giving glycerine suppositories or a phosphate enema.

Associated medical diagnoses

Angina pectoris
Bronchitis
Deep vein thrombosis
Myocardial infarction
Hepatic failure
Hepatitis
Renal failure
Rheumatoid arthritis

Problem	**Unable to express anger**

Assessment findings

Emotionally very controlled
Denies feelings of anger
Denies feelings of frustration
Hands clenched
Sore or stiff shoulders
Sits in a hunched position
Tense
Bad news received recently

Information for the patient

One of the normal reactions to bad news is the feeling of anger — feeling 'it's not fair', or 'why did this happen to me, I haven't done anything wrong.' Those kinds of feelings, if bottled up, can lead to tension, headaches, stiff shoulders and painful muscles, as if the body wants to fight other people but the blows are held back. One of the helpful ways of dealing with these feelings is to displace the anger by taking it out on some inanimate object such as a pillow or punch-bag. Another way anger comes out is being horrid to someone else other than the person with whom you feel angry as in the expression 'kicking the office cat'.

Nursing action	1. Provide privacy and say to the patient 'you look angry — do you feel it?'. Try to get the patient to explain how he feels. Listen and prompt the conversation rather than offer advice.
	RE. Note what the patient says verbally and their body position during and after the talk. Relief of tension and anger may be shown by a more open, less hunched posture and relaxed facial and other muscles.
	2. Suggest the patient takes out their angry feelings by punching a cushion or pillow, or by shouting. Provide privacy so that they feel safe to do so without being embarrassed at letting go in front of other people.
	RE. Relief of anger may be followed by weeping. Ask the patient if they are ready for company after letting go. Check the patient has recovered composure before returning to the company of others.
	3. If the patient cannot bring himself to act out the anger, suggest writing it down. An angry letter which can be torn up once it is written may provide a sufficient release.
	RE. Check that the staff are aware of the patient's feelings of anger and understand they may be on the receiving end of displaced anger.
Further action	1. Psychiatric advice or help from a trained counsellor may be sought if the repressed anger is intense and produces physical symptoms. Provide privacy for meetings with the counsellor.
	RE. Note whether the patient's mood indicates a need for privacy to continue for a while after the counselling sessions. If so, revise the care plan to provide such private time for thought and reflection.
Associated medical diagnoses	Acute leukaemia Alcoholism Carcinoma Drug overdose Hypertension Self-mutilation

---

Problem	**Unable to express fear**

Assessment findings	Restless Feels unable to settle to anything Feels tense Feels anxious Feels shaky Cold sweats Palpitations Rapid pulse Raised blood pressure Denies feeling worried Startles easily Unable to sleep Unable to grasp or remember information Repeatedly asks the same questions Constant complaints about minor things Overeating Loss of appetite

Information for the patient	When we are worried the body's flight or fight system swings into action, the heart beats faster, we sweat (the clammy palms before an exam or interview) and feel shaky and restless. Many patients in hospital feel the same way while waiting to see the doctor or to have X-rays or other tests. Sometimes illness and drugs can produce the same feelings. They are not unusual, and talking about the feelings may be helpful.
Nursing action	1. Provide privacy before saying to the patient, 'You seem anxious; can you tell me about how you feel?'. Provide information if asked to, but in small amounts, as anxiety makes it difficult to take things in. Write down a summary of the information for the patient to keep.
	RE. Record what was said to the patient. Note if questions are repeated later. Note whether talking about feelings leaves the patient looking more relaxed. Check if a raised pulse rate or blood pressure decreases.
	2. If the patient keeps asking the same questions, point this out and ask if they are worried about the subject. Try to explore how they feel. If the patient cannot talk about the topic, ask if there is someone else with whom they might feel more comfortable when talking about it.
	RE. Note what the repeated question is. Discuss the difficulty with the patient's doctor or social worker.
	3. Offer to make changes in the care plan, and provide opportunities for the patient to make decisions about their care.
	RE. Note how much decision making the patient seems to feel comfortable with; in some patients it may increase anxiety.
	4. Suggest more activity to reduce the need to think about problems. Suggest taking up hobbies, visits to the garden or listening to soothing music on cassette or radio. Review the care plan.
	RE. Note whether patient is able to concentrate on an activity for more than a few minutes.
Further action	1. Estimate blood glucose level for hypoglycaemia. Test the patient's urine for ketones.
	RE. Normal blood sugar levels lie between 3 and 9 mmol per litre. Lower blood sugar levels should be treated with 15 grams glucose in fruit juice if the patient can swallow.
	2. Review drug therapy for the presence of caffeine, thyroxine or epinephrine.
	RE. Record response of patient if drug dose is reduced.
Associated medical diagnoses	Alzheimer's disease Anoxia Carcinoma Diabetes mellitus Hypoglycaemia Hypoparathyroidism Myocardial infarction

Problem	Unable to control anger

Assessment findings

Agitated
Irritable
Suspicious of others
Delusions
Hallucinating
Raises hand as if to hit out
Throws things at others
Swears
Threatens to hurt or kill
Raises a clenched fist
Points a stiff forefinger at others
Swings legs as if to kick
Manipulates others
Seeks attention

Information for the patient

Physical anger should be controlled when other people are around; it is better to take it out on objects than on people, and better still to find a way of talking about feelings of anger. Then the feelings can be dealt with and perhaps the cause removed. Hurting other people is against the law; if violence is shown to others, then it may be necessary to involve the police.

Nursing action

1. Remain calm, and take a deep breath before speaking to reduce any tremor in the voice. Ask the patient politely to tell you what is troubling them. Avoid touching the patient until they have calmed down.

RE. Note whether the patient's posture relaxes slightly and threat postures decrease. Consider whether the patient is likely to listen to reason, and if not, summon help. Report the possibility of violence to the senior nurse manager, so that contingency plans can be made.

2. Speak calmly and firmly, suggest the patient sits down; if they do, ask if you too can sit with them to discuss the problem which appears to be making them angry. Listen carefully to what is said.

RE. Assess how much insight the patient has about how unacceptable their threats are to others. Note any abnormal thoughts expressed.

3. Discuss which particular events upset the patient. Ask how the patient usually deals with angry feelings and praise any redirected anger activities. Suggest other ways of expressing anger and dealing with frustrations.

RE. Note which events cause anger or frustration. Review the care plan. Check the other staff are aware of the hospital procedure for handling and reporting violent incidents.

4. If restraint is needed to prevent injury to others, at least three staff, preferably five, should be present. One should act as leader and the team should act in unison. Remind the team to remove ties and spectacles. One person should try to hold the patient's arms against the body with a bear hug from behind. The other staff should grasp the patient's legs from behind and at the knee to prevent kicking. The patient can then be lifted on to the bed or to the floor, face down, pressure being applied at shoulders, hips and knees to keep them there. The minimum of force should be used, the

intention being to restrain. Remove the patient's shoes to reduce the chance of injury. One person should stay at the patient's head, explaining quietly what is happening, to try to reduce further aggression resulting from fear of injury.

RE. Record the incident on the hospital's form and in the patient's records. Arrange for any clearing-up to be completed to reduce further hazards. Check if other patients and staff have been upset by the incident. Provide an opportunity for those involved to talk through their feelings about the incident.

5. If the patient tries to choke someone, grasp his little finger and pull it back until they release their grip. An alternative measure is to stamp on the instep sufficiently hard to cause pain and surprise so the grip is released.

RE. Anyone who is injured, however slightly, should be seen by a doctor and an incident form completed. Staff may claim through the Industrial Injuries Scheme and the Criminal Compensation Scheme if appropriate. Damage to clothing or property should be reported.

Further action

1. Chlormethiazole or diazepam may be prescribed; their action is increased by alcohol. Explain to the patient the tablets will help in relaxation.

RE. Record whether the patient's behaviour becomes more acceptable. Chlormethiazole may cause tingling in the nose, sneezing or itching, runny eyes or a headache. High doses of diazepam may produce double vision, ataxia, confusion, headache or a depressed respiratory rate.

Associated medical diagnoses

Alcoholism
Alzheimer's disease
Attempted suicide
Depression
Manic-depressive psychosis
Paranoid schizophrenia
Psychopathic personality
Senile dementia

Problem | **Loss of contact with family or friends**

Assessment findings

Does not have visitors
No telephone enquiries about patient's welfare
No letters or cards
Unable to name next of kin
Expresses annoyance at others' visitors

Information for the patient

It can be very boring to be ill and not have much contact with people outside hospital. If a patient would like help in making contact with local visitors they should let one of the staff know. It may be possible to arrange for someone to visit regularly, as many people enjoy the opportunity of doing this.

Nursing action

1. Spend time talking with the patient when other patients nearby are being visited. Discuss hobbies and interests. Ask if the patient would like to make contact with the local church members or a volunteer visitor.

RE. Note if the patient has any hobbies which involve other people, such as belonging to a club or writing to a pen pal. Keep an up-to-date list of contacts of volunteer visitors and local churches with members willing to see people in hospital or at home. Discuss whether the local or hospital chaplain could visit more often.

2. Discuss whether the care plan could be changed so that the patient can be occupied away from the visitors, for example with wound dressings, physiotherapy, occupational therapy or watching the television.

RE. Discuss suitable changes with other members of the health care team.

3. Consider introducing the patient to others in the ward who do not receive many visitors.

RE. Note the patient's reaction to the suggestion.

4. Ask the patient if they would like the staff to telephone or write to relatives on their behalf to inform them that the patient is in hospital.

RE. Note how the patient reacts. Some people feel very embarrassed at being unable to write or at being unsure in using the telephone. There may be gratitude for the suggestion, or the patient may resent the interference.

Further action	1. Socially isolated people may have other difficulties on transfer home, especially if they will need help during a period of convalescence. Consider requesting an assessment visit by the social worker so that plans can be made to provide services.
	RE. Check the medical staff are aware of the possible difficulties so that transfer home can be planned for an agreed date.
Associated medical diagnoses	Cardiac failure Chronic bronchitis Chronic obstructive airway disease Pneumonia Rheumatoid arthritis

---

Problem	**Unable to share information about diagnosis/prognosis**
Assessment findings	Patient has been told diagnosis and probable prognosis Refuses permission for relatives to be told by staff Feels unable to tell relatives personally
Information for the patient	Many people find it very hard to share bad news with those they love. Some people feel very hurt if the secret is kept from them; they become suspicious when staff do not answer their questions very fully and this can increase anxiety. The staff can try and help the patient work out the best way to break the news. However, they will not tell the relatives about the diagnosis without the patient's knowledge or permission.
Nursing action	1. Provide privacy and time for the information about the diagnosis and prognosis to be thought through by the patient. Ask them how they feel about the news.
	RE. Note any change in behaviour and whether the patient is able to discuss their feelings. Consider if there is any other member of the staff who has

established a particularly good rapport with the patient and with whom they might feel more comfortable discussing the news.

2. Discuss how much the patient understands and wishes to know about the illness. Try to identify if there are feelings of guilt or disgrace at being ill. Note any misunderstanding about the disease. Ask how the patient visualizes it within the body.

RE. Note how the patient views the illness. Some people see diseases such as cancer as a punishment for leading an 'unclean life'. If the patient or family members hold this view it may be difficult for the patient to admit to such an illness.

3. Suggest that a representative from the patient's religion visits to talk with the patient if they feel they would like this.

RE. Note whether the visit is accepted and if it appears to help the patient cope with their fears.

4. Ask whether a visit from someone suffering with the same disease or from the relevant association would be helpful. Consider if information leaflets from the associations or societies would help the patient's understanding and give them moral support.

RE. Note the patient's response to the offer.

Further action

1. Consider if skilled help from a trained counsellor or social worker would help the patient work through their feelings about the diagnosis and how it will affect the family.

RE. Plan sessions so that there is privacy and time afterwards to reflect on the discussion.

Associated medical diagnoses

Alzheimer's disease
Ankylosing spondylitis
Carcinoma
Cerebral tumour
Hepatic cirrhosis
Huntingdon's chorea
Leukaemia
Lung cancer
Multiple sclerosis
Myasthenia gravis
Paraplegia
Parkinson's disease
Renal failure
Tertiary syphilis

Problem

Poor housing

Assessment findings

Complains of damp in home
Complains of lack of heating
No running water
No facilities for hot water
No inside w.c.

Shares bathroom with other families
Shares toilet with other families
Inadequate cooking facilities

Information for the patient

It is often necessary to have a period of convalescence after illness in order to build up strength and stamina. Many people are able to go home for this period. If a patient is unsure whether their home is suitable, it may be possible for the community nurse to assess the facilities and make arrangements for the return. A stay at a convalescent home has to be arranged in advance, so the patient needs to discuss their home conditions a little while before they are due to leave hospital.

Nursing action

1. Discuss how much activity the patient will be fit to undertake when first at home. Identify which aspects of the home conditions may prove to be a problem.

RE. Record the potential problems with the home conditions and discuss the implications with the doctor.

2. Discuss any problems foreseen with the home facilities with the community nurse and agree possible courses of action to help the patient.

3. Review the care plan for the need to modify new skills or health teaching in the light of the home circumstances. Consider whether the occupational therapist or physiotherapist may be able to provide suitable aids or to teach the patient new skills to help in coping at home.

RE. Replan teaching and set realistic new goals. Review the patient's progress prior to transfer.

Further action

1. Council house tenants may request medical help in obtaining different accommodation. Most local authorities operate on a points system for setting priorities in allocating housing. Some request a statement of medical need from the doctor, others ask for a form to be completed.

RE. Record if a letter is requested from the doctor.

2. Advice in rehousing applications and in getting landlords to undertake essential repairs may be available from the local Citizens Advice Bureau. They may also guide individuals through the steps leading up to legal action if the landlord fails to fulfil his responsibilities.

RE. Note how much guidance the patient needs in dealing with the bureaucratic system. Those who have little self-confidence and education may find the experience very disheartening.

3. The medical social worker should be asked to arrange accommodation for the homeless prior to discharge. Liaison with local hostels or working men's hotels may be necessary to ensure the patient admitted as an emergency does not lose his room.

RE. Note whether the patient indicates any unwillingness to accept the accommodation arranged for them following their discharge.

4. A home assessment visit by the occupational therapist and physiotherapist may be requested for elderly people likely to be able to return to their own

home. The permission of the patient must be obtained, preferably in writing. A second person should be present during the visit so that there is a witness, should accusations of damage or theft be made later.

RE. Record when the visit took place. Review the recommendations and amend the care plan if appropriate.

5. Social work help may be needed to arrange special cleaning of dirty rooms by the local authority. Financial grants and benefits may be available to pay for replacement furniture. Charities may provide finance for special equipment such as a washing machine to aid a patient at home.

RE. Note the arrangements requested and made so that transfer home may be planned to fit in with them.

Associated medical diagnoses	Asthma Carcinoma Chronic bronchitis Chronic obstructive airway disease Colostomy Congestive cardiac failure Dementia Epilepsy Ileostomy Multiple sclerosis Rheumatoid arthritis Tuberculosis

---

Problem	**Change in home environment desired**

Assessment findings	Unable to climb stairs Confined to a wheelchair Unsteady when walking Unable to reach toilet Chronic illness
Information for the patient	Preparing the home so that the patient will be able to manage more easily and safely takes time. Local authorities will help in modifying council housing and may take a lenient view towards temporary buildings which otherwise might not get planning permission. The occupational therapist has a lot of expert advice to give when helping the patient decide the most effective aids and changes to the rooms. The nurses and the physiotherapists will help the patient learn the physical skills they will need once they get home.
Nursing action	1. Discuss the layout of the patient's home and the kind of facilities which would help the patient to compensate for their physical disabilities. Ask which, if any, of the family should be the main coordinator on behalf of the patient. RE. Note the major changes which may be needed, and the physical skills the patient will need to develop in order to be as independent as possible. Note how willing the patient appears to be in making decisions about the change. Ramps, rails and hoists make obvious the presence of disability and change the person's view of themselves. This may be resented, and the decision avoided so that the full implications can be denied.

2. Seek the help and advice of the occupational therapist in joint discussions with the patient and family.

RE. Note any tension or disapproval shown by the family. Building alterations on behalf of the patient will physically alter the environment for all those who share the household. The patient may become the focus of family disagreements and get blamed for problems highlighted by the need for change.

3. Plan the changes with the patient, family and health care professionals. Provide advice on the financial help available or request the information from the social worker.

RE. Review the care plan and the length of the patient's hospital stay; consider replanning activities if there will be delays.

4. Provide opportunities for the patient and family to learn to use hoists and other mechanical aids which are to be provided at home.

RE. Consider visits to a centre displaying aids so that different brands can be considered.

5. Consider contacting the community nurse and health visitor once the likely programme of changes has been agreed. An assessment of the facilities at home for nursing a chronically ill patient may be needed. A variety of aids and equipment can be obtained from the Community Health Service or the local branch of the British Red Cross.

Further action

1. Wheelchairs may be supplied by the NHS on the request of a doctor. The decision about the type of chair prescribed and its dimensions may be delegated to the occupational therapist. A home visit may need to be arranged if there is doubt about the ease with which it can be manoeuvered through doorways in the home.

RE. Consider the need for a pressure-relieving cushion, or a gel or sheepskin pad for use in the chair. Such items may need to be ordered at the same time.

2. Home dialysis may be recommended by the medical staff. Large units usually have one or more staff able to advise and organise the changes needed to the home. In some areas a portable unit which can be sited in the back garden may be offered.

RE. Note the patient's and the family's reactions to the proposed changes. It may be helpful to provide time for them to express their doubts and concerns to staff who are not directly involved in the project.

3. Weekend leave at home may be used to help the patient and family adjust to the changes and to practise new skills.

RE. Ask the patient to report on the events of the weekend away. Note the time the patient returned and their mood. Adjustment to home after several weeks in hospital may be difficult, as the old role cannot be resumed without modifications. Consider delaying the final transfer if either the patient or the family express concern at their ability to cope.

Associated medical diagnoses

Amputation
Cerebral vascular accident
Chronic obstructive airway disease

Chronic renal failure
Multiple sclerosis
Myasthenia gravis
Paraplegia
Parkinson's disease
Poliomyelitis
Spinal tumour

Problem	Socially unacceptable habits
Assessment findings	Uses fingers to eat cooked food Spits on the floor Sniffs loudly and repeatedly Eats noisily Rarely washes Smells strongly of stale sweat Takes other peoples' property Fails to repay borrowed money Disturbs other people's possessions
Information for the patient	As people grow up, they learn how to behave in a way that does not upset other people. It depends on the behaviour of the adults around them that they admire. If the behaviour acceptable to some adults is disliked by others, it can lead to friction.
Nursing action	1. Tell the patient exactly what behaviour upsets fellow patients or visitors. Ask them their reaction to the news, and what they intend to do about the problem.
	RE. If the patient does not intend to change their eating habits, arrange for them to eat their meals away from other people. Negotiate a more frequent wash, at least sufficient to make close proximity to the patient bearable.
	2. Consider moving the patient to an area away from the people who are unable to accept his behaviour. Explain to the patient the proposed move.
	RE. Record the reaction of the patient. Negotiate a continued change in behaviour to at least a minimum level acceptable to others if the patient rejects the idea of the move.
	3. If the patient accepts the need to change their behaviour then consider what rewards for success should be offered. Trips out, extra food or praise from respected staff may be suitable.
	RE. Record how the patient's behaviour changes.
	4. If the change in behaviour results from mental deterioration, consider planning a programme of habit training. Each step should follow the same pattern each day. Prepare a set of detailed instructions for staff so there is continuity between different shifts.
	RE. Review progress in the development of the new habit at least once a week. Amend the plan in the light of progress achieved.

Further action	1. Discuss with the doctor how long the patient needs to stay in hospital. Ask if out-patient treatment could be considered if the unsocial behaviour is creating major friction with other people.
	RE. Record that the discussion has taken place and the proposed action.
	2. Help from a clinical psychologist may be requested for difficult behaviour which does not respond to the planned actions. A detailed assessment of the frequency and sequence of the behaviour may be requested.
	RE. Amend the care plan to include the programme proposed, consider the need for extra supervision and practise to establish the new habit.
Associated medical diagnoses	Alzheimer's disease Dementia Space occupying lesions

---

Problem	**No fixed address**

Assessment findings	No address given No accommodation fixed for discharge Known vagrant No next of kin given No family contacts No visitors Few personal possessions
Information for the patient	When a patient is ready to leave hospital, there is no obligation on the staff to find them somewhere to stay. However, if they would like help from the social worker in finding a place in a hostel, it can be arranged. The decision belongs with the patient. Without a fixed address, it is not possible to claim Social Security benefits. If the patient needs further nursing care from the community nurse, this will be difficult to arrange unless the nurse knows where to find the patient, and what facilities there are for nursing them. Some hostels have clinic sessions provided by a nurse or doctor.
Nursing action	1. Discuss with the patient what their plans are when discharged. Advise them on the level of activity and the diet they will need to follow to help regain full health. Discuss what facilities they will need to look for when choosing accommodation.
	RE. Record the patient's decisions. Note if they try to play 'Isn't it awful, you only get help when you're ill.' Suggest to other staff that the problem is treated in a matter of fact way and that they do not join the game. If they do, it is quite likely that the patient will at the last moment refuse all the help arranged, so getting 'one up' on people who, the patient thinks, help others in order to feel good themselves.
	2. Review the patient's other problems to identify any which may reduce the possibility of acceptance into a hostel, hotel or home, such as incontinence, limited ability to walk or climb stairs, a colostomy or ileostomy or urinary conduit, mental confusion or socially unacceptable habits.
	3. Offer to arrange for the social worker to visit the patient. It may be possible to put the patient in touch with a charity or agency specializing in the

problems of the homeless. If the patient agrees, provide the social worker with information about the likely date of discharge and the kind of accommodation needed to support the patient's return to full health. Discuss the presence of factors likely to reduce acceptance and whether these are expected to be present on discharge.

RE. Record the offer and the patient's response. Review the care plan to identify any outcomes which need revision if the patient is to achieve acceptance at a suggested location. Replan the action to help the patient achieve them.

Further action	1. Discuss with the doctor the need for convalescence or continued medical supervision.
	RE. Note whether the patient is registered with a general practitioner. Record the doctor's advice and the patient's reaction to it.
Associated medical diagnoses	Alcoholism Chronic bronchitis Cirrhosis of the liver Epilepsy Head injury Hepatic failure Hypothermia Leg ulcers Peripheral vascular disease Pneumonia Severe burns

Potential problem

Potential problem	**Risk of aggression towards staff or other patients**
Assessment findings	Shouts verbal abuse Hits out at staff Confused Shouts and swears Threatens violence towards others
Information for the patient	People in hospitals are expected to conform to certain expected standards of behaviour. Any aggression shown towards staff or other patients will not be tolerated, and the police be involved, at the hospital's discretion. Treatments will not be forced upon anyone; the patient has the right to object or refuse treatment.
Nursing action	1. Consider the possible cause of the aggression; could it be due to fear, the influence of drugs, drink, mental illness, a head injury; or is it a usual pattern of coping when faced with people seen as being in authority? Review the resources available for summoning help if the aggression continues.
	RE. Confirm that all the staff know the location of any emergency buzzer or bell, and know how to use it to call for help.

2. A calm, cheerful approach with explanations for each step of a nursing procedure may be sufficient to reduce aggression. Give the patient time to understand and to give consent to each step of the treatment.

RE. If it appears that the patient fears loss of his control over decisions, which will make him aggressive, then provide as many opportunities as possible for the patient to decide on the next step. Review the care plan to see if there are other areas of treatment in which the patient can have a say.

3. Remove potential weapons from the patient's bed area. Each person has an invisible 'space bubble' around them, and discomfort is felt if others invade it by standing too close. It varies in area, so assess at what distance the patient shows signs of discomfort. Avoid invading the patient's personal 'space bubble' when possible, as this will decrease tension as well as limiting risk to the nurse.

RE. Observe for increased agitation or facial tension when moving close to the patient. When a person feels their personal territory being invaded, there may be a feeling of discomfort and threat.

4. Assess the reaction of other patients in the bed area and whether the stress will have an adverse effect on their medical condition. Consider moving them or the aggressive patient. They will feel less under threat if the staff appear calm and in control.

RE. Listen out for the patient who threatens the aggressive one on the staff's behalf, as this behaviour will increase rather than decrease the tension.

Further action

1. Blood alcohol levels may be taken if it is thought the patient has been drinking. Emergency admissions tend to have a high association with alcohol abuse, and aggression 24 to 48 hours after admission may indicate a falling blood alcohol in an alcoholic.

RE. Normal blood contains no alcohol. Levels over 50 mg per 100 ml indicate earlier intoxication (Table 4.2, section 4).

2. Intramuscular diazepam may be prescribed as a sedative, but its administration requires cooperation from the patient. It may be advisable for two staff to go to the patient, one to explain each step and give the injection, the other to calm the patient and provide assistance should violence appear imminent. On no account try to restrain the patient, as this will trigger aggression.

RE. The drug will take about twenty minutes to have its full effect.

3. Paraldehyde by intramuscular injection is rarely prescribed. It must be given with a glass syringe as it destroys plastic. It has a strong smell and may trigger fear and aggression in patients with previous mental hospital experiences.

RE. The drug acts within minutes. It is partly excreted on the breath.

Associated medical diagnoses

Drug overdose
Head injury
Paranoia
Psychopathic personality
Toxic confusion
Post-epileptic fit

References and further reading

Argyle, M. (Ed.) (1981). *Social Skills and Health.* Methuen & Co. Ltd. London.

Berne, E. (1964). *Games People Play.* Ballantine Books. New York.

Berne, E. (1975). *What Do You Say After You Say Hello?* Corgi Books. London.

Bond, J., Bond, S. (1980). Changing images. *Nursing Mirror,* March. **6**, 28−31.

Littlewood, R. Lipsedge, M. (1982). *Aliens and Alienists − Ethnic Minorities and Psychiatry.* Penguin Books. Harmondsworth, Middlesex.

Patients' Association, The. (1986). (10th edn.). *Self-help and the Patient − A Directory of National Organisations Concerned with Various Diseases and Handicaps.* The Patients' Association, London.

Priestly, P. McGuire, J. (1983). *Learning to Help − Basic Skills Exercises.* Tavistock Publications, London.

Smale, G.H. (1977). *Prophesy, Behaviour and Change.* Routledge, Kegan Paul. London.

Stockwell, F. (1984). *The Unpopular Patient.* Croom Helm, London.

Useful addresses

The Association of Carers
58 New Road, Chatham, Kent ME4 4QR
Tel. Medway (0634) 813981/2

National Council for Carers and their Elderly Dependants
29 Chilworth Mews, London W2 3RG
Tel. 01-262 1451/2

The Patients' Association
Room 33, 18 Charing Cross Road, London WC2H OHR
Tel. 01-240 0671

General references and further reading

Jones, B. (1978). *Pharmacology for Student and Pupil Nurses.* William Heinemann Medical Books Ltd. London.

McLeod, J. (1977). (12th edn). *Davidson's Principles and Practice of Medicine.* Churchill Livingstone. Edinburgh.

Watson, J.E. (1979). *Medical-Surgical Nursing and Related Physiology.* W.B. Saunders Co. Philadelphia.